Recent Advances in
OTOLARYNGOLOGY
Head and Neck Surgery

Recent Advances in OTOLARYNGOLOGY Head and Neck Surgery

Vol. 5

Editors

Anil K Lalwani MD
Professor and Vice-Chair for Research
Director, Division of Otology, Neurotology and Skull Base Surgery
Director, Columbia Cochlear Implant Center
Columbia University College of Physicians and Surgeons
Medical Director of Perioperative Services
New York Presbyterian—Columbia University Medical Center
New York, New York, USA

Markus HF Pfister MD MBA
Associate Professor of Otolaryngology—Head and Neck Surgery
Affiliated with Klinik St Anna, Lucerne, Hirslanden Group
HNO Sarnen, Switzerland
Swisstinnitus, Switzerland
Kantonsspital Obwalden
Hirslanden Klinik Meggen, Switzerland

JAYPEE *The Health Sciences Publisher*
Philadelphia | New Delhi | London | Panama

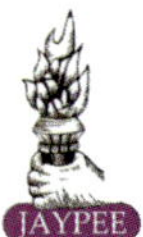 **Jaypee Brothers Medical Publishers (P) Ltd**

Headquarters
Jaypee Brothers Medical Publishers (P) Ltd.
4838/24, Ansari Road, Daryaganj
New Delhi 110 002, India
Phone: +91-11-43574357
Fax: +91-11-43574314
E-mail: jaypee@jaypeebrothers.com

Overseas Offices

J.P. Medical Ltd.
83, Victoria Street, London
SW1H 0HW (UK)
Phone: +44-20 3170 8910
Fax: +44(0)20 3008 6180
E-mail: info@jpmedpub.com

Jaypee Medical Inc.
325 Chestnut Street
Suite 412
Philadelphia, PA 19106, USA
Phone: +1 267-519-9789
E-mail: support@jpmedus.com

Jaypee-Highlights Medical Publishers Inc.
City of Knowledge, Bld. 237, Clayton
Panama City, Panama
Phone: +1 507-301-0496
Fax: +1 507-301-0499
E-mail: cservice@jphmedical.com

Jaypee Brothers Medical Publishers (P) Ltd.
17/1-B, Babar Road, Block-B, Shaymali
Mohammadpur, Dhaka-1207
Bangladesh
Mobile: +08801912003485
E-mail: jaypeedhaka@gmail.com

Jaypee Brothers Medical Publishers (P) Ltd.
Bhotahity, Kathmandu, Nepal
Phone: +977-9741283608
E-mail: kathmandu@jaypeebrothers.com

Website: www.jaypeebrothers.com
Website: www.jaypeedigital.com

Inquiries for bulk sales may be solicited at: jaypee@jaypeebrothers.com

Recent Advances in Otolaryngology—Head and Neck Surgery (Vol. 5)

First Edition: **2016**

ISBN: 978-93-5152-940-8

Printed at: Sanat Printers

Dedicated to

My parents—Madan and Gulab Lalwani
My in-laws—Rikhab and Ratan Bhansali
My children—Nikita and Sahil
And, most specially to my wife—Renu Bhansali Lalwani
A wonderful partner, friend, mother, community activist
and the smartest internist I know!

This book is also dedicated to Ms Ann Tenenbaum and Mr Thomas H Lee
for their commitment to supporting research in Otolaryngology that make
advances possible — the focus of this book.

Anil K Lalwani

My parents—Ingeborg and Hermann Pfister
My brother and sister—Stefan and Andrea
And, most specially to my beloved Doris
A wonderful partner and my center of inspiration.

Markus HF Pfister

Contributors

Jennifer Alyono MD MS
Department of Otolaryngology—
Head and Neck Surgery
Stanford University
Stanford, California, USA

Nikul Amin MRCS (ENT)
ENT Specialist Registrar
Department of Otolaryngology
University Hospital Lewisham
London, United Kingdom

Soly Baredes MD FACS
Professor and Chair
Director, Head and Neck Surgery
Department of Otolaryngology—
Head and Neck Surgery
Rutgers New Jersey Medical School
Newark, New Jersey, USA

Nikolaus Blin PhD
Part Time Professor
Department of Genetics
Wroclaw Medical University
Wroclaw, Poland

Rakesh K Chandra MD
Chief of the Division of Rhinology
Professor
Department of Otolaryngology—
Head and Neck Surgery
Vanderbilt University
Nashville, Tennessee, USA

Nipun Chhabra MD
Clinical Assistant
Professor of Surgery, University of
Illinois, College of Medicine
Rockford, Illinois, USA

Carleton Eduardo Corrales MD
Otology, Neurotology and
Skull Base Surgery
Division of Otolaryngology—
Head and Neck Surgery
Brigham and Women's Hospital,
Harvard Medical School
Boston, Massachusetts, USA

Alwyn D'Souza FRCS (ORL-HNS)
Consultant Head and Neck/Facial
Plastic and Reconstructive Surgeon
Department of Otolaryngology
University Hospital Lewisham
London, United Kingdom

Jean Anderson Eloy MD FACS
Professor and Vice Chair
Director, Rhinology and
Sinus Surgery
Director
Otolaryngology Research
Department of Otolaryngology—
Head and Neck Surgery
Neurological Institute of New Jersey
Rutgers New Jersey Medical School
Newark, New Jersey, USA

Brianna M Griffin BA
Medical Student
Columbia University College of
Physicians and Surgeons
New York, New York, USA

Oliver N Hausmann MD
Consultant in Neurosurgery
Neuro- and Spine Center
Hirslanden Klinik St. Anna
Lucerne, Switzerland

Steven Michael Houser MD
Associate Professor of
Otolaryngology
Case Western Reserve University
College of Medicine
MetroHealth Medical Center
Cleveland, Ohio, USA

Benjamin P Hull MD MHA
Clinical Housestaff Instructor
Department of Otolaryngology—
Head and Neck Surgery
Vanderbilt University
Nashville, Tennessee, USA

Ashutosh Kacker MBBS MS MD
Professor of Clinical Otolaryngology
Head and Neck Surgery
Weill Cornell Medicine
New York, New York, USA

Chin-Lung Kuo MD PhDc
Director
Department of Otolaryngology
Hsinchu Armed Forces Hospital
Taoyuan Armed Forces General
Hospital; Taipei Veterans General
Hospital; Institute of Brain Science
National Yang-Ming University
Taiwan, Republic of China

Anil K Lalwani MD
Professor and Vice-Chair for Research
Director, Division of Otology
Neurotology and Skull Base Surgery
Director
Columbia Cochlear
Implant Center
Columbia University College of
Physicians and Surgeons
Medical Director of
Perioperative Services
New York Presbyterian—Columbia
University Medical Center
New York, New York, USA

Valeria Silva Merea MD
Department of Otolaryngology—
Head and Neck Surgery
Weill Cornell Medicine
New York, New York, USA

Parwane P Pagano MD
Assistant Professor of
Anesthesiology at Columbia
University Medical Center
College of Physicians and Surgeons
of Columbia University
New York, New York, USA

Darlene M Parker RPR FAPR CAPM
Director of Steno Captioning and
Realtime Relations
National Captioning Institute
Chantilly, Virginia, USA

Rekesh Patel BSc MSc CCC
Principal Audiologist
The Tinnitus Clinic Ltd.
Harley Street
London, United Kingdom

Markus HF Pfister MD MBA
Associate Professor of
Otolaryngology—Head and
Neck Surgery
Affiliated with Klinik St Anna
Lucerne, Hirslanden Group
HNO Sarnen, Switzerland
Swisstinnitus, Switzerland
Kantonsspital Obwalden
Hirslanden Klinik Meggen
Switzerland

Steven D Rauch MD
Professor, Department of
Otolaryngology
Harvard Medical School
Chief, Vestibular Division
Massachusetts Eye and Ear
Boston, Massachusetts, USA

Steven D Schaefer MD FACS
Professor of Otolaryngology
New York Medical College
Director Sinus Surgery
New York Head and Neck Institute of
North Shore-Long Island Jewish
Health System
New York, New York, USA

Esther Schimanski MD
Center for Middle-Ear-Surgery
Brechtener Str. 57
44536 Lünen, Germany
HNO-Department,
Klinikum Westfalen

Goesta Schimanski MD
Center for Middle-Ear-Surgery
Brechtener Str. 57
44536 Lünen, Germany
HNO-Department,
Klinikum Westfalen

Ermioni Touli MD
Resident Neurosurgery
Neuro- and Spine Center
Hirslanden Klinik St Anna
Lucerne, Switzerland

Philip A Weissbrod MD
Director
Center for Voice and Swallowing
Assistant Professor
Division of Otolaryngology
UC San Deigo Health System
La Jolla, California, USA

Mark Williams BSc MSc Dip CCA
Chief Audiologist
The Tinnitus Clinic Ltd.
Harley Street
London, United Kingdom

Preface

Otolaryngology—Head and Neck Surgery is a dynamic medical and surgical specialty characterized by rapid advances in its scientific foundation and of its therapeutic armamentarium. Simultaneously, there are novel technical and technological innovations that positively impact on patient care. Consequently, Otolaryngology is constantly evolving as new knowledge comes forth and new technologies become available. Recent examples of advances in Otolaryngology include application of precision medicine in treating ENT disorders, management of laryngeal trauma, what to do about empty nose syndrome, technological advances in hearing aids, incorporation of genetics and gamma knife in the treatment of glomus tumors, and the use of glass beads for obliteration of mastoid cavity, among others. The challenge for the busy clinician in the 21st century is to remain abreast of these ever-expanding body of knowledge, surgical techniques, diagnostic test, imaging technology, and prosthetics, while deeply immersed in their clinical practice. Ironically, this has become even more difficult with the explosion of technologies designed to put information at one's fingertips. This annual periodical, *Recent Advances in Otolaryngology—Head and Neck Surgery,* covering all the subspecialties of Otolaryngology, is designed to make it easy for the clinician to keep current with what is new. Due to its rapid publication cycle, the material is current, topical, and immediately relevant to the clinician. Reviews emphasize clear artwork rendered in color to convey new concepts and surgical approaches. We have assembled an outstanding international editorial board to assist us in this exciting project. Similarly, invited authors are leaders in the field and have made seminal contributions in their topics. We hope that you will enjoy reading this 5th Volume as much as we have enjoyed assembling it.

Anil K Lalwani MD
Markus HF Pfister MD MBA

Acknowledgments

We would like to thank Ms Chetna Malhotra Vohra (Associate Director) and Sheetal Arora Kapoor (Development Editor) at Jaypee Brothers Medical Publishers (P) Ltd, New Delhi, India for their assistance with the 5th Volume of *Recent Advances in Otolaryngology—Head and Neck Surgery*.

Contents

Chapter 1

Precision Medicine in Otolaryngology

Markus HF Pfister, Nikolaus Blin

INTRODUCTION

Precision medicine proposes the customization of healthcare tailoring medical treatment to the individual characteristics of each patient. Diagnostic testing is used to classify individuals into subpopulations that differ in their susceptibility to a particular disease, in the prognosis of diseases they may develop, or in their response to a specific treatment. In addition, prevention or therapeutic approaches can be individualized based on the individual genetic information.

The area of the otolaryngology and head and neck surgery is especially demanded by today's communication society with the individualized diagnosis and treatment of hearing loss (HL) (congenital as well as age-related HL or syndromic HL), of tumors in the head and neck area, and of rare diseases such as hemorrhagic telangiectasia. The focus of this chapter is on aspects of precision medicine that already have an impact on the field of Otolaryngology and Head and Neck Surgery.

STATE OF THE ART OF MOLECULAR DIAGNOSTICS

The current medical evaluation of hereditary diseases involves a myriad of clinical and laboratory tests, many of them being costly, time-consuming, and stressful for the patient. Deoxyribonucleic acid (DNA) diagnostics for monogenic diseases have emerged and evolved over the last decades. At this moment, genetic tests are available for most frequent genetic diseases. The benefit of these tests for the patients is very large. They aid in determining prognosis (i.e. whether the condition will deteriorate), and provide the best intervention and recurrence risk to future children and other family members. As such they allow patients and clinicians to take appropriate measures in a timely manner. In addition, genetic diagnostics are being used to predict the occurrence of disease, both in adults for diseases with late onset and prenatally. Genetic testing is fundamentally different from other clinical tests in several aspects, and important ethical issues are involved.

It is beyond any doubt that genetic testing has taken a very important place in modern society, and it is to be expected that the demand for genetic testing will grow substantially. For some diseases, the current situation for DNA diagnostics is relatively favorable. For genetically homogeneous diseases (i.e. diseases caused by a single gene such as cystic fibrosis), it is clear which gene needs to be analyzed. Analysis of a single gene by current technology is feasible and affordable. Prices may range from <100 euros for small genes to several thousand euros for several large genes. However, for genetically heterogeneous diseases, where the same disease can be caused by many different genes, significant problems still arise.

Probably the most extreme example of a genetically heterogeneous disease is the hereditary HL. Hearing loss in children is in most cases caused by mutations in a single gene. Among these genetic cases, 70–80% are nonsyndromic, with HL being the only clinical abnormality. Most cases have an autosomal recessive inheritance. At this moment, already 70 different genes responsible for nonsyndromic HL have been identified. The rate of discovery of *HL* genes has been relatively constant over the last 10 years. The total number of responsible genes is unknown, but >100 different genes can be expected.

From the clinical side, there are almost no criteria to distinguish between genes. A large majority of early childhood HL shows profound hearing impairment, and little further clinical classification can be made. Newborns with HL are partly being picked up shortly after birth by neonatal hearing screening programs, but diagnostics have to be further improved and implemented. This is very important in terms of early intervention and rehabilitation. Hearing is critical to early development and if mutations and polymorphisms linked to HL could be detected at birth then learning and development would be facilitated in the formative early months and years of life. Genetic testing of a single gene, *GJB2*, explaining some 5–25% of cases, is nearly always part of the follow-up protocol, as it provides very valuable information in terms of early intervention and rehabilitation in case of a positive result. However, for a majority of cases no molecular cause can be identified. This creates a very frustrating situation for clinicians and parents. In order to be fully informative, molecular diagnostics directed to HL (as would be the case for other diseases with allelic heterogeneity) involve mutation scanning of entire coding regions including exon boundaries of all known genes. Clinical genetics centers that are carrying out genetic testing for HL are experiencing increased demand for more and better genetic testing by parents, audiologists, pediatricians, and other professionals involved in neonatal hearing screening, who are witnessing the successful identification of many *HL* genes.

New methods that allow for high throughput and affordable mutation scanning are now implemented and lead to improved diagnostic results.[1] The new diagnostic approaches provide answers in a much higher percentage of cases, creating a benefit for patients with severe HL. One particular example is Usher syndrome.

The genotypically and phenotypically heterozygous Usher syndrome is one of the most challenging diseases known. It is the second most common syndromic hearing impairment with an additional loss of vision and vestibular problems. Depending on the Usher syndrome type (I, I, III), patients suffer from a loss of the both most important senses known, the sight and hearing. Patients show a progressive visual loss due to retinitis pigmentosa and a congenital sensorineural HL, which is moderate in type II and profound in type I. Typically, type I patients show also an absent vestibular response during caloric testing. In addition to the two classic clinical types, a third type featuring progressive HL has been described.[2] This type is rare and has so far been found almost exclusively in Finland. Genetically, there are seven known loci for type I *(USH1B-H)*, three for type II *(USH2 A)*, and one for type III *(USH3 A)*.[2,3] The general speculation is that a defect in the cytoskeleton structure might be one reason for Usher syndrome. It has thus been speculated that the cilia of cochlear and vestibular hair cells could be the primary target structure in the inner ear, and that the nasal ciliary cells might also be defective, resulting in an olfactory loss. Due to the progressive visual loss, it is crucial to diagnose patients as early as possible in order to rehabilitate the hearing.

In type I patients, Cochlear implant surgery is the only option early in life to fully rehabilitate the hearing status. The genotype offers early additional information in subtyping the syndrome and allows an earlier integration in an implant program in order to use the visual input for rehabilitation.[4]

In types II and III patients, the situation is much more complex because a multitude of devices are possible including surgical implanted hearing devices. The progression of hearing in combination with the genotype allows a prediction of the phenotype. This knowledge is used regarding the choice of the hearing device, e.g. conventional hearing aids versus implantable hearing aids versus middle ear implants (Figs. 1.1A and B).[4]

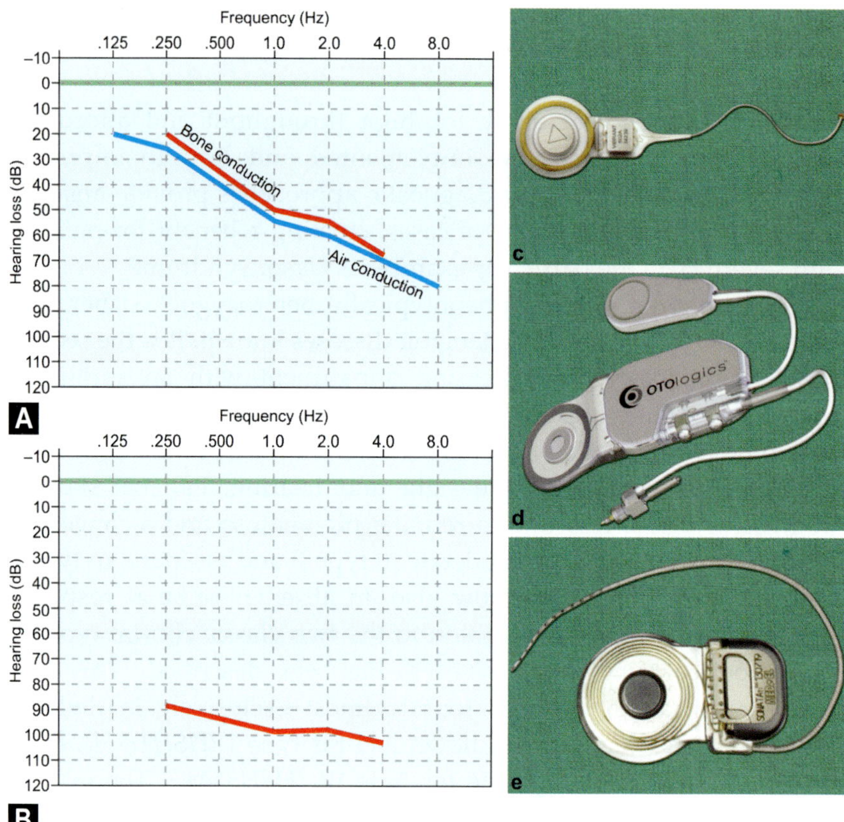

Figs. 1.1A and B: Part (A) represents moderate hearing impairment that can be progressive in type 3 Usher syndrome or stable in type 2 Usher syndrome. Possible implantable devices are represented by device c oder d showing a middle ear implant. Part (B) represents severe to profound hearing impairment. In this case, a cochlear implant fits best if implantation requirements are fulfilled device e.

SKULL BASE TUMORS/HEAD AND NECK TUMORS

Paraganglioma

Paragangliomas (*PGL*, OMIM 16,800) represent a group of generally benign tumors developing from extra-adrenal paraganglionic tissue. The majority of these tumors arise from the head and neck region with the carotid body being the most common site of origin. The incidence of paragangliomas is estimated to be between 1:100,000 and 1: 1,000,000.[5] Although paragangliomas usually occur sporadically, inheritance is observed in 10–50% of cases.[6]

Paragangliomas (Hereditary paraganglioma–pheochromocytoma) are genetically heterogeneous. To date at least four loci within one gene family are known to be involved in their development, namely *PGL1*

(11q23), *PGL2* (11q13), *PGL3* (1q21), and *PGL4* (1p36). The most frequently affected and, therefore, most important locus is *PGL1*, which was first demonstrated to co-segregate with the disease in a large Dutch family.[7]

Up to day, numerous mutations in the *SDHD* gene predispose an individual to hereditary paraganglioma–pheochromocytoma type 1; mutations in the *SDHAF2* gene predispose to type 2; mutations in the *SDHC* gene predispose to type 3; and mutations in the *SDHB* gene predispose to type 4.

Hereditary paraganglioma–pheochromocytoma is inherited in an autosomal dominant pattern. An additional mutation that deletes the normal copy of the causative gene is needed to cause the condition. This second mutation, called a somatic mutation, is acquired during a person's lifetime and is present only in tumor cells.

The risk of developing hereditary paraganglioma–pheochromocytoma types 1 and 2 is passed on only if the mutated copy of the gene is inherited from the father. The mechanism of this pattern of inheritance is unknown. The risk of developing types 3 and 4 can be inherited from the mother or the father.

Based on high throughput molecular testing, evaluation of relatives at risk as well as genetic counseling is possible and diagnostic as well as therapy can be tailored (*see* Chapter 9).[8]

HEREDITARY HEARING LOSS AND HEREDITARY HEMORRHAGIC TELANGIECTASIA[9]

Several published studies suggest that infection with oncogenic human papillomavirus (HPV) constitutes is a significant risk factor for the development of head and neck carcinomas. Prevalence of HPV positivity in oropharyngeal squamous cell carcinoma has increased significantly from 16.3% between 1984 and 1989 to 72.7% between 2000 and 2004 in the United States. The same trend can be seen in Europe. At least half of oropharyngeal carcinomas contain high-risk HPV. The significance in laryngeal carcinoma is less clear.

Human papillomavirus is today a proven genetic risk factor, particularly for oropharyngeal carcinoma. An HPV detection in tumor tissue of the oropharynx is now also associated with a better prognosis. Human papillomavirus-positive oropharyngeal carcinoma patients have a reduced risk of death (28% less) as well as a reduced risk of recurrence. Some evidence indicates that outcome benefits associated with HPV positivity are greater when patients are treated with radiotherapy, than when treated by other methods.[10,11-13]

Hereditary Hemorrhagic Telangiectasia or Rendu-Osler-Weber

Hereditary hemorrhagic telangiectasia (HHT) is a genetic disorder of the blood vessels, which affects approximately 1 in 5,000 people including males and females from all racial and ethnic groups. The disorder is also sometimes referred to as Osler-Weber-Rendu, named after several doctors who studied HHT about 100 years ago. In 1896, Dr Rendu first described HHT as a hereditary disorder involving nosebleeds and characteristic red spots that were distinctly different from hemophilia. Before Dr Rendu's work, doctors did not understand that individuals with what we now call HHT have abnormalities of their blood vessels, not a clotting problem in the blood itself. Dr Weber and Dr Osler reported on additional features of HHT in the early 1900s (Fig. 1.2).

Hereditary hemorrhagic telangiectasia is an autosomal dominant disorder affecting >1.4 million people worldwide. The main manifestations are epistaxis, telangiectasias in the oral and nasal aperture, and arteriovenous malformations in the internal organs, especially in the lungs, the brain, and the gastrointestinal tract. Vascular malformations of the heart and the blood supplying coronary arteries are also described. Two important genes have been identified whose mutations lead to the formation of HHT: endoglin *(ENG-HHT1)* and activin receptor-like kinase 1 *(ACVRL1-HHT 2)*. Changes in another gene, SMAD-related protein 4 *(SMAD4)*, cause a combined syndrome of juvenile polyps of the gastrointestinal tract and HHT. At least two other unidentified genes also appear to cause HHT in a smaller number of individuals. There are hundreds of different mutations in each of the three known genes that can cause HHT. Having a mutation in an HHT-associated gene causes some blood vessels to form improperly leading to symptoms of HHT.

A detection of a mutation in these genes leads to earlier diagnosis, the possibility of risk evaluation, and allows early interventional therapy of vascular shunts in the brain, the lung, the liver, or elsewhere.[14]

SUMMARY

This chapter highlights developments in the field of otolaryngology. These developments will be significantly expanded in the upcoming years. Based on the refinement of high throughput diagnostic procedures and the integration of phenotype data/retrospective outcome data with genotype data, new diagnostic as well as treatment approaches will be seen. This will ultimately lead to an interdisciplinary, comprehensive and thus more precise approach in the treatment of patients worldwide.

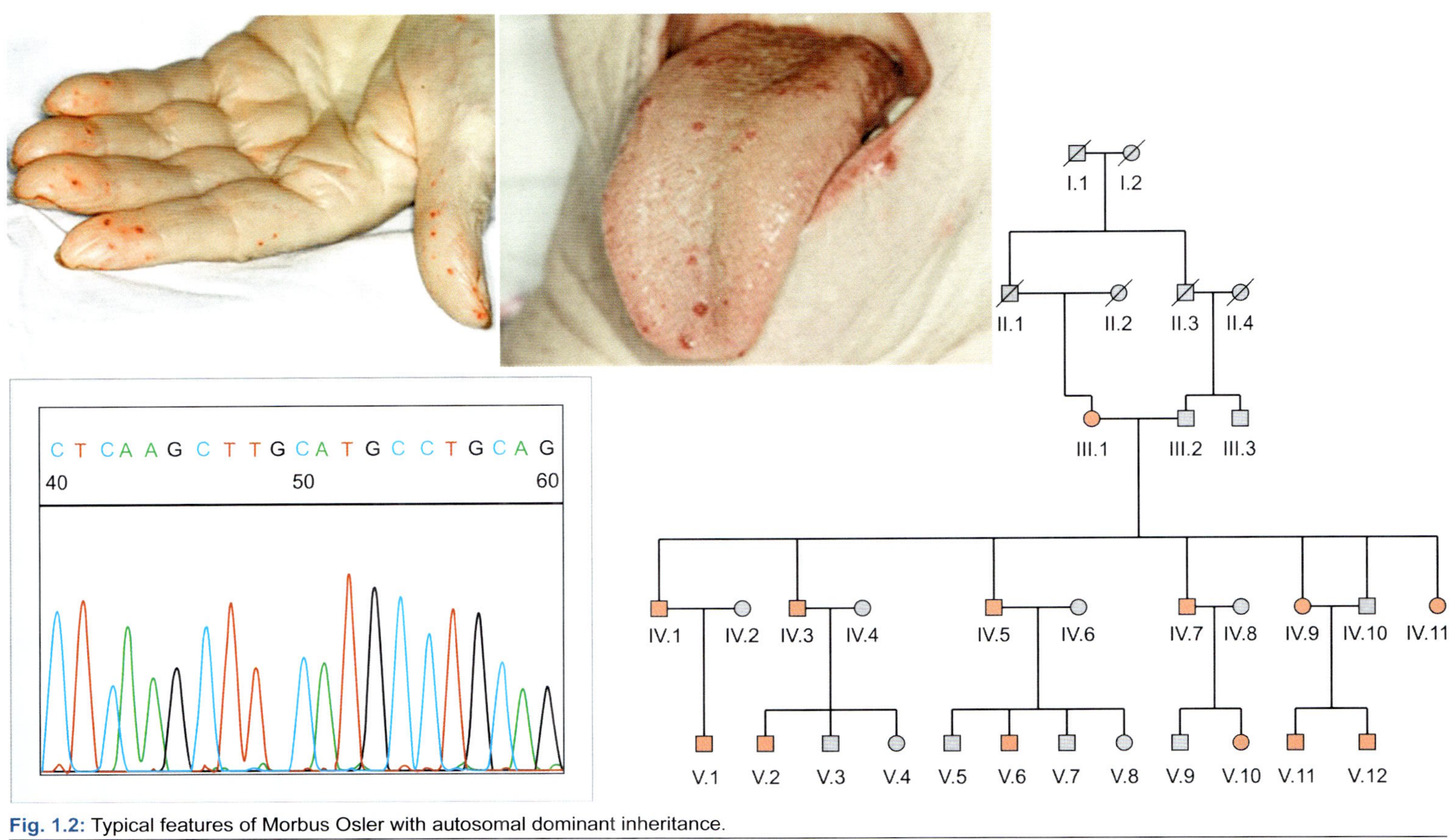

Fig. 1.2: Typical features of Morbus Osler with autosomal dominant inheritance.

REFERENCES

1. Gürtler N, Röthlisberger B. Genetics in otolaryngology. Recent Advances of Otolaryngology, Head and Neck Surgery, (Vol. 3). Jaypee Brothers.
2. Sankila EM1, Pakarinen L, Kääriäinen H, et al. Assignment of an Usher syndrome type III (USH3) gene to chromosome 3q. Hum Mol Genet. 1995;4(1):93-8.
3. Hereditary hearing Loss Homepage by Richard Smith and Guy van Camp. Available from http://hereditaryhearingloss.org, 2015.
4. Seeliger M, Pfister M. Usher syndrome: clinical features, diagnostic options, and therapeutic prospects. Ophthalmologe. 2009;106(6):505-11.
5. Baysal BE, Rubinstein WS, Taschner PE. Phenotypic dichotomy in mitochondrial complex II genetic disorders. J Mol Med. 2001;79:495-503.
6. Hoffmann J, Krober SM, Hahn U, et al. Polytopic manifestations of paragangliomas. Diagnosis, differential diagnosis and Indications for therapy. Mund Kiefer Gesichtschir. 2000;4:53-6.
7. Heutink P, van der Mey AG, Sandkuijl LA, et al. A gene subject to genomic imprinting and responsible for hereditary paragangliomas maps to chromosome 11q23-qter. Hum Mol Genet. 1992;1:7-10.
8. Carleton CE, Alyono J: Contemporary management of paraganglioma jugulare and tympanicum. Recent Advances of Otolaryngology, Head and Neck Surgery, (Vol.5), Jaypee Brothers.
9. Theurer J, Nichols. Human Papilloma virus in Head and Neck Cancer. Recent Advances of Otolaryngology, Head and Neck Surgery, (Vol. 2), Jaypee Brothers, pp. 78-99.
10. Chaturvedi AK, Engels EA, Pfeiffer RM, et al. Human papillomavirus and rising oropharyngeal cancer incidence in the United States. J Clin Oncol. 2011;29(32):4294-301.
11. Lindel K, Beer KT, Laissue J, et al. Human papillomavirus positive squamous cell carcinoma of the oropharynx: a radiosensitive subgroup of head and neck carcinoma. Cancer. 2001;92(4):805-13.
12. Mellin H, Friesland S, Lewensohn R, et al. Human papillomavirus (HPV) DNA in tonsillar cancer: clinical correlates, risk of relapse, and survival. Int J Cancer. 2000;89(3):300-304.
13. Schwartz SR, Yueh B, McDougall JK, et al. Human papillomavirus infection and survival in oral squamous cell cancer: a population-based study. Otolaryngol Head Neck Surg. 2001;125(1):1-9.
14. McDonald J, Wooderchak-Donahue W, VanSant Webb C, et al. Hereditary hemorrhagic telangiectasia: genetics and molecular diagnostics in a new era. Front Genet. 2015;6:1.

Chapter 2

Electronic Cigarettes

Valeria Silva Merea, Ashutosh Kacker

INTRODUCTION

Electronic cigarettes or e-cigarettes (ECs) are electronic nicotine delivery systems that were introduced to the US market in 2007, after they were first commercialized in China in 2003.[1,2] Electronic cigarettes are battery-operated devices that heat a liquid to produce a vapor that is then inhaled by the user. This liquid, called e-liquid, usually contains nicotine, flavoring and humectants such as propylene glycol or vegetable glycerin, and it may be contained in disposable ECs themselves, replaceable cartridges or refill liquids. Figure 2.1 illustrates the typical component of an EC. The heating of the solution may be initiated by the user's inhalation or by the pressing of a button. A key point is that there is no combustion involved. Table 2.1 contains important definitions about ECs.

Electronic cigarettes exist in a variety of brands and modifications. First-generation devices were designed to look and feel like tobacco cigarettes ("cigalikes"), but many newer ones do not resemble cigarettes and may look like pens, screwdrivers, or the tip of hookah pipes

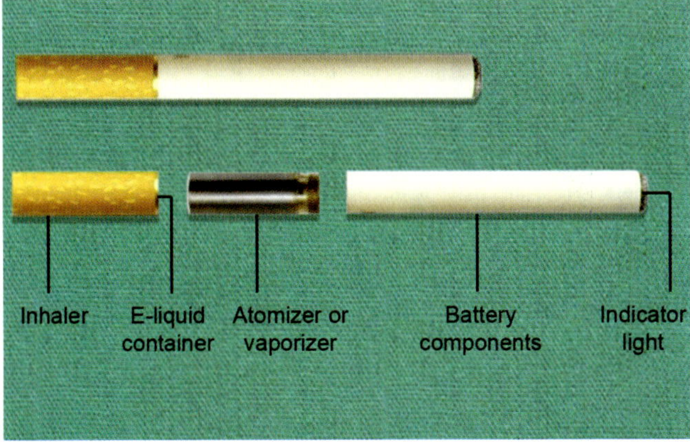

Fig. 2.1: Diagram with the typical components of an electronic cigarette.

Table 2.1: Important definitions.

Definitions

Vaping: The act of using electronic cigarettes

Active vaper: Electronic cigarette user

Passive vaper: Nonuser exposed to electronic cigarette vapor

E-liquid: Liquid inside an electronic cigarette; usually contains nicotine, flavoring, and humectants

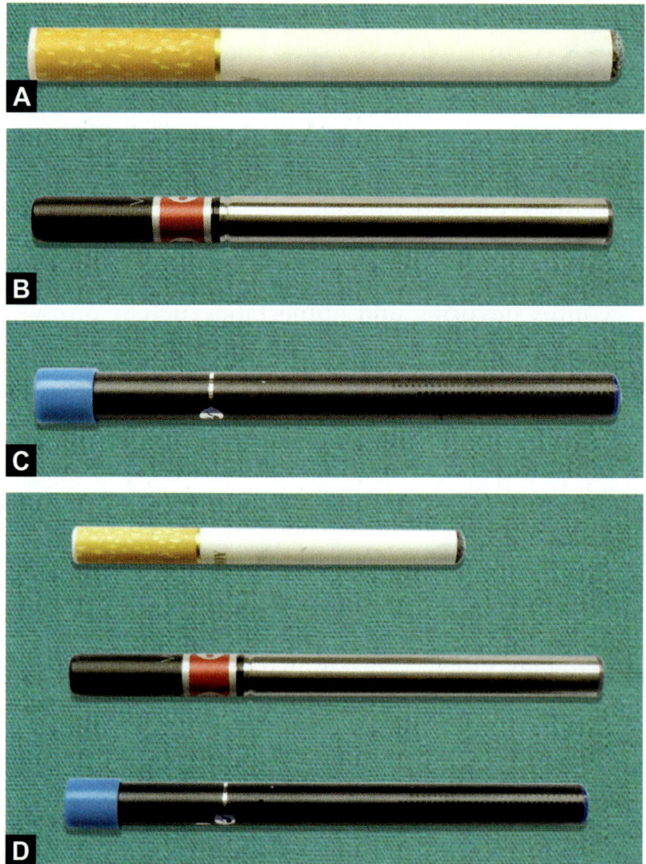

Figs. 2.2A to D: Three different brands of electronic cigarettes (A to C). Figure (D) provided for size comparison. Note the resemblance of (A) with tobacco cigarettes ("cigalike" electronic cigarette).

(Figs. 2.2A to D). They are widely available online and in retail outlets in many countries across the world.

Between May 2012 and January 2014, there was an increase of 10.5 brands of ECs and 242 of flavors per month, and by the end of this period there were 466 brands and 7,764 unique flavors.[3] With their increasing popularity, EC advertisement expenditure rose from $6.4 million in 2011 to $18 million in 2012[4,5] with resultant increase in sales in the US from $283 million in 2012 to $537 million in 2013.[6] The global EC market currently is estimated to be $6 billion.[7]

Results of an annual consumer-based web survey of US adults aged 18 and older indicated increases in EC awareness (40.9% vs. 79.7%), ever use (3.3% vs. 8.5%), and current use (1.0% vs. 2.6%) between 2010 and 2013, with the most prominent EC use among current tobacco smokers (36.5% in 2013).[8] An international survey found that vapers are often younger and more affluent than nonvaping cigarette smokers.[9] Patterns of EC use vary, and users report several reasons for EC use including the perception that it is less toxic than tobacco, to deal with tobacco cravings and withdrawal symptoms, to quit smoking or avoid relapsing, because it is less expensive than tobacco smoking, and to deal with situations in which smoking is prohibited.[10]

As the use and availability of ECs have expanded, they have generated considerable controversy. The primary issues that have been raised about ECs include questions about their safety, their efficacy as a smoking cessation tool, and the need for their regulation. In addition, there is growing concern about their use by youth.

SAFETY

Electronic cigarettes receive great criticism because of their unknown effects on health and their potential disease burden. Definitive statements about EC safety are not possible because of the large number of different devices and e-liquids, both of which continue to grow. In addition, no studies have looked at long-term effects of ECs past 12 months.

The US Food and Drug Administration (FDA) has received voluntary reports of adverse events involving EC from consumers, health professionals, and members of the public. The serious events include hospitalizations for illnesses such as pneumonia, congestive heart failure, disorientation, seizure, hypotension, second-degree burns to the face from a product that exploded in the consumer's mouth, and chest pain, among others.[11] Of course, causation cannot be established from these reports, as they may be related to pre-existing medical conditions.

Nicotine

Electronic cigarettes are used as nicotine delivery systems. Nicotine concentration in e-liquids is usually between 0 and 36 mg/mL. It is well known that nicotine is the major addictive chemical in tobacco cigarettes, and that at high doses, it has acute toxicity.[12] Importantly, nicotine was not associated with lung cancer on the Lung Health Study.[13]

Nicotine is readily absorbed by multiple routes of exposure: inhalational, gastrointestinal, dermal, intranasal, and ophthalmologic. Lethal poisoning may occur after ingestion of 1 mg of nicotine per kilogram of body weight in children, with lethal dose estimated to be 10 mg in children and 30–60 mg in adults.[14,15] The first signs of nicotine poisoning are gastrointestinal (e.g. vomiting and diarrhea), cardiovascular (e.g. tachycardia and hypertension) and neuropsychological (e.g. tremor of the extremities), and with higher doses, these effects are rapidly followed by loss of consciousness, convulsions, or respiratory failure.[15]

The amount of nicotine found in ECs varies with manufacturer, and the actual nicotine level may be different than that labeled.[14,16] Under laboratory conditions, EC users are not always exposed to measurable levels of nicotine.[17] Studies with automated smoking machines have shown that ECs require deeper inhalation than conventional tobacco cigarettes, and the need for deep inhalation increases as vaping progresses.[16,18] Moreover, there appears to be significant variability between and within brands in the airflow rate required to produce aerosol, pressure drop, length of time cartridges last, and production of aerosol.[18] Thus, it is not surprising that the user's experience and the device characteristics appear to influence nicotine delivery, with more experienced users showing higher plasma nicotine levels.[19]

E-liquids should be kept out of reach of children to prevent nicotine intoxication as generally, e-liquids are not sold in childproof containers.[20] Children may be drawn to e-liquids, because they are often brightly colored and sweet-flavored.[21] In December 2014, the death of a 1-year-old boy who ingested e-liquid was reported in New York State.[22]

In addition to accidental exposures, suicide attempts using e-liquids have also been reported.[23] Furthermore, liquid nicotine is also emerging as a drug of abuse in a modality known as "dripping," in which EC users drip the e-liquid onto the heating element of the EC and inhale the vapor, resulting in a larger dose of nicotine.[24] Other modalities to increase the amount of nicotine being inhaled include mixing of e-liquids, or increasing the voltage of the EC device.[24]

Indoor Air Quality and Secondhand Vapor Exposure

Studies have compared the carcinogenic content of smoke versus vapor. One study, which compared the composition of EC vapor and tobacco cigarette smoke in indoor air samples, showed that EC vapor posed a significantly lower risk than tobacco smoke under identical experimental conditions and methods.[25] Compounds covered in this analysis included volatile organic compounds (VOCs), carbonyls, polyaromatic hydrocarbons, tobacco-specific nitrosamines, nicotine, and glycols. Collected air samples were examined by expert toxicologists, who calculated the total cumulative hazard indices and excess lifetime cancer risks values. Overall, tobacco smoke was found to contain significantly more carcinogens and carcinogenic analytes than EC vapor, and the authors concluded that there seemed to be no recognizable health impacts from the vapor produced by any of the four e-liquids tested in the study.[25]

In a study aiming to identify the compounds that are released during vaping in order to estimate the effect of "passive vaping," Schripp et al. detected the emission of aerosols and VOCs such as 1,2-propanediol, flavoring substances, and nicotine, and noted that the aerosol size distribution of the vapor changes in the lungs, leading to exhalation of smaller particles. Upon exhalation, VOCs and ultrafine particulates are released, resulting in passive vaping by individuals who inhale the same air.[26]

Cardiovascular Effects

The cardiac effects of ECs have been examined and compared to those of tobacco cigarettes. Contrary to cigarette smoking, vaping does not appear to alter or impair left ventricular function.[27] Electronic cigarettes may increase heart rate and blood pressure, although in lower magnitudes than tobacco cigarettes, as expected secondary to nicotine absorption.[28] There are no reports of EC safety in patients with known cardiovascular disease.[29]

Effects on Complete Blood Count

An individual's complete blood count can provide an overview of his or her general health, as abnormal counts may indicate systemic problems including infection, inflammation, deficiency in the immune system, bone marrow disease, or other problems.[30] In a study comparing the effects of smoking, vaping, and secondhand exposure in both tobacco smokers and EC users, there was no increase in white blood cell, lymphocyte and granulocyte counts after EC use while active and passive tobacco cigarette smoking did increase these inflammatory markers.[31]

Cytotoxicity of Flavors

Studies have shown that flavoring molecules may be cytotoxic. A study that looked specifically at Cinnamon Ceylon found that two of its flavoring compounds (cinnamaldehyde and 2-methyoxycinnamaldehyde) were highly cytotoxic.[32] In addition, there are differences in the concentration of 2-methyoxycinnamaldehyde between identical bottles.[32]

SMOKING CESSATION

Since the first Surgeon's General report on smoking in 1964, more than 20 million premature deaths can be attributed to smoking and secondhand smoke, making smoking the leading preventable cause of death in the US.[12] A substantial number of head and neck malignancies can be attributed to tobacco and alcohol use, with tobacco associated with a greater risk than alcohol.[33] Not only does smoking cause cancer, but also persistent smoking after cancer diagnosis increases the risk of second primary tumors, cancer recurrence, other smoking-related illnesses, and mortality.[34-37] A significant number of head and neck cancer patients continue to smoke after diagnosis.[38] As physicians largely involved in the treatment of head and neck cancer, otolaryngologists have a responsibility in guiding patients toward effective smoking cessation methods.[39] Currently, ECs are not approved as smoking cessation devices.

Surveys

An important issue to be kept in mind when analyzing survey results is that self-reporting of cigarette smoking, when measured in cigarettes per day (as usually done in surveys), has been found to be unreliable.[40,41]

In a large survey of current and former smokers in Canada, the United States, the United Kingdom, and Australia ($N = 5,939$), although 85% of smokers who used ECs reported using them to quit, EC users did not quit smoking more frequently than nonusers at 12 months, but current EC use was associated with a greater reduction in cigarettes per day over time than nonusers.[9]

Another longitudinal survey with 1 year follow-up ($N = 949$) also found that EC use by smokers was not followed by greater rates of quitting or change in cigarette consumption. The variables that significantly predicted quit status were intention to quit and cigarettes smoked per day. The authors argued that the low number of EC users ($n = 88$), and in particular, those EC users who quit smoking

(n = 9) could have limited their statistical power to detect a significant relationship between EC use and quitting.[42]

An online 6-month follow-up survey of first-time purchasers of a particular brand of EC (N = 216), found a 31% prevalence of abstinence, with a larger percentage of respondents (66.8%) reporting reduction in the number of cigarettes they smoked.[43]

In a more recent survey of smokers making their first purchase at a vape shop (N = 71), 40.8% of participants were classified as quitters, 25.4% as reducers and 33.8% as failures at 12 months. Authors concluded that smokers purchasing ECs from vape shops in which professional advice is available, can achieve high cessation rates.[44]

Prospective Studies

In a randomized controlled study (N = 657) comparing ECs with (n = 289) and without nicotine (n = 73) with nicotine patches (n = 295), Bullen et al. found that ECs were only modestly effective at helping smokers to quit, and although nicotine-containing ECs had a higher rate of abstinence than nicotine patches, and nicotine-free ECs (7.3% vs. 5.8% vs. 4.1%, respectively), the differences were not statistically significant.[43] The authors attributed this lack of significance to lower rates of abstinence achieved in the study than those assumed in statistical power calculations.[45]

Another prospective randomized study comparing EC use in smokers not interested in quitting, studied the effect of varying e-liquid nicotine content. One group (n = 100) received 7.2 mg nicotine cartridges, a second group (n = 100) received 7.2 mg nicotine cartridges for 6 weeks and 5.4 mg cartridges for the remainder of the study, and a third group (n = 100) received no-nicotine cartridges. There were no statistical significant differences between groups. Overall, complete abstinence from tobacco smoking was documented in 10.7% at 12 weeks and 8.7% at week 52.[46]

A prospective study investigating the effects of ECs on smoking reduction and smoking cessation in smokers not intending to quit (N = 40) who had smoked at least 15 cigarettes for the past 10 years, found 50% reduction in 32.5% of participants while 22.5% of participants had quit smoking completely at 6 months.[47]

An ongoing prospective cohort study that is evaluating the safety and efficacy of EC as a tool for smoking cessation by directly comparing EC users (n = 236), tobacco smokers (n = 491) and dual smokers (n = 232), found that at 12 months, 61.9% of the EC users were still abstinent while 20.6% of tobacco smokers and 22% of the dual smokers achieved abstinence.[48] The addition of ECs to tobacco smoking did not enhance the likelihood of smoking cessation and did not reduce tobacco cigarette consumption. The study's expected completion date is 2019.[48]

Systematic Reviews

A systematic review by Pepper et al. found that in nonlongitudinal studies such as small surveys, focus groups, case studies, and interviews with dedicated EC users, participants often reported that using ECs helped them quit smoking or significantly reduce tobacco use, while large surveys did not find an association between successful quitting and EC use.[49] However, because smoking reduction may indicate dual use of ECs and tobacco cigarettes, the authors noted that smoking reduction, unlike smoking cessation, may not represent a positive public health outcome.[49]

A recent Cochrane systematic review with the goal of examining the efficacy of ECs in helping people who smoke achieve long-term abstinence or reduction, rated the quality of the evidence of the randomized studies as "low" by GRADE standards (Grading of Recommendations Assessment, Development and Evaluation)[50] because of the small number of trials, low event rates, and wide confidence intervals around the estimates.[51]

All in all, studies have shown that the use of ECs is associated with cessation or reduction of tobacco smoking for some individuals, but studies have yet to demonstrate that ECs are superior to an appropriate control condition.[52] Thus, current literature does not support EC use as a smoking cessation tool. Table 2.2 summarizes the studies mentioned above.

REGULATION

Although ECs are not federally regulated in the US, regulations have been developed in other parts of the world. Sales of ECs are prohibited in some countries including Australia, Brazil, Mexico, Panama, Singapore, and Switzerland. In Canada, electronic products that dispense nicotine by inhalation fall under the Food and Drugs Act of Health Canada, and thus, they cannot be imported, marketed, or sold without being approved as a new drug.[53] Furthermore, the delivery system of an EC containing nicotine must meet the requirements of the Medical Devices Regulations, and as a result, cartridges and liquids that contain nicotine are illegal while those that do not (and do not include a health claim) are not.[53] In Europe, there are organizations that have

Table 2.2: Summary of studies on effect of EC use on smoking cessation.

Year	First author	Study design	N	Location	Conditions	Findings
2011	Polosa[47]	6-month prospective pilot study	40	Italy	7.4 mg nicotine EC	22.5% quit smoking
2011	Siegel[43]	6-month follow-up online survey	216	US	First-time purchasers of a particular brand of ECs	31% quit smoking; 66.8% reduction
2013	Adkison[9]	12-month longitudinal survey	5,939	Canada, US, UK, Australia	N/A	EC users no more likely to quit smoking than nonusers
2013	Bullen[45]	6-month, 3-arm, randomized controlled trial	657	New Zealand	16 mg nicotine EC, 0 mg nicotine EC, 21 mg nicotine patch	Modest effect, no significant differences between conditions
2013	Camponnetto[46]	52-week, 3-arm, randomized controlled trial	300	Italy	7.2 mg nicotine EC, 5.4 mg nicotine EC, 0 mg nicotine EC	No significant differences; all reduced use; 8.7% quit smoking
2013	Pepper[49]	Systematic review	49 studies	US, Italy, UK, other	N/A	Successful quitting not associated with EC on large surveys. Small studies found ECs helpful
2014	Grana[42]	12-month longitudinal survey	949	US	N/A	EC use did not predict quitting
2014	McRobbie[51]	Cochrane systematic review	13 (2 RCT, 11 cohort)	New Zealand, Italy, US	N/A	EC users more likely to abstain than placebo users in RCT; GRADE; low
2015	Manzoli[48]	12-month prospective cohort study	959	Italy	EC users, tobacco smokers, dual users	61.9% of EC users still abstinent, 20.6% of tobacco smokers and 22% of the dual smokers quit
2015	Polosa[44]	12-month longitudinal survey	71	Italy	First-time EC purchasers at vape shops	40.8% quit smoking

(EC: Electronic cigarette; US: United States; UK: United Kingdom; N/A: Not applicable; RCT: Randomized controlled trials).

supported bans on EC sales,[54] others recommend regulation as tobacco products with lower nicotine content[55] or be submitted to medicinal regulation.[56]

While the FDA currently regulates cigarettes, cigarette tobacco, roll-your-own tobacco, and smokeless tobacco, there is no federal oversight of ECs at this time. Electronic cigarette manufacturing is unregulated, and their advertising is unrestricted. In April 2014, the FDA proposed a new rule that would extend its tobacco authority to additional products that meet the statutory definition of a tobacco product, including ECs, cigars, nicotine gels, pipe tobacco, waterpipe or hookah tobacco, and dissolvables.[57] Under the proposed rule, newly deemed tobacco products would be subject to the same provisions that regulated tobacco products are subject to, including the following:

- Required registration with the FDA, reporting of product and ingredient listings, and reporting of harmful and potentially harmful constituents.
- FDA review required prior to marketing new products.
- Direct and implied claims of reduced risk can only be made if the FDA confirms that scientific evidence supports the claim and issues an order permitting their use.
- Prohibition on distribution of free samples.
- Requirement for a minimum age of purchase to prevent sales to underage youth.
- Health warnings for product packages.
- Prohibition of vending machine sales unless in an adult-only facility.[57]

This is a good first step, but some issues such as sales of e-liquid cartridges in childproof containers, or restrictions in youth-appealing flavors would still not be addressed. If this proposed rule passes, it will likely be met with resistance, and may be challenged by EC manufacturers.

As of December 2014, 40 states have enacted laws that prohibit sale and use of EC in minors; 26 states and the District of Columbia have comprehensive smoke-free laws that prevent smoking in restaurants, worksites, and bars but only three states (New Jersey, North Dakota, and Utah) include restrictions of indoor EC use.[58]

YOUTH

Nicotine has been shown to uniquely alter adolescent brain development, and it may sensitize the brain to other drugs and prime it for future substance abuse.[59] Analysis of the 2011–2014 National Youth Tobacco Surveys (NYTS), a cross-sectional, school-based, self-administered questionnaire, showed statistically significant increases in the current use of ECs among middle and high school students, which tripled from 2011 to 2014.[60] Electronic cigarettes were found to be the most commonly used tobacco product: 3.9% of middle school and 13.4% of high school students used ECs in 2014. From these surveys, an estimated 4.6 million middle and high school students were using a tobacco product in 2014, of which 2.4 million were EC users.[60] Cross-sectional analyses from these surveys showed that the use of ECs was associated with higher odds of ever or current cigarette smoking, higher odds of established smoking, higher odds of planning to quit smoking among current smokers, and among experimenters, lower odds of abstinence from conventional tobacco cigarettes, concluding that EC use does not discourage and may in fact, encourage, conventional cigarette use among US adolescents.[61]

IMPLICATIONS FOR PHYSICIANS

It is imperative that physicians ask patients about EC use specifically, as vapers may not report EC use when asked about smoking history.[21] Both patients and providers should be aware that ECs are not approved as smoking cessation devices and that there is currently no federal oversight of ECs. This lack of regulation may result in product variability and potential for product contamination. Toxic compounds have been detected in the vapors of ECs but in concentrations much smaller than those of tobacco cigarettes. The impact of these exposures is still to be determined. Thus, prospective randomized controlled trials are needed to definitively answer questions about long-term safety and efficacy of EC as a smoking cessation tool. In the meantime, it is essential that physicians stay up to date on the current EC literature to allow for effective patient counseling.[21]

REFERENCES

1. Pauly J, Li Q, Barry MB. Tobacco-free electronic cigarettes and cigars deliver nicotine and generate concern. Tob Control. 2007;16:357.
2. Foulds J, Veldheer S, Berg A. Electronic cigarettes (e-cigs): views of aficionados and clinical/public health perspectives. Int J Clin Pract. 2011;65:1037-42.
3. Zhu SH, Sun JY, Bonnevie E, et al. Four hundred and sixty brands of e-cigarettes and counting: implications for product regulation. Tob Control. 2014;23 (Suppl 3):iii3-9.
4. Lowry JA. Electronic cigarettes: another pediatric toxic hazard in the home? Clin Toxicol. 2014;52:449-50.
5. Kim AE, Arnold KY, Makarenko O. E-cigarette advertising expenditures in the US, 2011-2012. Am J Prev Med. 2014;46:409-12.
6. Schipper EM, de Graaff LC, Koch BC, et al. A new challenge: suicide attempt using nicotine fillings for electronic cigarettes. Br J Clin Pharmacol. 2014;78:1469-71.
7. Besaratinia A, Tommasi S. Electronic cigarettes: the road ahead. Prev Med. 2014;66:65-7.

8. King BA, Patel R, Nguyen KH, et al. Trends in awareness and use of electronic cigarettes among US adults, 2010-2013. Nicotine Tob Res. 2015;17:219-27.

9. Adkison SE, O'Connor RJ, Bansal-Travers M, et al. Electronic nicotine delivery systems: international tobacco control four-country survey. Am J Prev Med. 2013;44:207-15.

10. Etter JF, Bullen C. Electronic cigarette: users profile, utilization, satisfaction and perceived efficacy. Addiction. 2011;106:2017-28.

11. Chen IL. FDA summary of adverse events on electronic cigarettes. Nicotine Tob Res. 2013;15:615-6.

12. National Center for Chronic Disease Prevention and Health Promotion. Reports of the Surgeon General. The Health Consequences of Smoking-50 Years of Progress: A Report of the Surgeon General. Atlanta (GA): Centers for Disease Control and Prevention (US);2014.

13. Murray RP, Connett JE, Zapawa LM. Does nicotine replacement therapy cause cancer? Evidence from the Lung Health Study. Nicotine Tob Res. 2009;11:1076-82.

14. Cameron JM, Howell DN, White JR, et al. Variable and potentially fatal amounts of nicotine in e-cigarette nicotine solutions. Tob Control. 2014;23:77-8.

15. Nicotine replacement products: poisoning in children. Prescrire Int. 2014;23:126-8.

16. Goniewicz ML, Kuma T, Gawron M, et al. Nicotine levels in electronic cigarettes. Nicotine Tob Res. 2013;15:158-66.

17. Vansickel AR, Cobb CO, Weaver MF, et al. A clinical laboratory model for evaluating the acute effects of electronic "cigarettes": nicotine delivery profile and cardiovascular and subjective effects. Cancer Epidemiol Biomarkers Prev. 2010;19:1945-53.

18. Williams M, Talbot P. Variability among electronic cigarettes in the pressure drop, airflow rate, and aerosol production. Nicotine Tob Res. 2011;13:1276-83.

19. Vansickel AR, Eissenberg T. Electronic cigarettes: effective nicotine delivery after acute administration. Nicotine Tob Res. 2013;15:267-70.

20. Cobb NK, Byron MJ, Abrams DB, et al. Novel nicotine delivery systems and public health: the rise of the "e-cigarette". Am J Public Health. 2010;100:2340-2.

21. Born H, Persky M, Kraus DH, et al. Electronic cigarettes: a primer for clinicians. Otolaryngol Head Neck Surg. 2015;153:5-14.

22. Mohney, Gillian. First Child's Death From Liquid Nicotine Reported as 'Vaping' Gains Popularity. ABC News Web. December 12, 2014. [Accessed June 15, 2015]

23. Schipper EM, de Graaff LC, Koch BC, et al. A new challenge: suicide attempt using nicotine fillings for electronic cigarettes. Br J Clin Pharmacol. 2014;78:1469-71.

24. Weaver M, Breland A, Spindle T, et al. Clinical case conference electronic cigarettes: a review of safety and clinical issues. J Addict Med. 2014;8:234-40.

25. McAuley TR, Hopke PK, Zhao J, et al. Comparison of the effects of e-cigarette vapor and cigarette smoke on indoor air quality. Inhal Toxicol. 2012;24:850-7.

26. Schripp T, Markewitz D, Uhde E, et al. Does e-cigarette consumption cause passive vaping? Indoor Air. 2013;23:25-31.

27. Farsalinos K, Tsiapras D, Kyrzopoulos S, et al. Acute and chronic effects of smoking on myocardial function in healthy heavy smokers: a study of Doppler flow, Doppler tissue velocity, and two-dimensional speckle tracking echocardiography. Echocardiography. 2013;30:285-92.

28. Yan XS, D'Ruiz C. Effects of using electronic cigarettes on nicotine delivery and cardiovascular function in comparison with regular cigarettes. Regul Toxicol Pharmacol. 2015;71:24-34.

29. Bhatnagar A, Whitsel LP, Ribisl KM, et al. Electronic cigarettes: a policy statement from the American Heart Association. Circulation. 2014;130:1418-36.

30. Michota FA, Frost SD. The preoperative evaluation: use the history and physical rather than routine testing. Cleve Clin J Med. 2004;71:63-70.

31. Flouris AD, Poulianiti KP, Chorti MS, et al. Acute effects of electronic and tobacco cigarette smoking on complete blood count. Food Chem Toxicol. 2012; 50:3600-3.

32. Behar RZ, Davis B, Wang Y, et al. Identification of toxicants in cinnamon-flavored electronic cigarette refill fluids. Toxicol In Vitro. 2014;28:198-208.

33. Hashibe M, Brennan P, Chuang SC, et al. Interaction between tobacco and alcohol use and the risk of head and neck cancer: pooled analysis in the International Head and Neck Cancer Epidemiology Consortium. Cancer Epidemiol Biomarkers Prev. 2009;18:541-50.

34. Doll R, Peto R, Boreham J, et al. Mortality in relation to smoking: 50 years' observations on male British doctors. BMJ. 2004;328:1519.

35. Duffy SA, Ronis DL, McLean S, et al. Pretreatment health behaviors predict survival among patients with head and neck squamous cell carcinoma. J Clin Oncol. 2009;27:1969-75.

36. Browman GP, Wong G, Hodson I, et al. Influence of cigarette smoking on the efficacy of radiation therapy in head and neck cancer. N Engl J Med. 1993;328: 159-63.

37. Kawahara M, Ushijima S, Kamimori T, et al. Second primary tumours in more than 2-year disease-free survivors of small-cell lung cancer in Japan: the role of smoking cessation. Br J Cancer. 1998;78:409-12.

38. Ostroff JS, Jacobsen PB, Moadel AB, et al. Prevalence and predictors of continued tobacco use after treatment of patients with head and neck cancer. Cancer. 1995;75:569-76.

39. Lee AH, Stater BJ, Close L, et al. Are e-cigarettes effective in smoking cessation? Laryngoscope. 2015;125:785-7.

40. Klesges RC, Debon M, Ray JW. Are self-reports of smoking rate biased? Evidence from the Second National Health and Nutrition Examination Survey. J Clin Epidemiol. 1995;48:1225-33.

41. Jena PK, Kishore J, Jahnavi G. Correlates of digit bias in self-reporting of cigarette per day (CPD) frequency: results from Global Adult Tobacco Survey (GATS), India and its implications. Asian Pac J Cancer Prev. 2013;14:3865-9.

42. Grana RA, Popova L, Ling PM. A longitudinal analysis of electronic cigarette use and smoking cessation. JAMA Intern Med. 2014;174:812-3.

43. Siegel MB, Tanwar KL, Wood KS. Electronic cigarettes as a smoking-cessation: tool results from an online survey. Am J Prev Med. 2011;40:472-5.

44. Polosa R, Caponnetto P, Cibella F, et al. Quit and smoking reduction rates in vape shop consumers: a prospective 12-month survey. Int J Environ Res Public Health. 2015;12:3428-38.

45. Bullen C, Howe C, Laugesen M, et al. Electronic cigarettes for smoking cessation: a randomised controlled trial. Lancet. 2013;382:1629-37.

46. Caponnetto P, Campagna D, Cibella F, et al. EffiCiency and Safety of an eLectronic cigAreTte (ECLAT) as tobacco cigarettes substitute: a prospective 12-month randomized control design study. PloS One. 2013;8:e66317.
47. Polosa R, Caponnetto P, Morjaria JB, et al. Effect of an electronic nicotine delivery device (e-Cigarette) on smoking reduction and cessation: a prospective 6-month pilot study. BMC Public Health. 2011;11:786.
48. Manzoli L, Flacco ME, Fiore M, et al. Electronic cigarettes efficacy and safety at 12 months: cohort study. PloS One. 2015;10:e0129443.
49. Pepper JK, Brewer NT. Electronic nicotine delivery system (electronic cigarette) awareness, use, reactions and beliefs: a systematic review. Tob Control. 2014;23:375-84.
50. Atkins D, Best D, Briss PA, Eccles M, Falck-Ytter Y, Flottorp S, et al. Grading quality of evidence and strength of recommendations. BMJ 2004;328:1490-4.
51. McRobbie H, Bullen C, Hartmann-Boyce J, et al. Electronic cigarettes for smoking cessation and reduction. Cochrane Database Syst Rev. 2014;12:CD010216.
52. Harrell PT, Simmons VN, Correa JB, et al. Electronic nicotine delivery systems ("e-cigarettes"): review of safety and smoking cessation efficacy. Otolaryngol Head Neck Surg. 2014;151:381-93.
53. Saitta D, Ferro GA, Polosa R. Achieving appropriate regulations for electronic cigarettes. Ther Adv Chronic Dis. 2014;5:50-61.
54. Bam TS, Bellew W, Berezhnova, et al. Position statement on electronic cigarettes or electronic nicotine delivery systems. Int J Tuberc Lung Dis. 2014;18:5-7.
55. European Parliament and Council of the European Union. Directive 2014/40/EU of the European Parliament and of the Council of 3 April 2014 on the approximation of the laws, regulations and administrative provisions of the Member States concerning the manufacture, presentation and sale of tobacco and related products and repealing Directive 2001/37/EC. 2014. Available from http://ec.europa.eu/health/tobacco/docs/dir_201440_en.pdf. [Accessed June 15, 2015].
56. Medicines and Healthcare products Regulatory Agency (MHRA). Press release: UK moves towards safe and effective electronic cigarettes and other nicotine-containing products. Available from http://webarchive.nationalarchives.gov.uk/20141205150130/http://www.mhra.gov.uk/NewsCentre/Pressreleases/CON286855. [Accessed June 15, 2015].
57. US Department of Health and Human Services UFaDA. Deeming tobacco products to be subject to the Federal Food, Drug, and Cosmetic Act as amended by the Family Smoking Prevention and Tobacco Control Act; Regulations on the sale and distribution of tobacco products and required warning statements for tobacco products. Periodical. 2014:23141-207.
58. Biyani S, Derkay CS. E-cigarettes: considerations for the otolaryngologist. Int J Pediatr Otorhinolaryngol. 2015;79:1180-3.
59. Yuan M, Cross SJ, Loughlin SE, et al. Nicotine and the adolescent brain. J Physiol. 2015;593:3397-3412.
60. Arrazola RA, Singh T, Corey CG, et al. Tobacco use among middle and high school students—United States, 2011-2014. MMWR. 2015;64:381-5.
61. Dutra LM, Glantz SA. Electronic cigarettes and conventional cigarette use among US adolescents: a cross-sectional study. JAMA Pediatr. 2014;168:610-7.

Chapter 3

Anesthesia for Otolaryngology

Parwane P Pagano

ANESTHESIA FOR SLEEP ENDOSCOPY

Drug-induced sleep endoscopy (DISE) aims to reproduce upper airway obstruction that occurs during natural sleep to assist in planning surgical intervention for obstructive sleep apnea (OSA) patients. Anesthesia protocols for DISE can be compared based on provision of a clinically adequate level of sedation to allow endoscopic evaluation of obstruction, safety (particularly avoidance of excess oxygen desaturation), and efficiency. Like other anesthesia cases, DISE is performed in the operating room or out-of-operating room location by qualified personnel with appropriate intravenous access, supplemental oxygen and standard monitoring. The overlap between a diagnosis of OSA and difficult mask ventilation or difficult endotracheal intubation requires availability of various airway management devices.

The intravenous benzodiazepine midazolam is used frequently for DISE. For example, an initial dose of 0.03 mg/kg is followed by additional doses of 0.015 to 0.03 mg/kg.[1] The relatively short duration of action facilitates outpatient DISE; if necessary, the competitive antagonist flumazenil may be administered to reverse benzodiazepine effects. Propofol, a rapid-onset nonbarbiturate hypotic agent, is administered for DISE using target-controlled drug infusions, other quantitative infusion methods and manual titration. In patients with severe OSA investigators found a median nadir for oxygen saturation of 81% when propofol for DISE was administered via a probability ramp control infusion scheme.[2] The lowest observed oxygen saturation during the procedure was better than the lowest saturation measured for these patients during sleep studies, and upper airway obstruction was accomplished reasonably quickly with this technique within a median time of 3.8 minutes. A prospective study of standardized manual titration compared to a target-controlled infusion of propofol for DISE in patients with moderate sleep apnea noted a 10% incidence of severe desaturation in the manual titration group.[3] Also, while the study time was longer in the target-controlled infusion group, this technique allowed the endoscopist to capture apnea events more frequently than with the manual titration technique.

Several combinations of agents have been evaluated for DISE, achieving the level of sedation required with a lower total dose of each individual agent. Remifentanil is an ultrashort-acting opioid that does not depend on hepatic biotransformation. In a prospective randomized study, patients undergoing sleep endoscopy with target-controlled infusions of propofol in combination with remifentanil had successful sedation, but a high incidence of desaturation (17 of 22 patients). Patients who received infusions of the centrally acting α-2 agonist dexmedetomidine with remifentanil had fewer desaturation episodes; dexmedetomidine minimizes ventilatory depression, but within this group several patients did not achieve a clinically adequate level of sedation.[4] Dexmedetomidine has been applied alone for sleep endoscopy using a loading dose of 1 mcg/kg and an infusion rate of 1.0 mcg/kg/hour; in this single patient case the endoscopic evaluation was completed without desaturation or significant hypotension.[5]

The bispectral index (BIS) is a dimensionless parameter derived from the electroencephalogram (EEG) signal that ranges from 0 for an isoelectric EEG to 100 in the awake state. To investigate the similarity of conditions achieved in DISE with natural sleep,6 BIS values of patients undergoing polysomnography were monitored, ascertaining average BIS levels for stages of non-REM sleep N1 (79.55), N2 (73.14), and N3 (53.21). In patients with OSA considered for surgical intervention, DISE with midazolam reproduced BIS levels seen in N1 and N2 sleep stages, offering ample opportunity to observe airway obstruction. During DISE with dexmedetomidine, the lowest BIS value observed was 75. With a combination of dexmedetomidine and remifentanil, the average BIS was 73, similar to that with propofol and remifentanil. Studies reporting BIS levels for propofol alone demonstrate average levels of 63–69 depending on the infusion technique. Based on the results of these studies, the BIS may be considered in addition to standard physiologic monitoring during DISE.

CARDIAC EVALUATION FOR PATIENTS UNDERGOING OTOLARYNGOLOGY PROCEDURES

Rationale and Outcomes

Cardiac evaluation aims to identify surgical patients at risk for perioperative major adverse cardiac events and institute interventions to lower this risk. Invasive tests and institution of cardiovascular medications should be critically examined for evidence of actual benefit in relation to the risks incurred. Well-organized perioperative cardiac management is an individualized process taking into account each patient's unique clinical situation.[7] A general approach to this problem is outlined in the American Heart Association/American College of Cardiology clinical practice guideline on perioperative cardiac evaluation for patients undergoing noncardiac surgery, in which evidence supporting various tests and interventions is reviewed.[8]

The incidence of adverse cardiac events accompanying otolaryngology procedures has been surveyed. Postoperative complications after major head and neck cancer surgery from 2006 to 2011 in England were identified from Hospital Episodes Statistics data. Adverse cardiovascular events occurred in 4.6% of patients, comprising myocardial infarction (MI), stroke or transient ischemic attack, and peripheral vascular complications.[9] A retrospective analysis of major head and neck surgery in a United States tertiary care institution over 5 years found 15% of patients developed elevated postoperative troponin I levels, and 2.6% were diagnosed with myocardial infarction postoperatively.[10] Patients with elevated postoperative troponin I levels had an increased risk of mortality at 30 days, 60 days, and 1 year after the surgical procedure.

Risk Assessment and Preoperative Testing

Perioperative cardiac evaluation takes into account the patient history and physical examination, surgical procedure-related risk, and the patient's functional status. High risk surgery, specifically intrathoracic, intraabdominal or suprainguinal vascular surgery was identified as one of the six predictors of major perioperative cardiac complications in the Revised Cardiac Risk Index (RCRI).[11] More generally, procedures associated with increases in heart rate and afterload, or significant decreases in preload and/or afterload can predispose a patient to cardiac events and various otolaryngology procedures have such features. In terms of hemodynamics, a retrospective study of over 30,000 patients having all types of noncardiac surgeries in a single institution found that intraoperative mean arterial pressure below 55 mm Hg was associated with myocardial injury and cardiac complications[12] probably due to ischemia-reperfusion injury.

A detailed history and physical examination will focus on the following: angina, previous MI, surgical or percutaneous interventions, smoking, diabetes mellitus, hyperlipidemia, hypertension, peripheral or cerebrovascular disease, chronic kidney disease, congestive heart failure, carotid bruit, and ventricular gallop.[13] Using a risk prediction index, the clinician may estimate whether the patient is low or high risk for perioperative adverse cardiac events. For example, the RCRI comprises six independent predictors of perioperative major cardiac complications: history of congestive heart failure, cerebrovascular disease, ischemic heart disease, preoperative treatment with insulin, preoperative creatinine >2.0 mg/dL, and high risk surgery (as listed previously). In the RCRI validation cohort, patients with zero risk factors had a 0.4% rate of adverse cardiac events, while the rate was 0.7% in the group with one risk factor.[11] In contrast, two risk factors resulted in a cardiac complication rate of 7% and the presence of three or greater risk factors was associated with an 11% rate. Major cardiac complications in the RCRI dataset included MI, pulmonary edema, ventricular fibrillation or cardiac arrest, and complete heart block.

Based on this information, stable patients at low risk generally do not need further cardiac testing before proceeding to surgery. Patients who have two or more predictors of adverse cardiac events may be stratified based on their functional capacity. Individuals who cannot perform activity expending at least four metabolic equivalents have poor functional capacity and can undergo preoperative stress testing to assess for myocardial ischemia. A low level of self-reported exercise tolerance (inability to walk four blocks or climb two flights of stairs) was associated with a greater incidence of perioperative myocardial ischemia and neurologic complications in a study of patients undergoing major noncardiac surgery.[14]

Limited functional capacity is a common sign of numerous diseases, including myocardial ischemia, heart failure, lung diseases (severe chronic obstructive pulmonary disease, pulmonary fibrosis, pulmonary hypertension), anemia, and deconditioning.[15] Heart failure and decreased left ventricular systolic function present significant perioperative risks. In a cohort of 174 patients previously diagnosed with heart failure requiring noncardiac surgery, severely reduced left ventricular ejection fraction (<30%) was an independent risk factor for perioperative MI, heart failure exacerbation, and 30-day mortality.[16] Echocardiography to assess left ventricular function yields useful information in patients with dyspnea associated with heart failure or without another obvious cause, and may be applied to reevaluate patients with reduced left ventricular function.[8]

Coronary Stents

An increasing number of patients scheduled for surgery have had coronary stents placed. Second-generation drug-eluting coronary stents release immunosuppressive agents (everolimus or zotarolimus) to block proliferation of vascular smooth muscle cells after stent placement.[17] In comparison with bare-metal stents, drug-eluting stents reduce the risk of repeat revascularization. To minimize the risk of stent thrombosis, current guidelines advocate treating drug-eluting stent patients with dual antiplatelet therapy, comprising aspirin and a P2Y12 inhibitor such as clopidogrel for at least 12 months.[18] Ongoing clinical trials aim to address the optimal duration of dual antiplatelet therapy to balance protection from stent thrombosis with the risk of hemorrhagic events.[19]

Occasionally, a patient presents for a surgical procedure that cannot be delayed while on dual antiplatelet therapy after recent drug-eluting stent implantation. Discontinuation of clopidogrel within the first 6 months after stent placement is significantly associated with stent thrombosis[20] often leading to MI. If the planned surgical procedure has low or moderate bleeding risk, it is optimal to continue both aspirin and clopidogrel through the perioperative period. For procedures with high bleeding risk for which clopidogrel is interrupted, aspirin should be continued through the perioperative period with intensive postoperative monitoring of the patient until the dual antiplatelet therapy is reinstituted.[21] In patients who must stop clopidogrel for surgery and present a very high ischemic risk due to clinical or angiographic factors, a short acting intravenous antiplatelet agent such as tirofiban or eptifibatide may be considered.[22]

Perioperative Biomarkers

Biomarkers associated with cardiac ischemic injury or volume overload such as natriuretic peptide and troponin are being explored for application in the perioperative period. In a large trial of noncardiac surgical patients, peak postoperative troponin levels correlated with 30-day mortality rates.[23] However, many of the events seen in studies of postoperative troponin elevation do not meet clinical criteria for MI and include mortality from a variety of causes. Accordingly, postoperative troponin measurement is supported if the patient presents a clinical picture consistent with myocardial ischemia or MI rather than as a general surveillance tool.[8] Higher postoperative natriuretic peptide levels were associated with an elevated risk of 30-day mortality or major cardiac events (MI or heart failure) in a meta-analysis of 18 studies of noncardiac surgical patients.[24] A well-defined clinical role for this biomarker in the perioperative period awaits further investigation.

RESPIRATORY COMPLICATIONS IN PATIENTS WITH OSA UNDERGOING SLEEP SURGERY

Patients with OSA undergoing noncardiac surgery have a higher incidence of postoperative cardiac complications, respiratory failure, oxygen desaturation, and postoperative intensive care unit (ICU) utilization, based on a meta-analysis of 13 studies comprising almost 4,000 patients.[25] A retrospective study of over 1 million records using the Nationwide Inpatient Sample database examined differences in postoperative cardiorespiratory outcomes between patients with sleep disordered breathing and those without after elective abdominal, cardiovascular, orthopedic, and prostatic surgery.[26] The investigators found a significant independent association between sleep disordered breathing and a greater odds ratio for application of continuous positive airway pressure (CPAP)/noninvasive ventilation, emergent intubation and mechanical ventilation, as well as atrial fibrillation. Among all patients who required emergent intubation, a higher percentage of sleep disordered breathing patients had this intervention early in their hospital course on postoperative day 0 or 1.

Obstructive sleep apnea patients undergoing sleep surgery present several concerns. The potential for upper airway obstruction in the postoperative period is significant as a result of postsurgical edema. Opioids, while effective in postoperative pain management, cause central respiratory depression and decreased tonic activity to the upper airway.[27] A review by the Cochrane Airways Group of randomized trials in adult OSA patients described lower oxygen saturation levels with short-acting opioids and specific benzodiazepines.[28] Postoperative disposition is a key decision as admission to a stepdown unit or ICU after sleep surgery provides close monitoring to rapidly detect cardiorespiratory complications but utilizes limited and costly intensive care resources.

Several studies have investigated the respiratory complication rate after sleep surgeries. Among 50 patients undergoing multilevel OSA surgery excluding major tongue-base surgery with an average apnea-hypopnea index (AHI) of 24.4, 22% were admitted to the hospital overnight based on a set of criteria applied in the postanesthesia care unit (desaturation, upper airway obstruction, witnessed apnea, opioid analgesic requirements) while the remainder were discharged.[29] No respiratory complications occurred in the group discharged home and only one hospitalized patient required a respiratory intervention in which CPAP was applied. A series of patients with an average AHI of 42 undergoing uvulopalatopharyngoplasty with or without septoplasty had no significant postoperative respiratory complications such as emergent reintubation.[30]

A retrospective study of 166 patients who had transoral robotic surgery for OSA included a single case of pulmonary embolism requiring anticoagulation.[31] Individuals in this study group had lingual tonsillectomy in conjunction with one or more additional procedures and all patients were admitted to the surgical ICU postoperatively. In a series of over 400 patients undergoing surgery for OSA, individuals who had nasal and palate procedures only and were stable after 6 hours observation in the PACU were discharged, while others were admitted to a step-down unit for 1 day.[32] One hospitalized patient developed upper airway obstruction requiring emergent awake intubation due to a floor of mouth hematoma. Overall few serious respiratory complications were reported with the level of postoperative care selected for these patients.

REFERENCES

1. DeVito A, Llatas MC, Vanni A et al. European position paper on drug-induced sedation endoscopy (DISE). Sleep Breath 2014;18:453-65.
2. Atkins JH, Mandel JE, Rosanova G. Safety and efficacy of drug-induced sleep endoscopy using a probability ramp propofol infusion system in patients with severe obstructive sleep apnea. Anesth Analg. 2014;119:805-10.
3. DeVito A, Agnoletti V, Berrettini S, et al. Drug-induced sleep endoscopy: conventional versus target controlled infusion techniques—a randomized controlled study. Eur Arch Otorhinolaryngol. 2011;268:457-62.
4. Cho JS, Soh S, Kim EJ et al. Comparison of three sedation regimens for drug-induced sleep endoscopy. Sleep Breath 2015;19:711-17.
5. Mathews AMV, Goh JPS, Teo LM. A case report on the anesthetic management of dexmedetomidine-induced sleep endoscopy and transoral robotic surgery for the treatment of obstructive sleep apnea. Proceedings of Singapore Healthcare. 2013;22:151-5.
6. Abdullah VJ, Lee DLY, Ha SCN, et al. Sleep endoscopy with midazolam: sedation level evaluation with bispectral analysis. Otolaryngol Head Neck Surg. 2013;148:331-7.
7. Eagle KA, Vaishnava P, Froehlich JB. Perioperative cardiovascular care for patients undergoing non-cardiac surgical intervention. JAMA Internal Med. 2015;175:835-9.
8. Fleisher LA, Fleischmann KE, Auerbach AD, et al. 2014 AHA/ACC guideline on perioperative cardiovascular evaluation and management of patients undergoing noncardiac surgery: a report of the American College of Cardiology/American Heart Association Task Force on Practice Guidelines. J Am Coll Cardiol. 2014;64:e77-137.
9. Nouraei SAR, Middleton SE, Hudovsky A, et al. A national analysis of the outcome of major head and neck cancer surgery: implications for surgeon-level data publication. Clin Otolaryngol. 2013;38:502-11.
10. Nagele P, Rao LK, Penta M, et al. Postoperative myocardial injury after major head and neck cancer surgery. Head Neck. 2011;33:1085-91.
11. Lee TH, Marcantonio ER, Mangione CM, et al. Derivation and prospective validation of a simple index for prediction of cardiac risk of major noncardiac surgery. Circulation. 1999;100:1043-9.

12. Walsh M, Deveraux PJ, Garg, AX, et al. Relationship between intraoperative mean arterial pressure and clinical outcomes after noncardiac surgery: toward an empirical definition of hypotension. Anesthesiology. 2013;119:507-15.

13. Pryor DB, Shaw L, McCants CB, et al. Value of the history and physical in identifying patients at increased risk for coronary artery disease. Ann Intern Med. 1993;118:81-90.

14. Reilly DF, McNeely MJ, Doerner D, et al. Self-reported exercise tolerance and the risk of serious perioperative complications. Arch Intern Med. 1999;159:2185-92.

15. Sweitzer BJ. Where do we make a difference? NYSSA 68th Annual Postgraduate Assembly in Anesthesiology SP-24, December 15, 2014.

16. Healy KO, Waksmonski CA, Altman RK, et al. Perioperative outcome and long-term mortality for heart failure patients undergoing intermediate- and high-risk noncardiac surgery: impact of left ventricular ejection fraction. Congest Heart Fail. 2010;16:45-9.

17. Stefanani GG, Holmes DR Jr. Drug-eluting coronary stents. N Engl J Med 2013;368:254-65.

18. Levine GN, Bates ER, Blankenship JC, et al. 2011 ACCF/AHA/SCAI guideline for percutaneous coronary intervention: a report of the American College of Cardiology Foundation/American Heart Association Task Force on Practical Guidelines and the Society for Cardiovascular Angiography and Interventions. J Am Coll Cardiol. 2011;58:e44-e122.

19. Price MJ. The optimal duration of dual antiplatelet therapy after drug-eluting stent implantation. J Am Coll Cardiol. 2015;65:1311-33.

20. Schulz S, Schuster T, Mehilli J et al. Stent thrombosis after drug-eluting stent implantation: incidence, timing, and relation to discontinuation of clopidogrel therapy over a 4-year period. European Heart Journal 2009;30:2714-21.

21. Savonitto S, Caracciolo M, Cattaneo M, et al. Management of patients with recently implanted coronary stents on dual antiplatelet therapy who need to undergo major surgery. J Thromb Haemost. 2011;9:2133-42.

22. Chassot PG, Marcucci C, Delabays A. Perioperative antiplatelet therapy. Am Fam Physician. 2010;82:1484-9.

23. Biccard BM, Devereaux PJ, Rodseth RN. Cardiac biomarkers in the prediction of risk in the non-cardiac surgery setting. Anaesthesia. 2014;69:484-93.

24. Rodseth RN, Biccard BM, Chu R, et al. Postoperative B-type natriuretic peptide for prediction of major cardiac events in patients undergoing noncardiac surgery: systematic review and individual patient meta-analysis. Anesthesiology. 2013;119:270-83.

25. Kaw R, Chung F, Pasupuleti V, et al. Meta-analysis of the association between obstructive sleep apnoea and postoperative outcome. Br J Anaesth. 2012; 109:897-906.

26. Mokhlesi B, Hovda MD, Vekhter B, et al. Sleep-disordered breathing and post-operative outcomes after elective surgery. Chest. 2013;144:903-14.

27. Chung F, Liao P, Yegneswaran B, et al. Postoperative changes in sleep-disordered breathing and sleep architecture in patients with obstructive sleep apnea. Anesthesiology. 2014;120:287-98.

28. Mason M, Cates CJ, Smith I. Effects of opioid, hypnotic and sedating medications on sleep-disordered breathing in adults with obstructive sleep apnoea. Cochrane Database Syst Rev. 2015;7:CD011090.

29. Rotenberg B, Theriault J, Cheng H, et al. Admission after sleep surgery is unnecessary in patients without cardiovascular disease. Laryngoscope. 2015;125: 498-502.
30. Talei B, Cossu AL, Slepian R, et al. Immediate complications related to anesthesia in patients undergoing uvulopalatopharyngoplasty for obstructive sleep apnea. Laryngoscope. 2013;123:2892-5.
31. Glazer TA, Hoff PT, Spector ME. Transoral robotic surgery for obstructive sleep apnea perioperative management and postoperative complications. JAMA Otolaryngol Head Neck Surg. 2014;140:1207-12.
32. Pang KP, Siow JK, Tseng P. Safety of multilevel surgery in obstructive sleep apnea: a review of 487 cases. Arch Otolaryngol Head Neck Surg 2012;138(4):353-57.

Chapter 4

Malpractice in Otolaryngology

Soly Baredes, Jean Anderson Eloy

OVERVIEW

Litigation associated with alleged medical malpractice has increased in the past three decades in the United States affecting the delivery of medical care and contributing to the cost of care through increasing liability insurance premiums, the cost of legal proceedings, and promoting the practice of defensive medicine.[1-6] Although malpractice premium rates may be plateauing, the cost of malpractice insurance for otolaryngologists in the United States averages $28,038, and can be substantially more in some localities.[7,8] In this chapter, we review some of the recent information regarding legal liability in otolaryngology-head and neck surgery.

In the current medical liability climate, it is generally accepted that medical negligence entails four elements: a duty to provide care, a deviation from the standard of care, an injury, and a direct relationship between the substandard care and the injury. In a clear review of the concept of the standard of care in medicine, Moffett and Moore[9] note that there has been an evolution in the legal definition of the standard of care. They note that the modern definition appears to increasingly be what a "minimally competent physician in the same field would do in the same situation, with the same resources". They also note that clinical practice guidelines are increasingly being used in litigation, but that their use is continuously changing and applied as the standard of care differently in individual cases, and that standards vary from state to state.

Recent investigations specifically related to otolaryngology have identified factors such as perceived deficits in informed consent and allegations of unnecessary procedures as important factors in litigation, in addition to procedure-specific complications.[10-17] In order to assess the overall current state of liability issues in otolaryngology, Svider et al. analyzed the results of trials dealing with alleged malpractice by otolaryngologists from 2008 to 2013 using the Westlaw legal database

(Thomson Reuters, New York, NY).[17] The 44 cases identified were studied to determine the procedures involved, the state in which the trial took place, alleged malpractice, specialty of co-defendants, and outcome. The most commonly litigated procedures and conditions involved endoscopic sinus surgery (21%), nasal surgery (18%), adenotonsillectomy (12%), thyroidectomy (11%), failure to diagnose cancer (11%), and ear surgery (9%). All other procedures or conditions comprised 18% of cases. Seven of the 44 cases involved the death of the patient. The deaths were associated with an alleged failure of a timely intubation, failure to diagnose cancer, complication of adenotonsillectomies, and hemorrhaging from tracheotomies. It is not surprising that litigation was most common in some of the most commonly performed procedures: rhinologic procedures, adenotonsillectomy, and thyroidectomy. In some procedures, such as endoscopic sinus surgery, the complications leading to litigation were often similar, with eye injury, cerebrospinal fluid (CSF) leak, brain injury, and meningitis being cited in most cases. In other procedures such as adenotonsillectomy and thyroidectomy, the causes leading to litigation were much more varied. Juries found in the physician's favor in 81.8% of the cases. Of the most commonly litigated conditions or surgeries, jury verdicts for the plaintiff only occurred in cases of endoscopic sinus surgery (three out of six cases), and thyroidectomy (two out of three cases). All missed cancer diagnosis, nonendoscopic sinus surgery rhinologic procedures, adenotonsillectomy, and otologic surgery cases were decided in the physician's favor. Of note was that the issue of a deficiency in informed consent was a factor in initiating litigation in >34% of cases. The litigation environment definitely varies from state to state, with New York State having 20.5% of cases, followed by Pennsylvania (11.4%), and Illinois and Kansas (9.1% each). The average jury award against otolaryngologists was $940,000, ranging from $148,000 to $3.6 million. Because a substantial number of cases against otolaryngologists involved surgical procedures, the most common codefendant physicians were anesthesiologists. Although the analysis by Svider et al.[17] provides an important snapshot of the most recent experience of litigation against otolaryngologists, it only deals with cases that have progressed to trial. It is not known how many cases are initiated against otolaryngologists, but do not progress to trial. One recent analysis not specific to otolaryngology estimated that only 15% of malpractice cases do eventually go to trial.[18] It can be safely assumed, therefore, that otolaryngologists were involved in more cases that were either dismissed or settled out of court than is represented by the jury trial experience recorded.

Hong et al.[19] reviewed the otolaryngology malpractice trial experience of the decade from 2001 to 2011. Although they found that results favored the otolaryngologists 58% of the time, they noted an increase in the percent of trials favoring otolaryngologists toward the end of the decade, consistent with Svider et al.'s review of more recent years. The average awards for cases settled was $1,149,451 compared to $1,782,514 for cases in which there was a jury award. Compared to more recent data, this may indicate an overall decrease in the average amount of awards in cases involving otolaryngologists, although these figures can often be influenced by a few outsized awards. Their data showed the settled amounts to be lower than jury awards in all categories of cases except pediatrics and head and neck surgery. As might be expected, failure to properly perform a procedure was among the two most frequently cited allegation; the other, perhaps less predictable but slightly more frequent, was failure to diagnose. In fact, the most common allegations in wrongful death litigation dealt with failure to diagnose or delay in diagnosis. As previously noted, failure of informed consent is a frequent allegation in medical malpractice cases. Hong et al., however, found that in cases where there was an allegation of lack of informed consent, the otolaryngologist defendants were clearly favored.

Despite recent data showing a trend for jury verdicts to increasingly favor otolaryngologist defendants, there are other unmeasured costs to the physician in the process. The opportunity costs in the time preparing for litigation, and the decreased productivity from the stress of the process, are difficult to measure, but can be significant.[18] Many physicians cite harm to professional reputation as an even greater concern than the direct financially related consequences of a malpractice suit.[20] Harm to reputation, of course, can also have long-term consequences in terms of income.

Below we review recent information on malpractice litigation in specific areas of interest to the otolaryngologist-head and neck surgeon.

PEDIATRIC OTOLARYNGOLOGY

Care of the pediatric otolaryngology patient presents unique challenges with regard to litigation. In a recent review of cases from 1994 to 2013 involving allegations of negligence in the care of pediatric otolaryngology patients by Rose et al.,[21] alleged negligence involved both operative and nonoperative cases, though otolaryngologists were defendants >90% of the time for alleged negligence related to surgery. Intraoperative negligence was alleged 76.1% of the time, and postoperative negligence 43.5% of the time. Unnecessary surgery, lack of informed consent, and bleeding constituted other significant allegations. Adenotonsillectomy was the most common procedure leading to litigation, with 25% of those cases having bleeding as a complication. Stevenson et al.[22] found that postoperative bleeding was the most common complication associated with tonsillectomy that led to allegations of negligence. Considering that 530,000 tonsillectomies are performed annually in patients under 15 years old,[23-25] the procedure represents a significant area of potential litigation risk.

Although the investigation by Rose et al.[21] found that few otolaryngologists are involved in litigation resulting from nonoperative management, other specialties, mostly pediatricians, were defendants in cases involving pediatric otolaryngologic disorders. The failure to diagnose a condition or a complication in a timely manner represented a significant number of cases. Situations that ultimately led to a diagnosis of meningitis posed a particular risk to ending up in litigation. As one might expect, situations that led to permanent deficits or death were also frequent causes of allegations of negligence. Of the 78 cases analyzed by Rose et al., 52.6% resulted in jury or out-of-court payments. The median payment was $450,000, though the range was $6,000–$24.3 million. Median jury awards were $874,190, and median settlements were $250,000. Airway complications and permanent deficits were most statistically associated with higher payments. Patients aged 1–5 years old were awarded greater payments, and patients over 11 years old lower payments compared to all other cases.

Stevenson et al.[22] specifically focused on tonsillectomy malpractice claims from 1984 to 2010. As with the study of Rose et al. bleeding was the most frequent complication leading to litigation, representing 33.7% of cases. It was the most frequent complication resulting in death. Bleeding was also responsible for the third highest median jury awards ($600,000), after anoxic events ($3,051,296), and medication-related complications ($950,000). The highest awards in cases of bleeding were associated with airway complications resulting from the bleeding, specifically anoxic brain injury or death resulting from aspiration of blood. Otolaryngologists will also be included in litigation for complications that are related to anesthesiology or nursing care; Morris et al.[26] noted that in the case of death or major injury, the otolaryngologist is almost always included in the litigation. Surgeons were dismissed as defendants in only half the cases of a purely anesthetic complication, and some jury awards were made against otolaryngologists in cases of purely anesthetic or nursing mishaps.

OTOLOGY

Otology often involves procedures where the margin of error is small and the consequences of iatrogenic injury may be immediately apparent to the patient in the form of facial paralysis, hearing loss or vertigo. Only recently has the area of malpractice litigation in otology in the United States been specifically examined.[27-29] Mathew et al.[30] performed a comprehensive study of otologic malpractice claims in the United Kingdom. Though their data is useful in identifying patient concerns, such as hearing loss and facial paralysis being the most frequent complications leading to litigation, the health care and legal systems in the United Kingdom differ substantially from those in the United States. Blake et al.[28] recently examined jury verdicts and settlements in otologic procedure complications in the United States from 1988 to 2011 using the Westlaw database. Of note is that of the 47 cases identified, only 28 cases involved otolaryngologists. The other cases involved primary care specialists, neurosurgeons, anesthesiologists, plastic surgeons, a radiologist, or nonmedical doctors. Cerumen removal was the most common procedure leading to litigation comprising 21.3% of claims. Most of these claims (80%) were against primary care physicians; only 20% were against otolaryngologists. At least half the cases involved lavage for cerumen removal. Other procedures frequently involved in litigation included acoustic neuroma resection, stapedectomy, mastoidectomy, tympanoplasty, myringotomy, ventilation tube placement, and ossiculoplasty. The most common complaint was hearing loss, mentioned in 53.2% of cases. Other common factors leading to litigation included facial nerve injury (27.7%), tympanic membrane perforation (23.4%), tinnitus (10.6%), and vertigo (23.4%). The majority of the cases (63.8%) resulted in a verdict for the defense, while the others were either a plaintiff verdict (25.5%) or settled (10.6%). The average award for plaintiff verdict was $446,697, ranging from $32,000 to $1.5 million. The average amount paid as a settlement was $372,607, ranging from $175,000 to $5 million. Cases that involved facial nerve injury, tympanic membrane perforation, and hearing loss were more likely to result in payment to the patient. Secondary injuries claimed that also increased the likelihood of payment included the need for additional surgery, lack of informed consent, and effect on an individual's career. The procedures that resulted in the greatest payments were acoustic neuroma surgery and stapedectomy; the injuries that resulted in the greatest payments were paralysis (other than facial nerve) and altered mental status.

Ruhl et al.[29] focused an analysis of malpractice cases specific to otologic surgery using two US databases, Westlaw and LexisNexis, for the period 1983–2012 (58 cases). This more expansive view of specifically surgical cases again showed hearing loss and facial nerve injury to be the most frequent complaints leading to litigation. Mastoidectomy was the most common surgery that reached the trial stage (48%), followed by ossiculoplasty including stapedectomy (21%), and tympanoplasty (16%). Fifty percent of the cases resulted in defense verdicts, 31% favored the plaintiff, and 19% were settled. The average jury award was $1,131,189, and the average settlement was $440,165. The average award for facial nerve injury was $693,775, for hearing loss $936,268, and for facial nerve injury with hearing loss $1,428,032. The most common factors that resulted in payment to the plaintiff were improper performance of the surgery (50%), failure to properly diagnose and treat (33%), inadequate informed consent (22%), and delay in diagnosis (22%). Of interest in the Ruhl et al. analysis was that outcomes were not significantly different for pediatric cases than adult cases, but adult cases received higher awards (it was not clear if the injuries were greater in adults). Also, the use of otolaryngologist expert witnesses versus other specialty expert witnesses did not seem to affect the outcome. The only case of facial nerve injury in their study where the lack of facial nerve monitoring was presented as the only argument for improper performance returned a defense verdict; the jury decided that intraoperative nerve monitoring was not the standard of care.

Reilly et al.[27] performed an analysis of 94 cases of hearing loss resulting in malpractice litigation using the Westlaw database. The most frequent causes of adult hearing loss resulting in litigation were drug toxicity, tumor, acoustic neuroma, ear infection, and ear flush. The most frequent causes of pediatric hearing loss resulting in litigation were meningitis, drug toxicity, ear infection, tumor, and jaundice. Although otolaryngologists were the most frequently sued specialists, they only represented 22% of the physicians involved in litigation for hearing loss. Pediatricians (13%), nurse/physician assistants (12%), emergency room physicians (10%), and family physicians (10%) were also frequently involved in litigation. Of the 13 cases against otolaryngologists, a defense verdict was reached in 9 cases, plaintiff verdict in 3 cases, and a settlement in one case. The types of cases were acoustic neuroma ($400,000), ossiculoplasty ($200,000), removal of facial mass ($549,000), and stapedectomy ($2,910,000).

FACIAL PLASTIC SURGERY AND CRANIOFACIAL SURGERY

Facial plastic surgery procedures are more often elective and cosmetic in nature. Svider et al.[16] performed an analysis specifically of facial plastic surgery procedures using the Westlaw database for the years 1984–2012 (88 cases). The procedures most commonly resulting in litigation were blepharoplasty and rhinoplasty, followed by rhytidectomy, facial fracture repair, cleft lip and/or palate repair, and laser procedures. The most common plaintiff complaints were excessive scarring/ disfigurement, difficulty closing one's eyes, and postoperative pain. The perceived lack of informed consent was a contributing factor in 38.6% of cases, and represented the single most common factor among the cases. Defendant specialties included plastic surgeons, otolaryngologists, ophthalmologists, oral surgeons, anesthesiologists, and dermatologists. Nearly half of the cases were against plastic surgeons and approximately a fifth against otolaryngologists. There was a defense verdict in 62.5%, and a plaintiff verdict in 28.4% of cases; 9.1% of cases were settled. The average jury award was $352,341, and the average settlement was $577,437. Why many of the cases occurred in California (38.7%) was not clear, but could be a reflection of the number of cosmetic cases performed in that state. Florida had the second most number of cases (10.2%).

Though there are overlapping aspects of cases that can be included in the categories of facial plastic surgery and craniofacial surgery, an investigation examining purely craniofacial patients, and not including cosmetic procedures such as rhinoplasty, blepharoplasty, and rhytidectomy, yielded interesting results.[31] Defendant verdicts were only achieved in 48% of cases, in large part because >83% of cases involving minors (representing 29% of the cohort studied) were resolved with payments. The remaining cases were evenly split between settlements, and plaintiff verdicts. Median settlements were $988,000, with a range of $32,400–$7.5 million. Median plaintiff verdict was $555,000, with a range of $7,000–$22.7 million. The median payment for minors (<18 years old) was $1.2 million, compared to $541,885 for adults. Cleft lip/palate repair were the most common cases represented, followed by ear reconstruction, Le Fort osteotomy, and mandible fracture repair. More than half the cases involved the need for additional surgery as a factor in the litigation, once again highlighting the importance of discussing this possibility or likelihood prior to surgery. Many of the cases of cleft lip/palate repair involved persistent oronasal fistula, emphasizing the need to include this possibility in the informed consent process. Approximately a fifth of cases involved a missed fracture on imaging studies, reinforcing the need to inspect one's own imaging studies, and to have good communication with radiologist colleagues.

RHINOLOGY

As previously noted, endoscopic sinus surgery and other nasal surgeries together comprise 39% of recent malpractice litigation in otolaryngology-head and neck surgery.[17] Winford et al.[32] performed an analysis of malpractice cases in sinonasal disease for the period 2004–2013. The most common symptoms or conditions that led to treatment were chronic sinusitis and nasal obstruction. Less frequent reasons for treatment were sleep apnea, headache, acute sinusitis, nasal polyps, and allergic fungal sinusitis. Negligent technique was alleged in 38% of the cases, and lack of informed consent in 27% of the cases. Multiple cases also included allegations of failure of the surgery to improve symptoms, wrongful death, surgery being unnecessary, and a failure to diagnose a condition such as cancer. Of the four wrongful death cases identified, only one involved a surgical complication (carotid artery injury). Two cases of wrongful death involved a missed diagnosis of sinonasal cancer, and a postoperative pneumonia. In this study, defendants were successful in 13 of 18 cases analyzed (72%), had jury awards in 3 cases, and settled 2 cases. The average of the known jury awards was $225,000, and the average of settlements was $212,500; these are low awards and settlements compared to other reported figures in otolaryngology.

Anosmia can have an effect on quality of life, including affecting taste and the ability to detect environmental cues. A recent study analyzed the role of anosmia as a complaint in malpractice litigation.[33] Otolaryngologists were defendants in 68% of cases where olfactory dysfunction was alleged as a cause of negligence. The most frequent procedure cited was endoscopic sinus surgery, followed by various other procedures performed by otolaryngologists and oral surgeons. The most frequent associated complaints were dysgeusia, CSF leaks, and meningitis. The lack of informed consent was an issue in 35% of the cases of iatrogenic injury causing the anosmia. Defendant verdicts were reached in 60% of the cases, plaintiff verdicts in 28% of cases, and settlements in 12% of cases. The median jury award was $300,000 (range $55,000–$2,000,000); the median settlement was $413,000 (range $250,000–$575,000). The amount of the payment appeared to be more related to injuries in addition to the anosmia. None of the cases in which anosmia was alleged as a factor in litigation involved objective testing of smell. Objective tests for olfactory function are available,[34,35] but have not been adopted in routine clinical care.[34,35]

Epistaxis is a common medical problem with potentially serious and life-threatening consequences; it accounts for 1 in every 200 emergency room visit in the United States.[36] In a study of epistaxis as a factor in malpractice litigation of 26 cases, Khan et al.[37] noted that a delay in the diagnosis of the underlying cause of the epistaxis led to litigation in 42.3% of the cases. Twenty-three percent of the cases involved cases of recurrent epistaxis in which there was a delay in obtaining a biopsy showing sinonasal cancer. A delay in noting a foreign body (battery) in a case of recurrent epistaxis, resulting in a septal perforation, was the basis of one case. A failed procedure in an attempt to control the bleeding was a factor in 30.8% of the cases. In three cases a failure to identify arterial anatomic variations prior to embolization resulted in complications including blindness and stroke. Iatrogenic cause of epistaxis was a factor in a minority of the cases (15.4%). In the majority of cases (76.9%), failure to recognize complications in a timely manner was alleged. Highlighting the potentially serious consequences of epistaxis, 30.8% of the cases in the Kahn et al.[37] study, were for situations in which the patient died either from complications of therapy or from having epistaxis as a complication of another procedure or pathology. Two of the deaths were related to patients aspirating the nasal packing. A malpositioned posterior nasal pack caused asphyxiation and coma in another patient, resulting in the largest payout in the study: $9,022,643. In the overall study, a defendant jury verdict was only reached in 42.3% of the cases, a settlement in 30.8% of the cases, and a plaintiff verdict in 26.9% of the cases.

Because of the critical structures surrounding the anatomy of the paranasal sinuses, image-guidance has been developed and frequently used in endoscopic sinus surgery. Critical examinations of the use of image-guidance in endoscopic sinus surgery have not shown definitive evidence of the benefit of its routine use, but have recommended its use based on a case-by-case evaluation, and the clinical judgment of the surgeon.[38,39] The American Academy of Otolaryngology—Head and Neck Surgery supports the use of image-guidance in defined situations, but ultimately recommends its use at the discretion of the operating surgeon. Image-guidance as a factor in endoscopic surgery litigation was evaluated by Eloy et al.[40] Of 30 cases evaluated between 2004 and 2013, only 4 cases (13.3%), mentioned image-guidance, and in no case was it a factor in the patient pursuing litigation. The other 26 cases (86.7%) did not mention the use of image-guidance, and the technology was not mentioned as a factor leading to litigation. The use or nonuse of image-guidance does not appear to be a significant factor in malpractice claims. The technology, therefore, should probably not be used solely as a medicolegal measure, but rather only at the discretion of the surgeon for its perceived advantages to conduct safer surgery.

Cerebrospinal fluid leak can result from endoscopic and nonendoscopic rhinologic surgery. Uncontrolled CSF leaks can be associated with severe consequences such as meningitis, and neurologic deficits. In an analysis of litigation in CSF leaks associated with sinonasal surgery, 77.8% of the cases were secondary to endoscopic sinus surgery.[41] The most frequent factors noted for litigation included the need for additional surgery (88.9%), developing meningitis (50%), and a failure to recognize complications in a timely manner (44.4%). Despite 55.6% of cases being decided in the physician's favor, the payments in jury awards (mean, $1,104,000; range, $300,000–$1,908,000) and settlements (mean, $966,887; range, $575,000–$1,800,000) were quite substantial.

In a study focusing on litigation for meningitis associated with management of otolaryngologic conditions, rhinologic (surgical and nonsurgical) cases accounted for nearly half of the cases, and only 35% were resolved in the defendant's favor.[42] The alleged failure to diagnose meningitis in a timely manner was the most common complaint leading to litigation. The failure to diagnose meningitis with sinusitis was more likely to result in a payment than an iatrogenic injury causing meningitis.

Rhinologic procedures represented 60% of cases of a recent analysis of litigation related to iatrogenic orbital injury that included all specialties.[15] Otolaryngologists were more subject to malpractice litigation for an iatrogenic orbital injury than ophthalmologists. The majority of injuries by otolaryngologists was caused during the performance of endoscopic sinus surgery (76.9%), almost exclusively related to compromise of the lamina papyracea. Though defendants in the study prevailed in 60% of cases, the payments for iatrogenic orbital injury were substantial. The mean plaintiff award was $472,661 (range, $75,000–$763,214). Out-of-court settlements were higher with the mean being $1.78 million (range, $487,500–$3.9 million). The largest settlement amount ($3.9 million) was in the case of a 45-year-old woman who suffered permanent diplopia and blurry vision related to breach of the lamina papyracea during endoscopic sinus surgery with transection of the medial rectus muscle and optic nerve and corneal injury. She also had subsequent glaucoma, disfigurement, and chronic pain.

HEAD AND NECK SURGERY

Head and neck surgery is a broad area within otolaryngology that encompasses a multitude of conditions and surgeries. More than other general areas within otolaryngology, procedures may deal with the management of malignancies, and affect vital functions such as speech, swallowing, and respiration. In a recent comprehensive review of litigation specifically related to the management of head and neck disease, Simonsen et al.[43] noted that perioperative complications and the delay in (or missed) diagnosis were responsible for the vast majority of malpractice claims (53.7% and 34.6% of cases, respectively). The most common litigated surgical complications were related to nerve injuries (20.3%). Other significant though less common surgical complications involved the loss of the airway (8.6%), esophageal injuries (4.4%), poor cosmesis (4.4%), vascular injuries (3.5%), and postoperative infections (0.6%). The most common nerve injury cases were related to the facial, spinal accessory, and recurrent laryngeal nerves. The most common procedures leading to litigation were excision of a neck mass (12.1% of cases), parotidectomy (7.9%), rigid endoscopy (5.4%), thyroidectomy (5.1%), and tracheostomy (4.8%). Most of the airway-related complications were due to the performance or postoperative care of tracheostomies. Payments to the plaintiffs resulted in 44.3% of the cases; the mean payment was $128,238, ranging from $1,000 to $1,000,000. The highest mean payments were for vascular and esophageal injuries, and the lowest for an undesirable cosmetic result. Analyzing their data, Simonsen et al. concluded that four factors increased the risk of litigation in head and neck surgery: young age, perioperative complications, delayed or missed diagnosis, and persistence or recurrence of disease.

Svider et al.[13] analyzed the results of malpractice trials associated with cranial nerve injuries. They noted an increasing number of cases litigated because of cranial nerve injuries over the period studied (1984–2011). The most common litigation was for injury to the facial nerve (24.4% of cases); parotidectomy and cosmetic procedures accounted respectively for 15.5% and 13.8% of those cases. Cranial nerve X injuries accounted for approximately 16% of cases, the vast majority for injury to the recurrent laryngeal nerve. Thyroid and parathyroid surgeries represented 47.4% of the cases that involved cranial nerve X injuries. Approximately 16% of cases were for spinal accessory nerve injuries. Lymph node excisions were responsible for 68.6% of these cases. Payments were awarded in 64.7% of thyroidectomy/parathyroidectomy-related cases. In contrast, payments were awarded in only 29.2% of cases of spinal accessory nerve injury. Failure to use a facial nerve monitor was only an issue in one trial that returned a verdict for the surgeon. This is consistent with a study of malpractice litigation in salivary gland surgery by Hong et al.[44] in which failure to use facial nerve monitoring in parotid surgery was not the cause of litigation in any case. The issue of recurrent laryngeal nerve monitoring was not brought out in any trial in the Svider et al. analysis. This is consistent with the Abadin et al.[12] study of malpractice litigation after thyroid surgery from 1989 to 2009 in which the use or nonuse of nerve monitoring was not an important factor in cases of recurrent laryngeal nerve injuries.

EXPERT WITNESSES

Our legal system relies heavily on the use of expert witness testimony for both the plaintiff and the defendant physician. The American College of Surgeons and the American Academy of Otolaryngology—Head and Neck Surgery have established guidelines, emphasizing obligations and ethical conduct expected of physicians serving as expert witnesses.[45,46] The American College of Surgeons has an affirmation document that highlights guidelines and acceptable behavior that it encourages surgeons offering expert testimony to sign.[47] The American College of Surgeons requirements for expert witnesses include having an active and unrestricted license to practice medicine, and demonstrating competence in the surgical procedures on which the surgeon is offering expert testimony.[45]

The American Academy of Otolaryngology—Head and Neck Surgery offers an online module on its expert witness guidelines and further includes these guidelines in an Ethics and Professionalism module for CME credit. The Academy does have a process in place for addressing concerns that a member's behavior may be unethical in offering expert testimony. Any member in good standing can request a review of a member's behavior as to whether there is a violation of the code of ethics. The executive vice president/CEO, the president, and the chair of the ethics committee are involved in a process to determine if the code of ethics has been violated and may propose censure, suspension, or expulsion for such violations. The respondent does have an opportunity to appeal and have a review by a panel appointed by Academy leadership.[47] The Academy also addresses the issue of compensation for providing expert testimony. Without offering specific guidance on the amount experts should be compensated, it notes that "compensation of the physician expert witness should be reasonable and commensurate with the time and effort given to preparing for deposition and court appearance".[46]

Eloy et al.[48] performed an analysis comparing the plaintiff and defendant expert witness qualifications in recent malpractice litigation in otolaryngology-head and neck surgery. Defendant expert witnesses were found to have a higher level of experience than experts testifying for the plaintiff, although both groups of experts were more often late-career practitioners. Hong et al.[19] found that 93% of expert witness otolaryngologists had at least 10 years of experience, and 81% had at least 15 years of experience, and that 41% had fellowship training. Eloy et al.[48] found that more of the defendant experts were full-time faculty in academic otolaryngology departments (49.3%) than plaintiff experts (31.7%), and had a higher scholarly impact as measured by the h-index (mean + SD 10.0 + 13.4 vs. 6.3 + 9.4). Plaintiff experts tended to testify in multiple cases more often than defendant experts; multiple practitioners testified for the same side multiple times. Interestingly, the amount of experience of the expert witness did not appear to influence the outcome of the proceedings. Cases in which the defendant expert had more experience than the plaintiff witness resulted in a verdict in favor of the defendant 73.7% of the time, whereas when the plaintiff witness had more experience, a verdict in favor of the defendant resulted in 77.2% of the cases. The Hong et al. study showed that when otolaryngologist defense expert witnesses were used in malpractice cases involving otolaryngologists, 70% of cases were decided in the otolaryngologist's favor, as opposed to 40% when otolaryngologist expert witnesses were not used.

Though it is not clear what the significance of voluntarily participating in the Maintenance of Certification (MOC) process for otolaryngologists achieving board certification prior to 2002 with regard to qualification, the vast majority of otolaryngologist expert witnesses in recent cases were board certified prior to 2002, and few chose to participate in the MOC process (1.9% of plaintiff witnesses and 4.6% of defendant witnesses, a nonstatistically significant difference).[49]

CONCLUSION

The majority of malpractice litigation cases are resolved in favor of otolaryngologist-head and neck surgeons. Nevertheless, circumstances leading to litigation are distressful to both patients and physicians. For the physician, the anxiety, stress, and potential loss of reputation and income are all nonquantifiable factors that are part of the process. In this chapter, we have reviewed some of the recent data available regarding malpractice litigation in various areas of otolaryngology-head and neck surgery. Rhinology, particularly endoscopic sinus surgery, appears to be an area of particular risk to the otolaryngologist. Unfortunately, there is no comprehensive database of malpractice litigation from which one can draw firm conclusions. Databases such as Westlaw and LexisNexis used in many analyses are useful, but selective, and do not include cases that are dropped or settled without going to court.[43] The Physician Insurers Association of America, an association of medical liability insurance companies, has provided valuable data for excellent studies on malpractice claims,[43,50] but its database still only represents a quarter of claims in the United States.[50] Nevertheless, examining available databases helps to highlight problematic areas for the otolaryngologist, and areas that can be addressed to improve outcomes and patient safety, and reduce litigation.

Given the complexity of otolaryngologic conditions and procedures, all otolaryngologists can expect to have some less than desirable results in their practice. Needless to say, meticulous clinical evaluation and taking steps to maximize patient safety can result in improved results, and decrease the possibility of litigation. Stankiewicz and Hotaling,[51] for example, recommend preparing a checklist for endoscopic sinus surgery of items to check off before, during, and after surgery. Other factors beside the level of care and complications, however, can lead to malpractice claims. Many of the recent studies identify the lack of informed consent, for example, as an allegation in malpractice litigation. The value of effective communication with patients in the avoidance of litigation cannot be overemphasized.[52] A well-documented informed consent process that explains potential complications, assures realistic expectations, explains the potential need for additional surgery and for recurrence of disease, is an invaluable tool in minimizing litigation.

REFERENCES

1. Lynn-Macrae AG, Lynn-Macrae RA, Emani J, et al. Medicolegal analysis of injury during endoscopic sinus surgery. Laryngoscope. 2004;114:1492-5.
2. Anderson GF, Hussey PS, Frogner BK, et al. Health spending in the United States and the rest of the industrialized world. Health Aff (Millwood). 2005;24:903-14.
3. Terry K. Exclusive Survey. Malpractice premiums: dropping, but still high. Medical Economics. 2008;85:36-8.
4. Brenner RJ, Smith JJ. The malpractice liability crisis. J Am Coll Radiol. 2004;1: 18-22.
5. Medical malpractice litigation raises health-care cost, reduces access, and lowers quality of care. J Med Pract Manage. 2004;20:44-51.
6. Hermer LD, Brody H. Defensive medicine, cost containment, and reform. J Gen Intern Med. 2010;25:470-3.
7. Hertz BT, Arthurs J. Malpractice rates plateauing. The only thing to fear may be fear itself. Med Econ. 2011;88:24-5, 28-9, 32.
8. 2004 Socioeconomic Facts and Figures, 8th Annual Survey. American Academy of Otolaryngology—Head and Neck Surgery.
9. Moffett P, Moore G. The standard of care: legal history and definitions: the bad and good news. West J Emerg Med. 2011;12:109-12.

10. Lydiatt DD. Medical malpractice and facial nerve paralysis. Arch Otolaryngol Head Neck Surg. 2003;129:50-3.
11. Lydiatt DD. Medical malpractice and the thyroid gland. Head Neck. 2003;25: 429-31.
12. Abadin SS, Kaplan EL, Angelos P. Malpractice litigation after thyroid surgery: the role of recurrent laryngeal nerve injuries, 1989–2009. Surgery. 2010;148: 718-22;discussion 722-13.
13. Svider PF, Sunaryo PL, Keeley BR, et al. Characterizing liability for cranial nerve injuries: a detailed analysis of 209 malpractice trials. Laryngoscope. 2013;123:1156-62.
14. Svider PF, Pashkova AA, Husain Q, et al. Determination of legal responsibility in iatrogenic tracheal and laryngeal stenosis. Laryngoscope. 2013;123:1754-8.
15. Svider PF, Kovalerchik O, Mauro AC, et al. Legal liability in iatrogenic orbital injury. Laryngoscope. 2013;123:2099-103.
16. Svider PF, Keeley BR, Zumba O, et al. From the operating room to the court-room: a comprehensive characterization of litigation related to facial plastic surgery procedures. Laryngoscope. 2013;123:1849-53.
17. Svider PF, Husain Q, Kovalerchik O, et al. Determining legal responsibility in otolaryngology: a review of 44 trials since 2008. Am J Otolaryngol. 2013;34: 699-705.
18. Jena AB, Chandra A, Lakdawalla D, et al. Outcomes of medical malpractice litigation against US physicians. Arch Intern Med. 2012;172:892-4.
19. Hong SS, Yheulon CG, Wirtz ED, et al. Otolaryngology and medical malpractice: a review of the past decade, 2001–2011. Laryngoscope. 2014;124:896-901.
20. Burkle CM, Martin DP, Keegan MT. Which is feared more: harm to the ego or financial peril? A survey of anesthesiologists' attitudes about medical malprac-tice. Minn Med. 2012;95:46-50.
21. Rose C, Svider PF, Sheyn A, et al. Protecting the most vulnerable: litigation from pediatric otolaryngologic procedures and conditions. Laryngoscope. 2014;124:2161-6.
22. Stevenson AN, Myer CM, 3rd, Shuler MD, et al. Complications and legal outcomes of tonsillectomy malpractice claims. Laryngoscope. 2012;122:71-4.
23. Traeger N, Schultz B, Pollock AN, et al. Polysomnographic values in children 2–9 years old: additional data and review of the literature. Pediatr Pulmonol. 2005;40:22-30.
24. Boss EF, Marsteller JA, Simon AE. Outpatient tonsillectomy in children: demographic and geographic variation in the United States, 2006. J Pediatr. 2012;160:814-9.
25. Shah UK, Theroux Z, Shah GB, et al. Resource analysis of tonsillectomy in chil-dren. Laryngoscope. 2014;124:1223-8.
26. Morris LG, Lieberman SM, Reitzen SD, et al. Characteristics and outcomes of malpractice claims after tonsillectomy. Otolaryngol Head Neck Surg. 2008; 138:315-20.
27. Reilly BK, Horn GM, Sewell RK. Hearing loss resulting in malpractice litigation: what physicians need to know. Laryngoscope. 2013;123:112-7.
28. Blake DM, Svider PF, Carniol ET, et al. Malpractice in otology. Otolaryngol Head Neck Surg. 2013;149:554-61.

29. Ruhl DS, Hong SS, Littlefield PD. Lessons learned in otologic surgery: 30 years of malpractice cases in the United States. Otol Neurotol. 2013;34:1173-9.
30. Mathew R, Asimacopoulos E, Valentine P. Toward safer practice in otology: a report on 15 years of clinical negligence claims. Laryngoscope. 2011;121:2214-9.
31. Svider PF, Eloy JA, Folbe AJ, et al. Craniofacial surgery and adverse outcomes: an inquiry into medical negligence. Ann Otol Rhinol Laryngol. 2015;124: 515-22.
32. Winford TW, Wallin JL, Clinger JD, et al. Malpractice in treatment of sinonasal disease by otolaryngologists: a review of the past 10 years. Otolaryngol Head Neck Surg. 2015;152:536-40.
33. Svider PF, Mauro AC, Eloy JA, et al. Malodorous consequences: what comprises negligence in anosmia litigation? Int Forum Allergy Rhinol. 2014;4:216-22.
34. Dalton P, Doty RL, Murphy C, et al. Olfactory assessment using the NIH Toolbox. Neurology. 2013;80:S32-S36.
35. Doty RL, Shaman P, Kimmelman CP, et al. University of Pennsylvania Smell Identification Test: a rapid quantitative olfactory function test for the clinic. Laryngoscope. 1984;94:176-8.
36. Pallin DJ, Chng YM, McKay MP, et al. Epidemiology of epistaxis in US emergency departments, 1992 to 2001. Ann Emerg Med. 2005;46:77-81.
37. Khan MN, Blake DM, Vazquez A, et al. Epistaxis: the factors involved in determining medicolegal liability. Int Forum Allergy Rhinol. 2014;4:76-81.
38. Smith TL, Stewart MG, Orlandi RR, et al. Indications for image-guided sinus surgery: the current evidence. Am J Rhinol. 2007;21:80-3.
39. Ramakrishnan VR, Orlandi RR, Citardi MJ, et al. The use of image-guided surgery in endoscopic sinus surgery: an evidence-based review with recommendations. Int Forum Allergy Rhinol. 2013;3:236-41.
40. Eloy JA, Svider PF, D'Aguillo CM, et al. Image-guidance in endoscopic sinus surgery: is it associated with decreased medicolegal liability? Int Forum Allergy Rhinol. 2013;3:980-5.
41. Kovalerchik O, Mady LJ, Svider PF, et al. Physician accountability in iatrogenic cerebrospinal fluid leak litigation. Int Forum Allergy Rhinol. 2013;3:722-5.
42. Svider PF, Blake DM, Sahni KP, et al. Meningitis and legal liability: an otolaryngology perspective. Am J Otolaryngol. 2014;35:198-203.
43. Simonsen AR, Duncavage JA, Becker SS. Malpractice in head and neck surgery: a review of cases. Otolaryngol Head Neck Surg. 2012;147:69-73.
44. Hong SS, Yheulon CG, Sniezek JC. Salivary gland surgery and medical malpractice. Otolaryngol Head Neck Surg. 2013;148:589-94.
45. American College of Surgeons. Statement on the physician acting as an expert witness. Available from http://wwwfacsorg/fellows_info/statements/st-8html. [Accessed August 30, 2015].
46. American Academy of Otolaryngology—Head and Neck Surgery. Statement on Qualifications and Guidelines for the Physician Expert Witness. Available from http://wwwentnetorg/aboutus/Ethicscfm. [Accessed August 30, 2015].
47. Svider PF, Eloy JA, Baredes S, et al. Expert witness testimony guidelines: identifying areas for improvement. Otolaryngol Head Neck Surg. 2015;152:207-10.
48. Eloy JA, Svider PF, Patel D, et al. Comparison of plaintiff and defendant expert witness qualification in malpractice litigation in otolaryngology. Otolaryngol Head Neck Surg. 2013;148:764-9.

49. Eloy JA, Svider PF, Patel D, et al. In response to "comparison of plaintiff and defendant expert witness qualification in malpractice litigation in otolaryngology". Otolaryngol Head Neck Surg. 2013;149:649-50.

50. Singer MC, Iverson KC, Terris DJ. Thyroidectomy-related malpractice claims. Otolaryngol Head Neck Surg. 2012;146:358-61.

51. Stankiewicz JA, Hotaling J. Medicolegal issues in endoscopic sinus surgery and complications. Otolaryngol Clin North Am. 2015;48:827-37.

52. Carroll AE. To be sued less, doctors should consider talking to patients more. The New York Times, 2015.

Chapter 5

Captioning: How, When, and Why

Darlene M Parker

INTRODUCTION

Captioning is the process of converting all audible components of video — the dialogue, narration, and sound effects — into words that appear on a screen. Like subtitles, captions display as on-screen text, but they appear as white letters on a black background (Fig. 5.1). Captioning presumes that the viewer cannot hear, so sound effects, song lyrics, speaker identifications, etc., must be added. Today captioning allows millions of deaf and hard-of-hearing people to watch national and local newscasts, be alerted during times of weather and other life-threatening emergencies, and to fully enjoy media across various platforms — television, DVDs, the Internet, and even mobile devices.

Captioning can be traced back to a joint corporate and United States government effort in the 1960s to develop improved technology for translating Russian into English. That project was abandoned, but it allowed for the eventual evolution of computer-aided transcription that enabled court reporters to more efficiently produce court or deposition transcripts. After a court case or deposition was finished, a court reporter's phonetic notes, taken down on a stenotype machine, had to be translated into full English words. The new software automated this process, eliminating the need for the court reporter to read their notes and retype the transcript word for word — or dictate

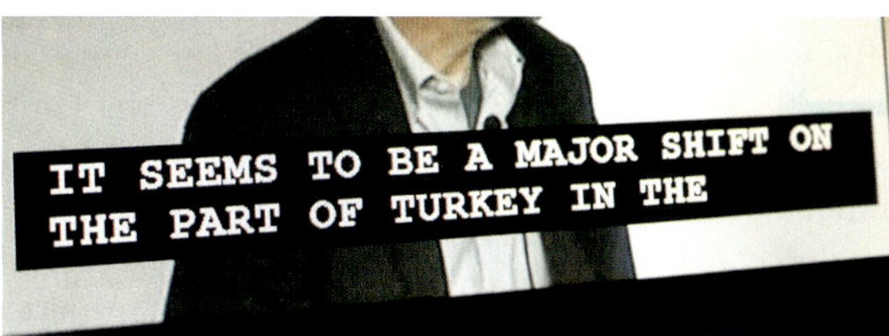

Fig. 5.1: Closed captions displayed on a television screen. Appearing as white letters on a black background distinguishes closed captions from subtitles.
Courtesy: National Captioning Institute, 2015.

their notes to a typist. However, court reporters still had to review and make corrections to the transcript. Not all court reporters could avail themselves of the new technology, as it was costly. This computer-aided transcription laid the groundwork for real-time captioning, the instantaneous method of converting the spoken word into text.

Captioning for the deaf and hard-of-hearing debuted in 1972 on the prerecorded program *The French Chef*, hosted by Julia Child. The captions were prepared in advance and appeared as open captions, meaning they could not be turned off. Many in the hearing audience found the captions distracting.

In 1973, *The Captioned ABC News* debuted. For almost a decade, it was the only accessible timely news program offered. "Timely" in this circumstance meant that it was rebroadcast approximately 5 hours after it originally aired. The original uncaptioned newscast was recorded, open captions were added, and then the same broadcast re-aired, this time with captions. WGBH, The Caption Center, produced both *The French Chef* and *The Captioned ABC News*. Although captioning was a welcomed breakthrough, it was felt that the captions should be visible to only those who wanted to view them.

Therefore, the National Captioning Institute (NCI) was established in 1979 in cooperation with ABC, NBC, PBS, and the federal government as a 501(c)(3) nonprofit corporation. Its mission: to promote and provide access to television programs for the deaf and hard-of-hearing community through the technology of closed captioning. "Closed" in this context means that the captioned information is transmitted within the broadcast signal in encoded (or closed) form. A caption-decoder connected to a television, or the caption-decoding television that became available in 1993, is necessary to "open" the captions and display the words on the TV screen. The "closed" nature of the captions would satisfy the wants and needs of both hearing and non-hearing audiences.

On March 16, 1980, the first closed-captioned television programs were broadcast: *The ABC Sunday Night Movie* (ABC), *Disney's Wonderful World* (NBC), and *Masterpiece Theatre* (PBS). A silence had been broken. For the first time ever, deaf people across the United States could turn on their caption decoder-connected television sets—and finally understand what they had been missing on television. Caption decoders were available for $250 from Sears (Fig. 5.2). Today there are approximately 37.5 million deaf and hard-of-hearing Americans[1] who benefit from this service.

Prerecorded (offline) captioning was the method used to caption these programs and refers to the post-production process of adding

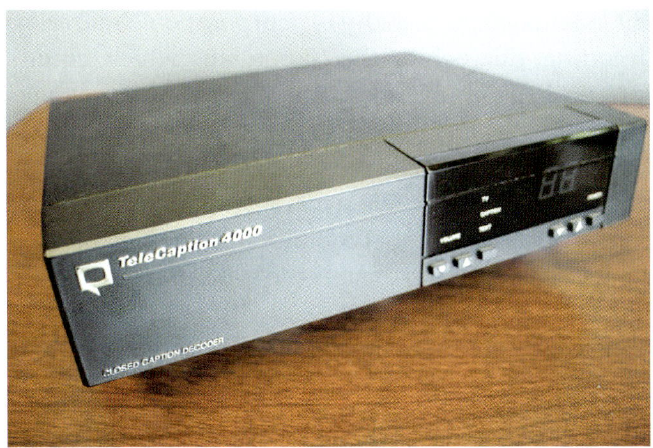

Fig. 5.2: Telecaption decoder, a device that was required to view closed captions prior to the availability of televisions with a built-in decoder chip.
Courtesy: National Captioning Institute, 2015.

captions to a program *after* it has been recorded but *before it airs*. A full explanation of prerecorded (offline) captioning will be provided later in the chapter.

The closed captioning television service was an overnight sensation. Suddenly, thousands of people who had been living in a world of silence could enjoy the shared experience of television.

Although the success of the initial prerecorded closed captioning was profound, the available offerings were very limited in scope. It was only natural that this preliminary introduction would cultivate the audience's desire to access a wider range of programming, including, primetime series, soap operas, talk shows, game shows, sports events, children's programming, cartoons, and home videos—the same diverse variety of programming that hearing people take for granted. Most importantly, deaf and hard-of-hearing viewers wanted *instant* access to live national and local newscasts. NCI responded.

In 1982, NCI developed real-time captioning services, a process for captioning newscasts, sports events, specials, and other live broadcasts as the events are being televised. There was some testing under the radar, but the first advertised real-time captioning on television occurred during the 1982 Academy Awards broadcast (ABC). Then in June of 1982, the first live news event was captioned in its entirety— the launch of the Space Shuttle *Columbia* (ABC).

Later that year, the first regularly-scheduled 30-minute newscast was captioned in real time—*ABC World News Tonight*. Then in 1984, *Good Morning America* and other live programs were added to the list of real-time captioned programs.

In 1989, NCI partnered with ITT Corporation to develop the first caption-decoding microchip, the Superchip, which could be built directly into new television sets at the manufacturing stage. This led to the introduction and subsequent passage in the United States of the Television Decoder Circuitry Act of 1990,[2] which mandated that, effective July 1, 1993, all new television sets 13″ or larger manufactured for sale in the United States must contain caption-decoding technology. Now millions of people have access to captions with the push of a button on their remote controls.

Real-time captioning was and still is performed by court reporters or recent court reporting graduates trained to take down the spoken word on a stenotype machine at extremely high rates of speed. The machine is similar to one used in a courtroom. Only the most proficient court reporters were hired to become real-time captioners. Once hired, trainees undergo intensive training to improve their skills to be able to caption news at a high accuracy rate.

Real-time captioners enter data at speeds up to and often exceeding 250 words per minute to allow viewers instantaneous access to live news, sports, and vital information. The result is that the viewer at home sees the captions within three to four seconds of the words being spoken.

Transitioning from court reporter to real-time broadcast captioner is extremely challenging, and that makes for a small universe of potential captioners. Graduation rates from court reporting schools for stenotype reporters are a mere 15%. The labor pool is narrowed even further by the high standards of industry-leading closed captioning companies. For example, at NCI, only one in seven real-time captioner applicants is deemed skilled enough to be hired.

In the early 2000s, in response to a shortage of qualified stenotype candidates, NCI developed proprietary speech recognition software designed specifically for live captioning. This captioning software was pioneered in order to access a broader group of captioners so that more live captioning would be available to end users. Professionals of varying backgrounds are trained to use their strong listening, communication, and grammar skills to "echo" or repeat what they hear into a computer profile that has been trained to recognize their unique voice. Voice writers then go through an intensive training program that guides them through the process of developing a strong voice profile, allows them to develop their articulation abilities and breathing techniques, and teaches them about the technical, stylistic, and grammatical components of closed captioning. In 2004, NCI slowly started to introduce voice writing into its real-time captioning model. Since then, voice writing has expanded tremendously and has allowed NCI to keep pace with the growing demand for captioned programming.

A full explanation of both types of real-time captioning will be provided later in this chapter.

Captioning has grown from a little known service for people who are deaf to a truly global communications service that touches the lives of millions of people every day. Because of the efforts of NCI, the television industry, the federal government, and so many others, people who are deaf or hard-of-hearing will never again be isolated. Most importantly, they will be informed immediately of important, possibly life-saving information delivered by their local news stations during severe weather or other emergencies. Captions will also be present on most local stations' live simultaneous webcasts.

HOW CAPTIONING WORKS

Prerecorded (Offline) Captioning

Prerecorded (offline) captioning is the post-production process of adding captions to a program after it has been recorded or produced. This includes prime time television series, movies, and a vast array of online video content. To give the viewer the full experience of the video, care is taken to include ambient noises, such as a dog barking or a door bell ringing.

Captions can be prepared in three different styles:
- Standard pop-on captions are timed and placed to synchronize with the program.
- Center placement pop-on captions are centered at the bottom third of the TV screen and moved as necessary to avoid covering graphics. Speakers are identified whenever possible.
- Timed roll-up captions scroll on and off the screen in a continuous motion and identify speakers by name whenever possible.

There are four steps involved in producing prerecorded captions (Fig. 5.3):
- *Log-in, preview, and digitalization*: The broadcaster provides a digital video file or DVD of the program that includes time code that exactly matches the master.
- *Caption preparation*: Caption editors watch and transcribe media at their networked computers. Using a standard computer keyboard, they enter a verbatim transcription of the dialogue, sound effects, and other essential non-verbal features into the captioning system. The editors break the text into individual captions, assign

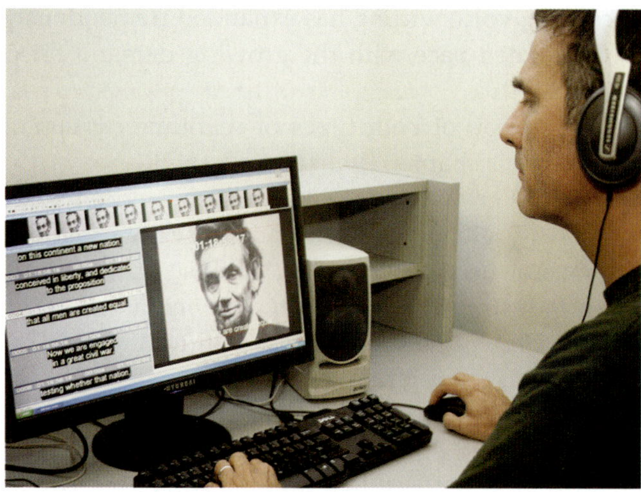

Fig. 5.3: Offline captioner creating prerecorded captions for a television program. *Courtesy*: National Captioning Institute, 2015.

appropriate screen placement to each caption, and time each caption to the associated audio.

- *Editor review*: The completed caption file is checked and corrected for accuracy, spelling, and timing. Unfamiliar terms are researched.
- *Ready for encoding to DVD or digital media*: The completed caption file is transmitted to the client or designated encoding facility via email, FTP, or other media. The client or encoding facility then integrates the caption data with the video portion of the program. The caption company provides encoding for some types of media.

Depending upon the captioning style, it can take 6–8 hours to produce a 1-hour program.

REAL-TIME CAPTIONING—STENO CAPTIONING AND VOICE WRITING (FIGS. 5.4 TO 5.6)

For real-time (live) captioning, caption data is added to the television signal using a piece of hardware at the broadcast site called an encoder. A real-time broadcast captioner will use a modem or Internet connection to send captions to a client's encoder. As the captioner listens to the spoken audio being broadcast, he or she transcribes what is being said using specialized equipment while simultaneously adding speaker identifications and punctuation. A steno captioner will phonetically key the information onto the stenotype machine. A voice writer will echo (repeat) the information into a microphone. This process transforms the spoken audio of a broadcast into grammatically correct words on the screen. Since the captioner cannot

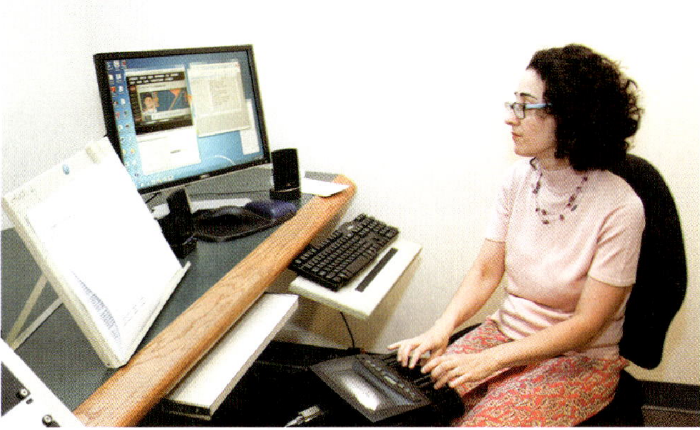

Fig. 5.4: Steno captioner creating closed captions for a live television program in real time. *Courtesy*: National Captioning Institute, 2015.

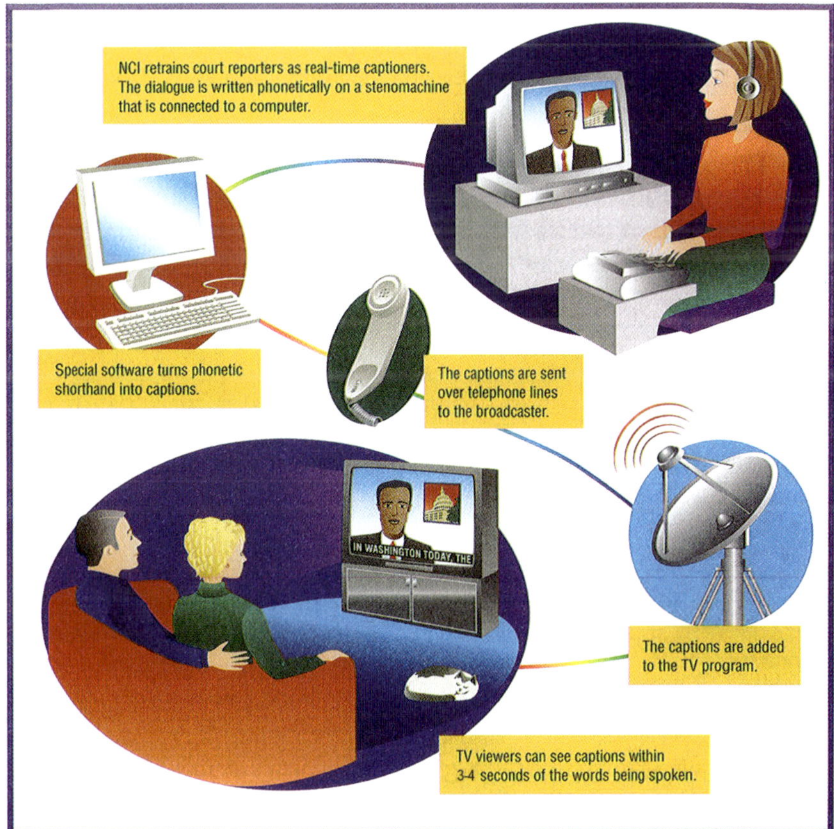

Fig. 5.5: An illustrated view of real-time captioning. *Courtesy*: National Captioning Institute, 2010.

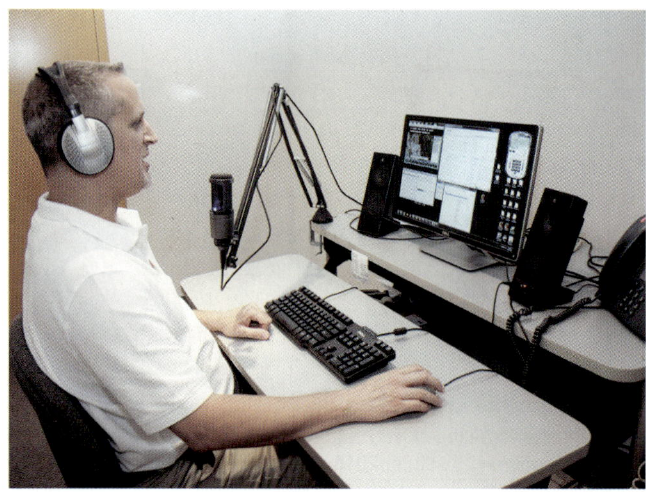

Fig. 5.6: Voice writer creating closed captions for a live television program in real time. *Courtesy*: National Captioning Institute, 2015.

input or echo a word until it is spoken, real-time captions typically lag behind the audio by 3–4 seconds.

Live captions are generated as the program is being broadcast, which means that there is no opportunity to proofread them in advance. As a result, errors do occur, usually in the form of incorrect, though phonetically similar, words. Captioners continually assess their work so that accuracy rates of 98% or better can be maintained. Captioners also engage in rigorous research prior to all broadcasts in order to prepare for the names, proper nouns, and terminology they may encounter.

Steno Captioning

Real-time steno captioners initially attend court reporting school for approximately 2–3 years and obtain an Associate's degree. Some schools award Bachelor's degrees. They undergo the same training as a court reporter that works in court or takes depositions. Some schools offer captioning training, but many people receive that specialized training on the job. Students are trained to take down the spoken word at speeds in excess of 225 words per minute on a stenotype machine (Figs. 5.7A and B). The machine is not like a computer keyboard. It has only 22 keys, which means not all 26 letters of the English alphabet are represented, so combinations of keys are stroked to equal certain individual letters. The stenotype theory is based on phonetics and syllables. Because of that, more than one key is usually stroked at a time. It's more akin to playing chords on a piano than typing on a computer

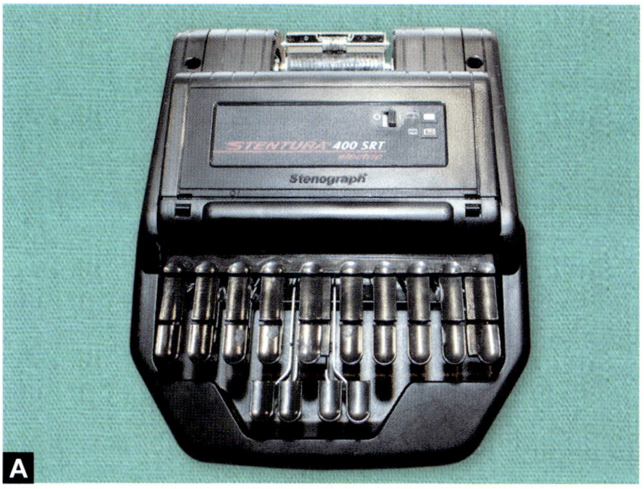

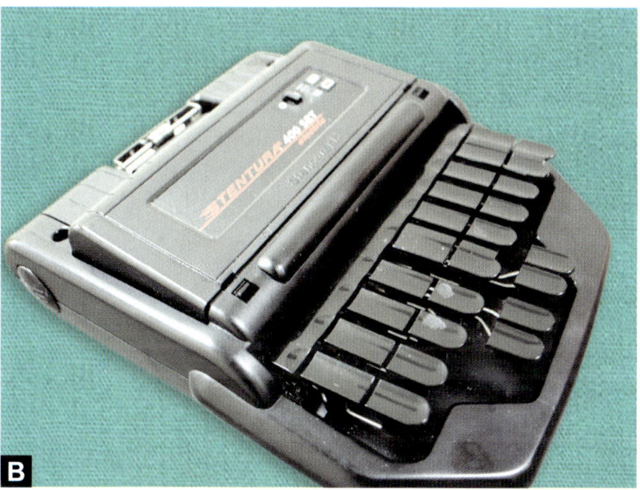

Figs. 5.7A and B: Stenotype machine used by steno captioners to create closed captions in real time.
Courtesy: National Captioning Institute, 2015.

keyboard. The name Darlene on the computer keyboard would be seven distinct strokes, D-a-r-l-e-n-e. On the stenotype keyboard, it would be only two strokes—TKAR/HRAOEPB/. The reason it looks so strange is because there are only 22 keys, and combinations of keys must be used to equal individual letters. As the captioner listens to the broadcast, s/he inputs phonetic codes onto the stenotype machine. Brief forms are also used for some words and proper names. Brief forms can be thought of as macros. Because the broadcasts are live, there is no chance to correct errors once a certain number of strokes have been hit. Once the captioner strokes the word or words, his/her individual dictionary is searched for the correct English match. That caption data then travels via modem or Internet connection to the encoder at the broadcast origination site and is merged with the video signal.

As you can imagine, since stenotype is a very difficult skill to learn and master, especially at high speeds, captioners comprise a very small and elite group. Many captioners are experienced court reporters. A few are outstanding recent graduates. Once hired, captioners undergo 3–4 months of intensive training before they are allowed to caption on the air. The length of training depends on the ability of the captioner. Training continues for another 18 months to 2 years to ensure that captioners are knowledgeable of and can caption all sports, including fast-paced sporting events, such as hockey games, and sports talk shows.

As the captioner listens to the program, their steno strokes are translated against the captioner's personal dictionaries. The dictionaries contain steno strokes and the corresponding English translation. Generic words and common proper nouns are contained in all captioners' dictionaries. To help ensure that unusual or technical terminology and proper names translate correctly, it is most helpful when the broadcaster provides as much information as possible about the program so that the captioner can make appropriate dictionary entries.

Errors can occur for many reasons—difficult terminology, including strange proper names the captioner did not receive in advance, the extremely fast pace of some programs, difficulty in understanding audio in general or understanding some speakers in particular, and speakers talking over each other. At high rates of speed, the captioner may simply make a mistake and hit an extra key or omit a key. Think of it this way: how many people can write emails all day long and never make a typo? Also, two steno strokes can stack and be read as one, resulting in a jumbled, unreadable word. At times the errors can be unintentionally humorous. During the weather segment of a newscast during a heat wave, instead of the captions reading, "Tomorrow will be smoking hot," the captions read, "Tomorrow will be smoking pot." This is an "equal-opportunity" error that can easily be committed by a steno captioner or a voice writer. On the steno keyboard, the "h" and "p" keys are right next to each other. In the case of voice writing, the software can simply misinterpret what the captioner said.

Finally, transmission errors can cause strange-looking errors. Transmission errors occur when there is any disruption on the line carrying the caption data and can appear as two characters dropping out, garbling, white boxes, captions moving around the screen, or changing colors. Captioners cannot cause these errors. Sometimes disconnecting and reconnecting the modem clears up the problem. Captions may also be adversely affected as they are passed along by cable or small dish distributors, or if a viewer receives their signal by antenna.

VOICE WRITING

Many people use Siri or other types of voice recognition software every day with mixed success. It is one thing to use this technology to dictate texts or emails using deliberate enunciation, but relying on it to provide at least 98% accurate captioning of rapid-fire newscasts or fast-paced sports talk programs is not feasible. Also, consider all of the accents, not only from around the world, but regional accents in the United States. Voice recognition technology on its own is not advanced enough to correctly translate multiple random voices with various, unpredictable accents. A human intermediary is necessary to interpret exactly what is being said and who is saying it.

Several court reporting/captioning software companies manufacture voice writing software. National Captioning Institute voice writers are trained to manipulate their proprietary software to publish what they want through the use of verbal shortcuts, keyboard integration, and other captioning-specific features. National Captioning Institute voice writers learn the importance of how to do research so that they and the software are both adequately prepared for the varying subject matters and current events items they will encounter. At the direction of the voice writers, the software can also be programmed to learn from its errors, recognize context, understand specific vocabulary, and respond to verbal cues. Then they use superior articulation skills, verbal commands, and software tools to produce high-quality real-time captions by "echoing" or repeating the broadcast audio into their microphones. While listening and repeating, they simultaneously add speaker identifications and punctuation. As the technique of voice writing has spread throughout the industry, a wide range in voice writing quality has resulted. High-quality captioning companies invest ample time and resources in selecting, training, and testing voice writers and do not rely on the basic capabilities of off-the-shelf software.

Voice writers transmit captions the same as steno captioners, via modem or Internet connection, and hence, can also experience technical transmission errors. However, the linguistic and contextual errors that result from voice writing are often different. Although voice writers train the software to recognize their voices, on occasion the software will misinterpret a word. For instance, the voice writer may echo the word "lacrosse," but the software may translate it as "across." In some cases, voice writing can be more accurate than steno captioning, depending on the specific content. For example, highly technical content, such as medical or financial material, can be captioned more accurately than steno, due to the specialized vocabulary base that is present in some voice software. This is also due to the fact that speech recognition software does especially well translating longer, technical words because they are less likely to be mistaken for another similar word. Shorter words that sound alike are more problematic and require trained personnel to guide the software in the right direction. However, when captioning medical and technical material, the playing field is leveled when the steno captioner is provided adequate preparation materials for the program, allowing them to make the necessary dictionary entries in advance.

CART CAPTIONING

CART stands for Communication Access Real Time. CART captioning is provided in educational settings, in the workplace, at conferences and conventions, and anywhere it may assist a deaf or hard-of-hearing person. It is usually provided by a steno captioner, but if a voice writer is adept at using a "mask" so that s/he cannot be heard, that works as well. The voice captioner whispers or speaks at a very low volume into the mask to avoid disturbing any hearing participants in close proximity. CART captioning can be provided onsite or remotely. If onsite, the CART captioner may sit next to their student or client, and the student or client will read off of the CART captioner's computer screen. In some instances, the person receiving the CART services may ask the CART captioner to sit in another part of the room if they do not wish to draw attention to him or herself. The recipient of the service would then view the captions on a wireless device. In a conference or convention setting, the captions appear on one or more large screens. A CART captioner in Maryland recently had an unusual and satisfying assignment. Thanks to wireless technology, one of her clients was able to attend and participate in the conversations at a dinner party, preceded by a cocktail hour—without the CART captioner needing to be right next to her. The client wore a small wireless microphone and carried a small tablet. The CART captioner was literally sitting in a corner behind a very large plant. Wearing wireless headphones, the captioner could clearly hear the conversations picked up by the wireless microphone, caption them for the client, and have them appear on her tablet within a few seconds. The client was delighted because she was able to enjoy and fully participate in the dinner party. And no one ever suspected, or asked, "Who is that woman sitting in the corner behind the plant?"

MOVIE THEATER AND PERFORMING ARTS CAPTIONING

Assistive devices are now available in movie theaters. The devices range from closed-captioned "eyeglasses" to devices that can attach to the cup holder.

In the live theater setting, an LED sign system may be used to display captioning. The sign is 4 feet long and scrolls 2–3 lines with 2–3-inch lettering in a choice of colors on a black background. The sign is positioned near the stage. In the larger theaters, there is a designated captioned seating section from which the captioning is easily visible.

STADIUM AND ARENA CAPTIONING

In 2006, a lawsuit was brought against the Washington Redskins of the National Football League, alleging that they were in violation of the Americans with Disabilities Act of 1990.[4] The Redskins lost the suit and were required to display captions of everything spoken or sung over the public address system, which they accomplished by hiring a former captioner. It was decided that the captions would be displayed on the small "out-of-town" scoreboards on the 50-yard line on both sides of the stadium. Since then, a multitude of stadiums and arenas have instituted captioning. Some stadiums display their captions on the "out-of-town" scoreboard, some on the Jumbo Tron, and some others offer their fans hand-held devices.

THE MANY BENEFITS OF CAPTIONING

As mentioned earlier, there are approximately 37.5 million deaf and hard-of-hearing people in the United States. This figure is growing rapidly, due to the large Baby Boom population, those people born between 1946 and 1964. The first wave of Baby Boomers turned 65 in 2011.

Imagine if you were a deaf or hard-of-hearing person on September 11, 2001. Imagine seeing the events of that day unfold on your television set and not having the same information as the hearing audience. Or, imagine how it would feel to watch your local newscast's coverage of an impending weather emergency, and then all of a sudden, the audio cuts out. Captioners know that times of crisis are when their unemotional professionalism and skills are needed the most, and they rise to the occasion—sometimes with tears streaming down their faces as they caption.

With prerecorded programming, such as prime time dramas, captioning allows the deaf and hard-of-hearing community to feel included in pop culture and allows them to be full participants in discussions about such topics as the exciting season finale of their favorite TV show.

Captioning also benefits the ELL (English Language Learner) population. There are approximately 47 million non-native English speakers in the United States.[3] In addition to obviously being helpful to learn the language, captions are especially helpful in learning slang and idioms because they are spoken in context and the video also assists in understanding.

Numerous research studies have shown that captioned television provides a successful learning environment for deaf and hard-of-hearing students. The benefits of captioning also extend to siblings of children who are deaf and hard-of-hearing students with special educational needs. Among the many benefits of captioned television and online content are improved reading skills, listening comprehension, and vocabulary skills, as well as increased self-confidence.

Captioned television and captioned online content helps all children and illiterate adults learn to read. It helps them to comprehend video content, understand new terminology, increase their vocabulary, improve spelling and punctuation, recognize large numbers, and, finally, increase their reading rate.

In many ways, captions also benefit the general population in places such as restaurants, bars, airports, and gyms. Many hearing people prefer to watch TV with the captions on so that if they do not hear or understand a word or phrase, they merely look at the captions. So as to not disturb someone else in the room, people often mute the sound and only watch the captions. Many find it helpful to understand dialogue that is whispered or is drowned out by a crescendo of very loud music.

Recently, a proposed ordinance has been heard by the Portland, Oregon City Council to mandate that all televisions in public places have the captions turned on.[5] The backers of the proposed ordinance hope that the movement will spread to other large cities across the United States.

THE FUTURE

Captioned television continues to be a vital means of receiving information and entertainment for the deaf and hard-of-hearing audience, but in the 21st century the demand for captioning online content has exploded. This includes television programs aired later online, and in some instances, clips posted online, as well as original online content. The 21st Century Telecommunications and Video Accessibility Act, passed in 2010, ensures the deaf and hard-of-hearing audience will have access to broadband, digital and mobile innovations — the emerging 21st century technologies for which the act is named.[6]

As media distribution and content development companies place greater emphasis on the web as a way to connect with viewers, the value of closed captioned files continues to increase. Once viewed as an isolated asset of limited use, the caption file (which is the complete text of a program with time code) has evolved to become a major component within the media delivery chain. Closed captioned files are now a valuable tool through which content providers increase their program's visibility via tagging, redirects, and metadata, helping them achieve greater ad revenues and viewership.

The leaders of the captioning industry will continue to ensure that the needs of the 21st century are met so that the deaf and hard-of-hearing audience will never again experience the isolation that they endured more than 35 years ago.

REFERENCES

1. Blackwell DL, Lucas JW, Clarke TC. Summary health statistics for U.S. adults: National Health Interview Survey, 2012. National Center for Health Statistics. Vital Health Stat. 2014;10(260). http://www.nidcd.nih.gov/health/statistics/pages/quick.aspx.
2. https://transition.fcc.gov/Bureaus/OSEC/library/legislative_histories/1395.pdf. 1990.
3. US Census Bureau. 2010.
4. http://nad.org/news/2011/3/deaf-washington-redskins-fans-win-stadium-access-case.
5. https://www.portlandoregon.gov/oni/article/526602.
6. https://www.fcc.gov/encyclopedia/twenty-first-century-communications-and-video-accessibility-act.

Chapter 6

Management of Acute External Laryngeal Trauma

Philip A Weissbrod, Steven D Schaefer

INTRODUCTION

Over the past 40 years, we have witnessed a decrease in the incidence of laryngotracheal trauma in the United States, largely due to automobile safety regulations including mandatory use of seatbelts and airbag placement. While motor vehicle accident induced injury incidence has dropped, it still remains the most common mechanism for laryngeal fracture, followed by sports-related injury and penetrating trauma. Despite improved prehospital care allowing for increased acuity of injury being treated in the ED and hospital systems,[1] incidence of laryngeal trauma decreased in the 1980s from 1 in 5,000 emergency visits[2] to 1/30,000–137,000 emergency visits in the 1990s.[3,4] Other, less common mechanisms of injury include clothesline injury, strangulation, animal bites, fracture induced by cough and sneeze, and various forms of projectile injury.

While some of the details regarding management have changed, the basic tenets remain the same: airway control, early intervention, stabilization of fractures, repair of mucosal injury, and stenting for complex injury. These concepts account for the goal of reestablishing basic laryngeal function: breathing, talking, and protection during deglutition.

Laryngeal trauma, even in busy centers is a rare event. The larynx is protected by the mandible cranially, muscular structures laterally, and sternum caudally. In young individuals, the cartilage is soft and the larynx is positioned cranially, allowing for reduced susceptibility to injury. As individuals age, the larynx calcifies and migrates caudally increasing the likelihood of direct impact.

Early recognition of injury is important given that repair becomes increasingly difficult as inflammation, scar, and fibrosis set in. Delayed repair can have significant deleterious consequences with respect to voice and airway outcomes. While laryngeal injury can be complex and challenging at times, we hope to provide a basic framework of understanding to allow for effective treatment.

EVALUATION

Evaluation of laryngeal trauma begins with assessment of airway stability and consideration of the mechanism of injury. Full body assessment, Glasgow Coma Scale, measures of hemodynamic stability, and careful evaluation of the cervical spine need to be included as part of the initial evaluation and should be treated appropriately. If there is significant airway trauma and intraluminal airway hemorrhage, immediate airway control is essential and should be prioritized.

Assessment of anterior neck and laryngeal trauma proceeds with examination for signs of impending airway obstruction: stridor, dyspnea, shortness of breath, aphonia, or use of accessory respiratory muscles. If present, one must be prepared to establish a safe airway at any given time. There has been debate in the literature regarding the method used to secure the airway. If airway symptoms are present requiring emergent intervention, tracheotomy provides the safest means for control. With obvious thyroid cartilage deformity, worsening airway obstruction, or evidence of significant airway hemorrhage, it is advisable to proceed directly to a surgical airway under local anesthesia to avoid additional laryngeal airway injury that could precipitate complete obstruction.

If intubation is attempted, one must be prepared for emergent tracheotomy or cricothyrotomy. Orotracheal intubation can potentiate airway obstruction by worsenING endolaryngeal soft tissue injury. In the case of tracheal separation, the distal trachea can retract inferiorly, therefore, incorrect tube placement can have catastrophic consequences. Intubation should only be considered in cases where there is a grossly intact larynx without mucosal avulsion, adequate visualization, and performed by a physician experienced in complex airway management.[2,5] Data suggests that less experienced practitioners misplace endotracheal tubes anywhere from 4% to 26% depending on the study.[6]

Tracheotomy supplies should be present during evaluation and if tracheotomy is not performed immediately, supplies should travel with the patient as he or she navigates through the hospital during diagnostic workup.

If airway symptoms are stable, flexible laryngoscopic examination of the upper airway should be a priority to evaluate for intraluminal swelling, exposed cartilage, lacerations, hematoma, or vocal fold paralysis. Endoscopy should be done delicately in an effort to reduce additional airway trauma, which could precipitate cough and obstruction.

Concurrent bedside evaluation of the head and neck should be performed. Evidence of laryngeal trauma includes anterior neck swelling, crepitus, bruising, step-off deformity of the cartilaginous structures, loss of normal landmarks, change in voice, dysphagia, respiratory change, or displacement of structures.[7] Voice change, subcutaneous emphysema, hemoptysis and dyspnea rank as the most common signs of injury regardless of etiology.[8] Lack of external evidence does not eliminate the possibility of fracture given that a majority of patients do not have evidence of external deformity.[9] Evaluation of cranial nerves should be performed. Specifically, the vagus and its branches, spinal accessory, and hypoglossal nerves run in the vicinity of the larynx and should be considered carefully.

If the patient and airway are stable, imaging is the next step in evaluation. Computed tomography (CT) is the gold standard imaging modality for assessment of cartilaginous framework injury. It is widely available and images can be acquired quickly. It is appropriate for all patients with significant anterior neck blunt force trauma irrespective of physical exam findings.[10] Computed tomography of the neck often suffices but thin cut CT imaging of the cartilaginous airway can give a detailed account of the extent of injury and provide an excellent roadmap for surgical exploration and repair. Given the proximity of the larynx to the great vessels, CT angiography can also easily be added if vascular injury is suspected, especially in the case of penetrating trauma. Computed tomography is an excellent modality for evaluation of fractures. If the inferior horns of the thyroid cartilage are fractured, one must rule out cricothyroid joint dislocation and cricoid fracture.[11]

While outside of the scope of this chapter, brief discussion of penetrating neck trauma is relevant when discussing laryngeal trauma. The neck is divided into three zones: zone I extends from the clavicles to the cricoid, zone II from the cricoid to the angle of the mandible, and zone III from mandible to skull base. The larynx lies completely within zone II.

Most important in penetrating trauma of the anterior neck is assessment of vascular structures. Classically, any wound that extends beyond platysma warrants further evaluation. As many as 25% of vascular injuries are asymptomatic, so absence of bleeding does not preclude vascular injury.[12-14] Evaluation of zones I and III vascular injuries with CT angiography is 100% sensitive and 93% specific.[15] Unless there is obvious significant hemorrhage, these areas are not explored surgically due to anatomic challenges with access. For zone II injury, classic teaching dictates surgical exploration for sub-platysmal injury. In recent years, CT angiography has been used effectively to reduce the number of exploratory surgeries needed to evaluate injury of zone II.[16]

If no surgical intervention is necessary based on imaging and flexible endoscopy, esophagram should be completed to rule out pharyngeal, hypopharyngeal, or esophageal perforation prior to initiating oral intake. Perforation is present in as high as 3% of cases of penetrating trauma.[4,17] If surgery is indicated, both flexible and rigid esophagoscopy are highly sensitive (80–90%) for evaluation for perforation.[18] Both carry the potential for morbidity: rigid endoscopy can worsen a small tear due to mechanical injury and flexible endoscopy can increase subcutaneous emphysema from insufflation. When endoscopy is used in conjunction with fluoroscopic imaging, sensitivity nears 100%.[15] Oral contrast-enhanced CT is another option for assessment of leak; however, it is equivalent to traditional barium swallow in sensitivity.[19]

MANAGEMENT

Over the years, there have been a number of classification systems that have helped guide management strategy. The most commonly used classification of laryngeal trauma, by Schaefer, divides injury into four groups of increasing severity (Table 6.1).[20] A fifth category was added by Fuhrman et al. to allow for inclusion of laryngotracheal separation in the classification system.[21]

In general, management approaches can be broken down into five categories: (1) observation/nonoperative management, (2) endoscopic management alone, (3) neck exploration including fracture repair with or without tracheotomy, (4) neck exploration with thyrotomy and tracheotomy, and (5) exploration, thyrotomy, and stent placement with tracheotomy.

Group I injuries, as defined by Schaefer, can be managed conservatively. If there is any question about the extent of injury, microdirect laryngoscopy allows for improved visualization via rigid telescopes, and allows for palpation of cricoarytenoid joints to assess for dislocation.

Table 6.1: Schaefer-Fuhrman classification system.

Group	Findings
I	*Fracture*: None
	Soft tissue: Minor laceration or hematoma
II	*Fracture*: Nondisplaced fracture
	Soft tissue: Edema, hematoma, minor mucosal disruption with no exposed cartilage
III	*Fracture*: Displaced fracture
	Soft tissue: Significant edema, large mucosal lacerations, exposed cartilage
IV	*Fracture*: Two or more fractures, unstable framework
	Soft tissue: Same as group III with severe mucosal injury or anterior commissure disruption
V	Complete laryngotracheal separation

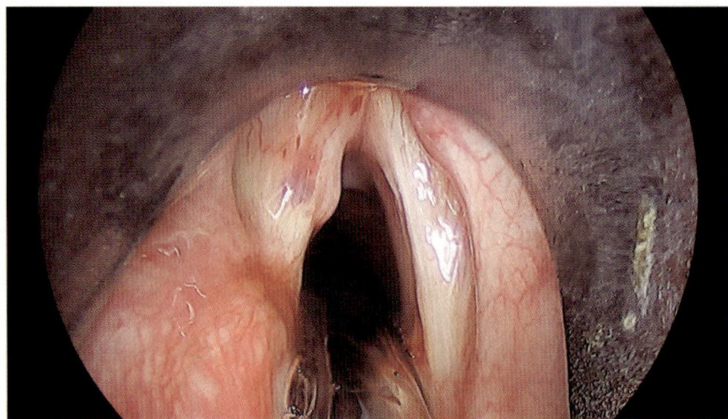

Fig. 6.1: This is a 22-year-old male with persistent voice change after a motorcycle accident. He was evaluated at the time of injury at an outside hospital for nondisplaced fracture and vocal fold laceration. Laceration was not repaired. Now, 5 months later, he has persistent voice change and left-sided paralysis. Note the anterior retraction of the left thyroarytenoid muscle.

Missing a significant mucosal injury can have profound consequences in regards to long-term function because of suboptimal wound healing leading to scar, contractures, and associated dysfunction (Fig. 6.1). Group I strangulation injuries should be carefully observed, even if asymptomatic, due to late onset edema and airway obstruction up to 24 hours postinjury.[22]

Nonoperative and postoperative cases should be observed in a monitored setting for at least 24 hours. It is the authors' practice to use steroids, antibiotics, anti-reflux medication, head of bed elevation, and humidified air to prevent progression of edema, infection, and mucosal irritation. Most patients undergo bedside evaluation by a speech pathologist if there is any dysphagia or odynophagia present. Modified barium swallow is ordered on an as needed basis and alternate feeding sources are utilized as indicated.

Traditionally, as with Group I, straightforward Group II injuries without signs of airway edema or distress, can be managed conservatively and observed. There is some thought that any identified fracture should be plated due to risk of developing displacement days to weeks postinjury. This treatment group remains controversial.[10,23] We have increasingly favored miniplating for any fracture.

For more complex injuries, as seen in Group III or IV, microdirect laryngoscopy should be done once the airway has been secured. In general, this means a surgical airway has been performed, often under local as apposed to general anesthesia.

In the hands of an experienced surgeon, select Group III patients without significant mucosal injuries can undergo fracture repair without a tracheotomy assuming there is no significant manipulation of the airway or development of edema. If a tracheotomy is present and open reduction and fixation of a fracture is indicated, maintaining separate incisions reduces risks of seeding secretions into the surgical field and subsequent infection of the field and hardware.

Repair of fractures can be done in a number of different ways. Regardless of the method, the priority is recreating cartilaginous continuity in the anterior-posterior dimension at the level of the true folds to reestablish vocal fold length and tension. This, typically, is at the level of the junction of the inferior and middle third of the thyroid cartilage. Failure to do so will result in a loss of tension of the vocal fold, shortening of the ipsilateral side, and pitch change. Realignment of the fracture in a caudal cranial dimension is also essential ensuring that the vocal folds align correctly.

Today, cartilage repair is commonly performed using titanium miniplates. Midface plates are of an appropriate size, can be shaped to approximate the native contours of the cartilage, and secured with 4–6 mm screws depending on cartilage thickness. If screws are too long and protrude transmucosally, they can cause endolaryngeal granulation and delay wound healing or cause granuloma formation. Absorbable miniplates are available but experience with them is limited.[24]

If plates are unavailable, cartilage can be repaired with suture or wire. If maintaining an anatomic position is difficult while plating, sutures can be used to secure the height at the inferior and superior margins prior to plate application. If there are multiple mobile fragments, multiple miniplates or mesh can be used to help stabilize segments.

In Group III or IV injury where there has been severe mucosal injury, repair of mucosal defects or skin grafting is necessary to prevent scar formation (Fig. 6.2). Usually, this entails a thyrotomy to access the endolarynx. Some lacerations are candidates for endoscopic repair, although this is technically challenging. If there is a vertical cartilage fracture present in the midline or paramedian, this can be used as an access point for the thyrotomy. Otherwise, one must be created with an oscillating saw or blade if the cartilage is soft. The mucosal incision should extend from the cricothyroid membrane, through the anterior commissure, to the thyrohyoid membrane. If a plate will be used for reconstruction, bending of the plate and making screw holes prior to the thyrotomy can speed reconstruction after the intralaryngeal work is completed and ensure accurate reconstruction of the cartilage.

Once the larynx is open, lacerations without tissue loss can be repaired primarily. If there has been significant tissue loss, mobilization

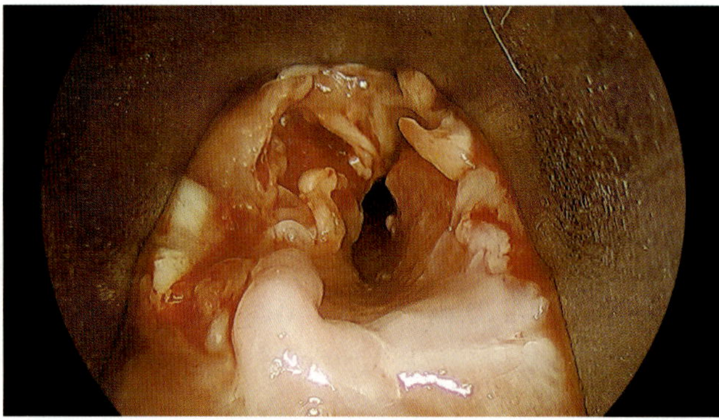

Fig. 6.2: This a 42-year-old male who was shot at close range with a small caliber bullet. The bullet entered the left infraglottis, passed through the airway, and exited the right infraglottis creating comminuted thyroid cartilage fractures and significant soft tissue injury. This 0' telescopic image was taken 10 days postinjury, shortly after being transferred for surgical exploration and repair.

of surrounding tissues, advancement flaps, and skin grafting are all options for covering defects.

If there is cartilaginous instability or concern for glottic web formation and stenosis, use of an intralaryngeal stent is prudent. Stents are suitable for stabilizing severely comminuted fractures or for scenarios where there has been significant tissue loss and plating options are limited. Also, if grafting is necessary, a stent can support a graft while it takes. They come premade in a number of different shapes, sizes, and materials, or can be fashioned by the surgeon by using xeroform packed glove tips or silicone tubing (Fig. 6.3).[25] If there is significant tissue loss that cannot be closed or covered, a skin graft can be sutured circumferentially to the stent, basal layer outward, which may facilitate wound healing (Fig. 6.4).[26]

Prior to closure of the thyrotomy, the anterior aspect of each vocal fold should be resuspended to the outer perichondrium on the ipsilateral side. Careful approximation with consideration of vocal fold height and tension is critical for postoperative voice quality. If a paramedian fracture is used as opposed to midline thyrotomy, the anterior muscle she be suspended to the anterior thyroid cartilage via suture passed through the cartilage or a drill hole. If a stent is placed, it needs to be secured by suturing to a button on the skin surface with at least two points of fixation should one fail. The miniplate can then be applied to stabilize the thyrotomy. As the screws are placed, gentle torsion should be applied, as they are prone to stripping.

In considering closure of the wound, coverage of the laryngotracheal complex with the anterior strap muscle reduces risk of skin tethering to the cartilaginous framework, which can be a nuisance

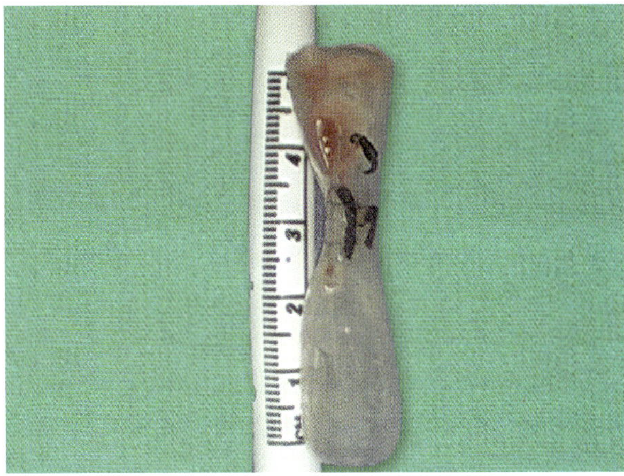

Fig. 6.3: This custom stent was fashioned similar to the method described by Schaefer and Carder. A soft silicone tube was clamped at the junction of the middle and upper third and sutured together to recreate the indentation of the vocal folds.

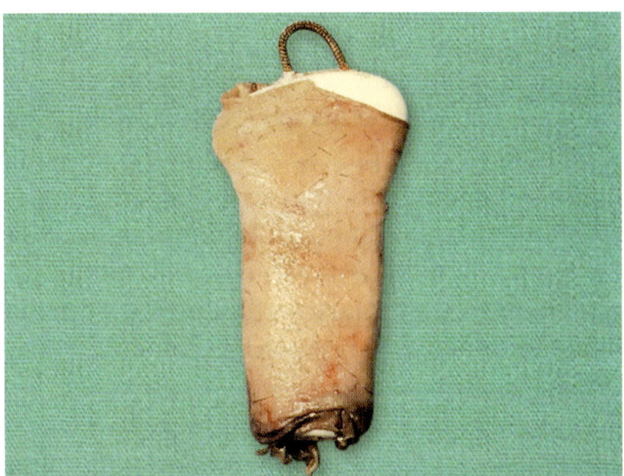

Fig. 6.4: This is a medium Montgomery laryngeal stent (Boston Medical Products, Westborough, MA) wrapped in a split thickness skin graft. It was placed due to extensive soft tissue loss and comminution postgunshot.

postoperatively during swallow. A drain should be left in place to allow for egress of accumulated secretions and air that may collect subcutaneously.

RESULTS

Assessment of laryngeal trauma outcome focuses on preservation of laryngeal function, mainly breathing and swallowing. In a review of the Nationwide Inpatient Sample encompassing 392 laryngeal trauma patients, 46% underwent direct laryngoscopy, 34% required tracheotomy, and 24% required some other additional surgical repair.[4]

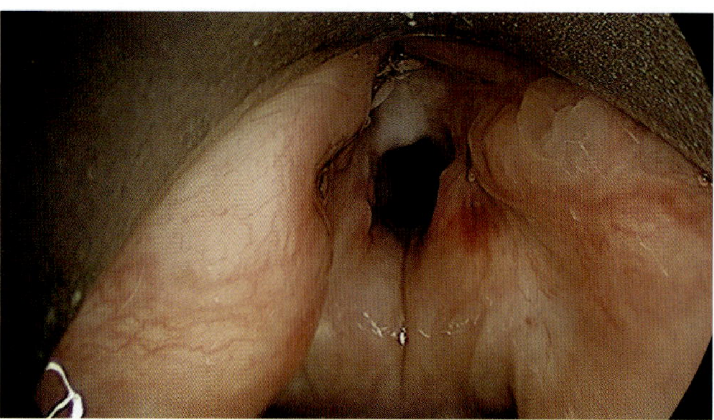

Fig. 6.5: This is a 17-year-old female who feel neck first onto a brick wall. She had comminuted thyroid cartilage fracture and mucosal injuries that were not evaluated at the time of injury. She presented 8 weeks postinjury with worsening voice and airway quality. The image is a 0' telescopic. Note the thick anterior glottic web that has formed.

As a single entity, laryngeal trauma has relatively good outcomes with 69–74% having good voice and 91–94% having good airway.[3] Typically, the more severe the injury, the poorer the voice quality and respiratory function of the larynx. For Group 1–3 injury, most if not all patients typically can maintain near-normal voice quality and live tracheotomy free lives. Group 4 and 5 injuries are less likely to maintain near-normal vocal function. In Schaefer and Close's series, 9/29 had "fair voice" with 2/28 requiring permanent tracheotomy.[7]

Management of Group 4 injury is clearly more complex than other groups. Given that the group represents a heterogeneous collection of soft tissue, cartilaginous framework, and neurologic injury, predicting outcomes and providing treatment algorithms for all situations is challenging. Based on anecdotal observations, injury to the recurrent laryngeal nerves (RLNs), cricoarytenoid, and posterior glottis all negatively impact voice quality and airway function.

Timing of intervention is important. There does seem to be consensus that early intervention is advantageous. While the definition of early varies, studies that stratify time of intervention support the notion that voice and airway outcomes are better with early intervention.[2,27] Delay in intervention/repair allows for maturation of scar, onset of fibrosis, leading to poor outcome (Fig. 6.5). Use of stents and length of stenting is also somewhat controversial. Duration of stenting can be from a week to a couple of months and type of stent varies considerably, presumably due to author preference. One must balance the virtues of laryngeal skeletal stability versus the potential harm to mucosal lining that comes with the stent. Comparing various practices within a group of heterogeneous injuries is challenging and accounts for the lack of consensus on approach. Anecdotally, in most cases somewhere in the vicinity of 2 weeks is advisable.

If unilateral RLN transection is identified at the time of initial presentation, reinnervation is ideal. Both primary anastomosis and ANSA-cervicalis to RLN are valid options. There are no data specific to trauma patients; however, reinnervation in younger patients provides equivalent or better function as compared to thyroplasty.[28]

SUMMARY

Over the past 25 years, the most notable advances in laryngeal trauma have been made in diagnostics. Specifically, improved endoscopic and imaging technology allows for better characterization of injury and categorization within treatment algorithms. Basic concepts of treatment in laryngeal trauma have not changed significantly. Reconstruction of the larynx, reapproximation of mucosal injury, and stenting in severe cases remain important principles in treating this complex group.

REFERENCES

1. Rossbach MM, Johnson SB, Gomez MA, et al. Management of major tracheo-bronchial injuries: a 28-year experience. Ann Thorac Surg. 1998;65:182-6.
2. Bent JP, Silver JP, Prorubsky ES. Acute laryngeal trauma: a review of 77 patients. Otolaryngol Head Neck Surg. 1993;109:441-9.
3. Schaefer, SD. Acute management of external laryngeal trauma: a 27 year experience. Arch Otolaryngol Head Neck Surg. 1992;118:598-604.
4. Jewett BS, Shockley WW, Rutledge R. External laryngeal trauma analysis of 392 patients. Arch Otolaryngol Head Neck Surg. 1999;125:877-80.
5. Schaefer SD. State of the art: the acute treatment of external laryngeal injuries. Arch Otolaryngol Head Neck Surg. 1991;117:35-9.
6. Adams BD, Cuniowski P, Muck A, et al. Combat airway management: the registry of emergency airways arriving at combat hospitals. J Trauma. 2008;64:1548-54.
7. Schaefer SD, Close LG. Acute management of laryngeal trauma: update. Ann Otol Rhinol Laryngol. 1989;98:98-104.
8. Mussi A, Ambrogi MC, Ribechini A, et al. Acute major airway injuries: clinical features and management. Eur J Cardiothorac Surg. 2001;20:46-52.
9. Fuhrman GM, Stieg FH, Buerk CA. Blunt laryngeal trauma: classification and management protocol. J Trauma. 1990;30:87-92.
10. Schaefer SD. Management of acute blunt and penetrating external laryngeal trauma. Laryngoscope. 2014;124:233-44.
11. Becker M, Leuchter I, Platon A, et al. Imaging of laryngeal trauma. Eur J Radiol. 2014;83:142-54.
12. Rao PM, Ivatury RR, Sharma P, et al. Cervical vascular injuries: a trauma center experience. Surgery. 1993;114:527-31.
13. Mansour MA, et al. Validating the selective management of penetrating neck wounds. Am J Surg. 1991;162:517-21.

14. Sclafani SJ, Cavaliere G, Atweh N, et al. The role of angiography in penetrating neck trauma. J Trauma. 1991;31:557-63.
15. Inaba K, Munera F, Mckenney M, et al. Prospective evaluation of screening multislice helical computed tomographic angiography in the initial evaluation of penetrating neck injuries. J Trauma. 2006;61:144-9.
16. Woo K, Magner DP, Wilson, MR, et al. CT angiography in penetrating neck trauma reduces the need for operative neck exploration. Am Surg. 2005;71:754-8.
17. Grewal H, Rao PM, Mukerji S, et al. Management of penetrating laryngotracheal injuries. Head Neck. 1995;17:494-502.
18. Noyes L, McSwain N, Markowitz I. Panendoscopy with arteriography versus mandatory exploration of penetrating wounds of the neck. Ann Surg. 1996; 204:21.
19. Gonzales RP, Falimirksi M, Holvar MR, et al. Penetrating zone II injury: does dynamic computed tomographic scan contribute to the diagnostic sensitivity of physical examination for surgically significant injury? A prospective blinded study. J Trauma. 2003:54:61-5.
20. Schaefer SD. Primary management of laryngeal trauma. Ann Otol Rhinol Laryngol. 1982;91:399-402.
21. Fuhrman GM, Stieg FH, Buerk CA. Blunt laryngeal trauma: classification and management protocol. J Trauma. 1990;30:87-92.
22. Stanley RB, Hanson DG. Manual strangulation injuries of the larynx. Arch Otolaryngol. 1983;109:344-7.
23. Pou AM, Shoemaker DL, Carrau RL, et al. Repair of laryngeal fractures using adaptation plates. Head Neck. 1998;20:707-13.
24. Sasaki CT, Marotta JC, Lowlicht RA, et al. Efficacy of resorbably plates for reduction and stabilization of laryngeal fractures. Ann Otol Rhinol Laryngol. 2003;112:745-50.
25. Schaefer SD, Carder HM. How I do it—fabrication of a simple laryngeal stent. Laryngoscope. 1980;90:1561-3.
26. Harris HH, Tobin HA. Acute injuries of the larynx and trachea in 49 patients. Laryngoscope. 1970;80:1376-84.
27. Maran AGD, Stell PM, Murray JAM, et al. Early management of laryngeal injuries. J R Soc Med. 1981;74:656-60.
28. Paniello RC, Edgar JD, Kallogieri D, et al. Medialization versus reinnervation for unilateral vocal fold paralysis: a multicenter randomized clinical trial. Laryngoscope. 2011;121:2172-9.

Chapter 7

Empty Nose Syndrome

Nipun Chhabra, Steven Michael Houser

INTRODUCTION

Empty nose syndrome (ENS) is a poorly understood iatrogenic disorder that may occur following turbinate reduction surgery. It is most recognized for paradoxical nasal obstruction despite a seemingly wide and patent nasal cavity. The term was initially coined to describe a spectrum of symptoms associated with anatomic tissue loss and corresponding radiographic findings. In the literature, ENS has often been interchangeably, but erroneously, described as a form or subset of atrophic rhinitis. As our understanding of ENS has evolved, it is important to appreciate the distinction from atrophic rhinitis as well as potential treatment options that may significantly improve the quality of life for patients afflicted with this rare and debilitating disorder.

DISTINGUISHING ATROPHIC RHINITIS FROM EMPTY NOSE SYNDROME

The term ENS was first coined by Eugene Kern and Monika Stenkvist in 1994 to describe certain symptomatology and the appearance of a lack of normal intranasal anatomy on a radiographic computed tomography (CT) scan (Fig. 7.1). However, our understanding of ENS has evolved over than last two decades, and it is now used to describe a debilitating complication that may occur following turbinate resection, most commonly as a result of inferior turbinoplasty techniques. Although atrophic rhinitis and ENS share some underlying similarities, they are separate entities arising from distinct origins. To better appreciate key differences between the two disorders, it is important to understand the background of atrophic rhinitis.

Atrophic rhinitis is a chronic, degenerative condition characterized by inflammation and atrophy of the nasal and paranasal mucosa.[1] As with ENS it is often a diagnosis of exclusion and should be considered in patients with chronic rhinosinusitis and significant crusting. The classic symptoms of atrophic rhinitis symptoms include thick and

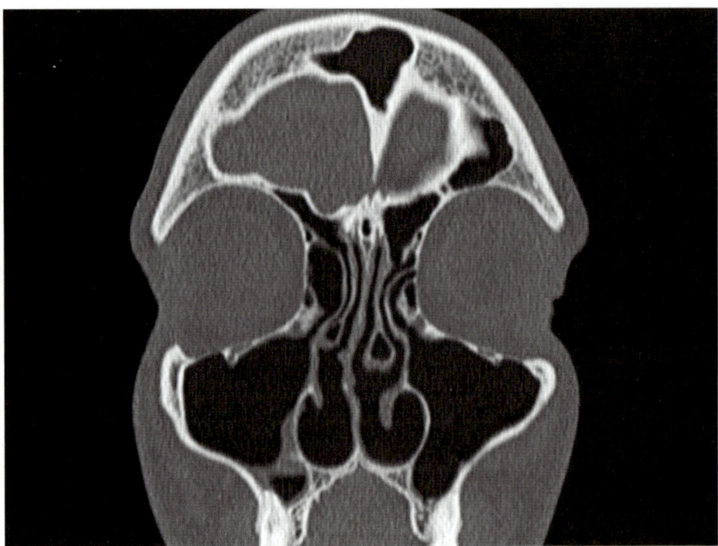

Fig. 7.1: Computed tomography (CT) scan of a patient with empty nose syndrome. Note the absence of bilateral inferior turbinate tissue.

adherent crusting known as *rhinitis atrophicans, cum foetore,* or *ozena,* foul odor (or *fetor*), and nasal obstruction.[1-3] The excessive and recurrent crusting is commonly a late sequela of a chronic underlying inflammatory state or repetitive nasal trauma or injury. While atrophic rhinitis is primarily a clinical diagnosis, histopathologic sampling through conservative biopsy or serum blood testing may be useful in certain cases to distinguish it from other inflammatory disorders or autoimmune conditions.

An important distinction is between primary and secondary atrophic rhinitis. The primary disorder is often spontaneous with unknown etiology and follows a very protracted and indolent course, thought to be due to prolonged microvascular or ischemic injury.[1-3] Secondary atrophic rhinitis is far more common and usually develops as a result of direct injury including trauma, irradiation, reductive nasal or sinus surgery, or in certain rare granulomatous diseases.[1] In this latter form, significant nasal crusting, nasal congestion, and atrophy of mucosal and turbinate surfaces are seen. Severe cases may present with complete absence of recognizable anatomic landmarks, septal perforations, or a formidable saddle nose deformity. Hyposmia, epistaxis, and facial pain or pressure may also be variably encountered. By far, the most common pathogen isolated in atrophic rhinitis is *Klebsiella ozaenae.* Other bacteria include *Staphylococcus aureus, Proteus mirabilis,* and *Escherichia coli.* Crusting is usually exuberant and covers the sidewalls and floor of the nose.

In atrophic rhinitis, the loss of normal mucosal and turbinate tissue together with its constellation of symptoms has erroneously been termed "the empty nose" in much of the literature. This is propagated by the paradoxical nasal congestion, which is the most common complaint of atrophic rhinitis patients. Nasal congestion in atrophic rhinitis may be caused by excessive crusting, but when the disease produces widened nasal cavities, the mechanism is more likely due to atrophy of olfactory epithelium, pain, temperature, and sensory receptors and neural endings.[1,4] In addition, the lack of anatomical barriers and adequate mucociliary clearance due to atrophic and damaged mucosa results in reduced nasal airflow resistance, which may contribute to a subjectively inadequate or unsatisfactory nasal breathing.[5-7]

The goal of treatment in atrophic rhinitis is to improve quality of life and reduce crusting and chronic sinusitis symptoms. Aggressive nasal hygiene with regular intranasal irrigation helps to restore nasal hydration and is considered the standard of conservative therapy.[1] Irrigations are most commonly composed of saline or a balanced salt solution, but in refractory or severe cases, a compounded formulation, topical antibiotic rinses, or nebulized medications with a high-powered irrigation device may be useful. Surgical approaches are limited by long-term efficacy and possible worsening or complications but include conservative and regular debridements, curettage, autologous or allogenic injections and implants, and complete or partial to staged closure of the nasal cavities.[3,8,9] These surgical approaches aim to reduce the volume of the nasal cavity, which will attenuate nasal airflow during inspiration, thereby resulting in less drying, crusting, and subsequent mucosal damage.[1,6] The shape and position of the nostrils, valvular action of the lateral nasal cartilages, amount of residual mucosal and turbinate tissue, and the biomechanical effects of implanted materials on vascular flow all play a significant and interwoven role in healing the atrophic nose.[5,6,10]

The most important distinction between ENS and atrophic rhinitis is the underlying pathophysiology. The resorption of turbinate or adjacent mucosal and nasal tissue in atrophic rhinitis reflects a chronic and often idiopathic inflammatory process, whereas ENS is an iatrogenic disorder. Secondary atrophic rhinitis has been described following turbinate reduction surgery; however, it is more commonly due to other factors such as trauma, infection, or immunologic disease. Atrophic rhinitis also has clear pathogenic associations based on nasal cultures, whereas no known or common pathogen is associated with ENS. Bacteria laden atrophic rhinitis patients usually suffer from heavy crusting, whereas ENS patients exhibit none or only minor crusting.

THE PATHOPHYSIOLOGY OF EMPTY NOSE SYNDROME

ENS is a rare but recognized late complication of turbinate excision, most often total inferior turbinectomy. In general, turbinate tissue in the nose should be conserved whenever possible, although inferior turbinate reduction is an accepted and common treatment for disorders such as allergic rhinitis, rhinitis medicamentosa, rhinitis of recumbency, and refractory nasal obstruction due to turbinate hypertrophy. Resection of the middle turbinate is more controversial, and routine removal should be avoided, except when clearly or significantly diseased, traumatized, or when involved with neoplasm or in extended endonasal approaches to sinonasal and skull base lesions. Ultimately, whether to resect a turbinate and the choice method is left to the surgeon's discretion but prior to undertaking any type of turbinoplasty or turbinate reduction, the operator should be aware that ENS is an iatrogenic disorder resulting from the loss of excessive turbinate tissue.

Although the underlying pathophysiology and exact mechanism of ENS is poorly elucidated, several hypotheses exist. Most likely a "two-hit" phenomenon takes place: (1) the tissue is excised/damaged, (2) neural sensory components and receptors regenerate poorly. As the turbinates are a known source of nerve growth factor, it is possible that damage to turbinate tissue containing neural components may result in sensory alterations in airflow.[11] Nerve damage and long-term hypoesthesia or paresthesias may occur with any surgical procedure, and the nose can be similarly affected. Several studies have demonstrated cutaneous sensory alterations almost 1 year postoperatively.[12,13] As the nose is involved in the critical function of sensing airflow and since nasal breathing is far more satisfactory than oral breathing, it follows that significant quality-of-life issues often arise from derangements in nasal breathing. The possible mechanism of underlying nerve damage in ENS should not be underemphasized. This may help explain why most patients undergoing total turbinectomy never develop ENS and those with lesser damage to turbinate tissue, and seemingly normal anatomy, may still go on to develop ENS. This can also explain the development of unilateral ENS in patients who underwent parallel turbinate reduction observed in three patients by the senior author. The location and extent of damage to sensory afferents may play a central, albeit poorly understood, role.

Another theory relates to trigeminal thermoreceptors and their cooling effect on the nasal mucosa. Transient receptor potential cation channel subfamily M member 8 (TRPM8) is a nonselective voltage-dependent cation channel that is activated in the presence of menthol and increases the perception of coolness.[14] Normal and satisfactory nasal breathing is dependent on an adequate number of functioning TRPM8 receptors. Research has demonstrated that the primary physiological mechanism that produces the sensation of nasal patency is activation of such thermoreceptors by nasal airflow.[15] Damage and loss to these receptors may increase the sensation of nasal fullness or blockage, which in turn may result in an increased respiratory drive. In addition, the turbinates help direct laminar airflow throughout the nose by serving as 'contact points' and eliciting some degree of turbulent airflow. When turbinates are absent, particularly the inferior turbinates, poor or reduced thermoreceptor activation will compromise nasal mucosal cooling and thereby affect the sensation of nasal patency.

Paradoxical nasal obstruction is a perplexing, yet central, symptom of ENS patients. This complaint describes a subjective sense of poor nasal breathing despite an objectively patent nasal fossa. The mechanism likely relates to a malfunction of resistance patterns within the nose. The nasal resistor has been cited as critically important for enhancing alveolar ventilation, gas exchange, and adequate pulmonary backflow.[16] Normal rates of nasal resistance help to maintain expiratory lung volumes and may also indirectly determine arterial oxygenation.[17] Although cool thermoreceptors are poorly activated in the ENS patient, air still reaches the lungs and stimulates pulmonary stretch receptors.[16,18] As the body strains to sense airflow through a lack of nasal resistance, poor pulmonary function may result, and the symptoms may be so severe that the patient experiences dyspnea and may relate a sense of "suffocation". Also, neural messages from the nose suggesting absent airflow contradicts information from pulmonary stretch receptors, which may contribute to anxiety.

In general, the turbinates define and are intimately related to the nasal meati through which air passes. The middle and superior meati are narrow airspaces, which limit the total amount of airflow through the nose and paranasal sinuses. They also serve to increase the velocity of airflow and ensure a mostly laminar pattern. This conductive air–mucosal interface provides maximum cooling function and sensation while also directing nasal airflow and olfactory particles toward certain regions.[14,19,20] Loss of turbinate tissue ultimately disrupts meatal anatomy, and computational modeling of nasal airflow patterns after inferior turbinate resection demonstrates turbulent, inefficient, hyposmic, and less sensate airflow through the nose.[14,19,20-22]

The ENS patients usually suffer from dryness that likely results from impaired cooling and humidification. Mucociliary clearance, immunoglobulin A secretion, and humidification capacity are significantly disrupted following total inferior turbinectomy.[22] Inferior turbinate resection alone reduces heat and water vapor flux in the nose by 16%, and when combined with middle turbinate resection, this results in an approximate 25% loss.[23,24] In summary, the pathophysiology of ENS is complex and multifactorial, and further research is needed to better elucidate contributory mechanisms.

THE PRESENTATION OF EMPTY NOSE SYNDROME

Although few patients develop ENS following turbinate resection, an astute suspicion and clinical awareness of this rare disorder is necessary to alleviate patient anxiety and to help formulate a treatment algorithm. The hallmark complaint that accompanies ENS is paradoxical nasal obstruction.[4,25] On physical examination, a large and patent nasal cavity may be present due to the lack of turbinate tissue, but patients report a subjective feeling of "stuffiness" and congestion. This may be coupled with a sensation of "emptiness", which describes the inability to sense airflow. Dyspnea and shortness of breath may also be present as patients tend to compensate with excessive breathing, sometimes resulting in hyperventilation and a relentless need to over breathe. This is often worse with physical or strenuous activity and is the most severe symptom of ENS.

Chronic pain can follow any surgery, including nasal surgery. Irritation from dry mucosa is often seen in ENS, but unrelenting severe pain existing independent of breathing is a distinct pain entity that fails to respond to ENS therapy. Unfortunately, there is much misinformation suggesting that chronic nasal/facial pain is ENS, yet this is not the case.

The ENS patients typically become very preoccupied with their nasal symptoms and may relate fatigue, irritability, anxiety, depression, and the inability to concentrate (*aprosexia nasalis*).[4,26] Often times, the confounding constellation of symptoms accompanying ENS is overlooked, because the physician has difficulty accounting for the paradoxical obstruction in view of a widely patent nasal fossa. The symptoms may go undiagnosed for months, years, or even decades.

Patients undergoing any type of turbinate reduction surgery either independently or in conjunction with endoscopic sinus surgery or other nasal procedures should be followed closely in the postoperative period. A protracted period of crusting or pain, especially in the region of the operated turbinates, should be closely monitored through regular follow-up, nasal hygiene, and selective debridement. In its late stages, a constant feeling of congestion and persistent dryness may occur despite healed mucosa. Supportive therapy such as moisturization, a good diet, and exercise to encourage nasal blood flow should be advised. The ENS symptoms may fade over the course of a year but when persistent beyond that time, then permanent therapies can be considered.

THE DIAGNOSIS OF EMPTY NOSE SYNDROME

Although ENS was originally coined to describe radiographic findings that accompany a postoperative "empty" nasal cavity, the diagnosis relies heavily on clinical suspicion and physical examination. The onset of ENS varies widely, ranging from days to years following turbinate surgery. Late onset ENS is difficult to explain through nerve damage, although some patients do describe years of adequate nasal breathing after surgery followed by a slow decline into ENS symptoms. Most commonly, ENS is encountered following inferior turbinate resection. Still, it may occur following middle turbinate resection and rarely in patients who have seemingly normal turbinate tissue. Nonetheless, all patients afflicted with ENS have had some type of turbinate procedure performed during their lifetime.[25]

Overall, ENS appears most commonly following surgeries or procedures that are destructive to the overlying mucosa. It is estimated that approximately 20% of patients with inferior turbinate resection will develop fulminant ENS, and a greater percentage will suffer from at least dryness or some alteration in nasal airflow.[26,27] Procedures that are less aggressive than total inferior turbinate reduction would be expected to produce a lesser incidence of ENS. As endoscopic technology has advanced, so has our armamentarium of turbinoplasty techniques. Submucosal reductions with a microdebrider or other mucosal sparing operations (e.g. radio-frequency reduction and outfracture) are safer alternatives that may reduce the incidence of ENS by preserving the overlying mucosal surface.

Although ENS can be a challenging diagnosis, a modification on the validated 20-item Sino-Nasal Outcome Test (*SNOT-20*) is useful for identifying potential patients and narrowing the spectrum of symptoms. The standard 20-item questionnaire is scored from 0 (no symptoms) to 5 (severe symptom) and include the following: (1) need to blow nose, (2) sneezing, (3) runny nose, (4) cough, (5) postnasal discharge, (6) thick nasal discharge, (7) ear fullness, (8) dizziness, (9) ear pain, (10) facial pain/pressure, (11) difficulty falling asleep, (12) waking up at night, (13) lack of a good night's sleep, (14) waking up tired, (15) fatigue, (16) reduced productivity, (17) reduced concentration, (18) frustration/restless/irritable, (19) sad, and (20) embarrassed. The five additional ENS-specific questions (*SNOT-25*) added by Houser

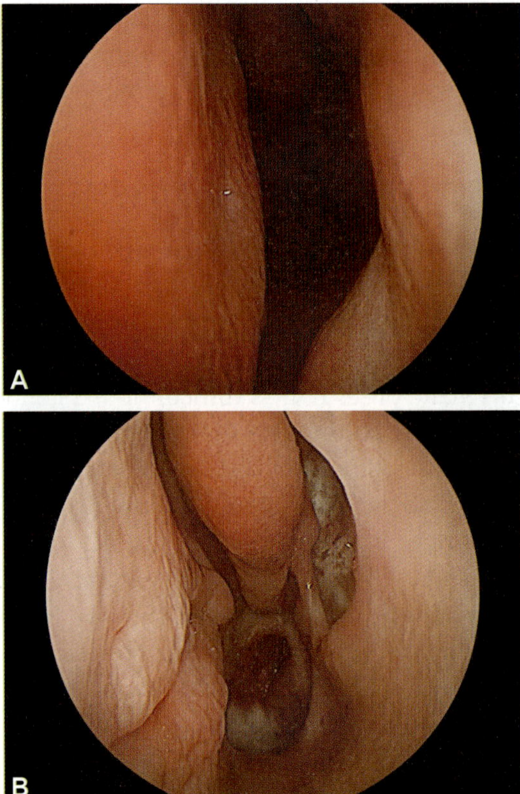

Figs. 7.2A and B: Endoscopic view of the left anterior (A) and posterior (B) nasal cavity in an empty nose syndrome patient. The inferior turbinate has been resected, and there is evidence of prior sinus surgery.

in 2001 include the following: (1) dryness, (2) difficulty with nasal breathing, (3) suffocation, (4) nose is too open, and (5) nasal crusting. Patients are also encouraged to free text or expand on their responses. The *SNOT-25* is a robust method for assessing both preoperative symptoms and quality of life and improvement following surgical treatment for ENS. It has high internal reliability, and patients have shown statistically significant improvements in the five axes of the questionnaire following implantation techniques aimed at restoring nasal volume.[28,29] Frequently, ENS patients are extremely or excessively preoccupied with their nasal symptoms. The combination of paradoxical airway obstruction, dyspnea, nasal or pharyngeal dryness, hyposmia, and often depression are very predictive of ENS. Nasal examination or endoscopy often demonstrates dry and pale mucosa, which may signify underlying squamous metaplasia, periodic crusting, and a lack or significant reduction of turbinate tissue (Figs. 7.2A and B).

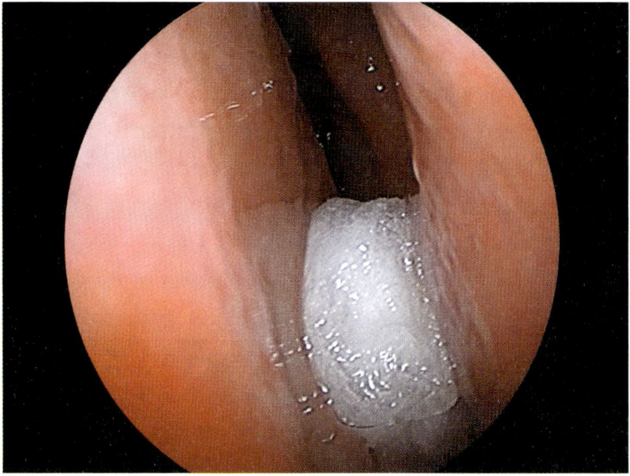

Fig. 7.3: Endoscopic view of the "cotton test". Moistened cotton is placed in the left nasal cavity to simulate absent tissue and determine the feasibility of an implant.

Houser developed the "cotton test" to aid in both diagnostic utility and surgical planning. This simple office-based procedure allows the physician to gauge the dimensions and ideal location of potential implants. Using isotonic sodium chloride solution, cotton is moistened and placed within the nasal cavity in a region where either there is an absence of turbinate tissue or where an implant may be feasible (Fig. 7.3). This is kept in place for approximately 20 minutes, and the patient is asked to breathe comfortably and report any changes in symptoms. The cotton serves to simulate both a nasal implant and existing mucosal tissue that has since been absent, thereby increasing intranasal volume and altering nasal airflow patterns. Patients, who report a definitive subjective improvement and whose symptoms and physical examination findings otherwise are consistent with ENS, are then offered submucosal implantation. If the patient feels no improvement, or feels worse, with cotton in place then plans for implantation should be aborted. The cotton test may not be reliable in the face of confounding or active inflammatory conditions, such as untreated allergic rhinitis or rhinosinusitis; repeat testing after therapy may be needed. Because ENS is such a challenging disorder, the otolaryngologist should be adept at not only identifying clinical cues but also by utilizing the *SNOT-25* and the cotton test to ascertain the diagnosis.

ENS SUBTYPES

Empty nose syndrome can be divided into several subtypes. ENS–inferior turbinate (ENS-IT) is by far the most common form and occurs only after resection of inferior turbinate tissue. The amount of lower turbinate loss may vary from complete or subtotal, and there is no agreed upon measure of quantifying the degree of tissue injury. Rhinometry may assist in detecting derangements in nasal airflow, but clinical findings and radiographic imaging is generally adequate for diagnostic purposes and treatment planning. When compared with other subtypes of ENS, paradoxical nasal obstruction is most often felt with ENS-IT. The reason for this is not well understood, although it may be due to alterations in nasal airflow as it relates to the lower turbinates. The inferior turbinates direct approximately 60% of airflow upward through the middle (50%) and superior (10%) meatus during regular steady nasal respiration.[30-32]

ENS–middle turbinate (ENS-MT) is a very rare and controversial disorder. In comparison with the inferior turbinate, the middle turbinate plays a smaller role in nasal breathing and obstructive disorders such as allergic rhinitis. The middle turbinate is more involved in inflammatory conditions such as chronic sinusitis and nasal polyposis.[33] In addition, abnormal aeration of the middle turbinate as a concha bullosa may further narrow the middle meatus and ostiomeatal complex. Lateralization, weakening, or ongoing involvement of the middle turbinate in inflammatory disease can predispose patients to recurrent symptoms and obligate revision surgery. In such cases or in endoscopic endonasal approaches to the skull base, the middle turbinate may be operatively resected or reduced. Albeit exceedingly rare, ENS can occur as a result of absent middle turbinate tissue. In addition to breathing dysfunction, ENS-MT patients may report pain associated with inspiration, which is more unique to this ENS subtype. This may be due to the effect of turbulent airflow striking exposed mucosa overlying the sphenopalatine ganglion.[34,35]

ENS-type refers to a small and select group of patients with symptoms that fully emulate ENS and who have undergone some type of turbinate procedure in the past but appear to have adequate turbinate tissue. Although the mucosa appears intact, the history of a mucosa damaging procedure (e.g. laser reduction or surface cautery) and significant crusting after surgery usually exists. These patients report significant improvement during the cotton test and may improve with surgical intervention.

ENS–both, as its name implies, involves loss of both inferior and middle turbinate tissue and is the most severe and debilitating form of ENS (Fig. 7.4). Patients are often crippled by their symptoms with higher rates of depression and olfactory derangements resulting from alterations in the delivery of odorant particles to the olfactory

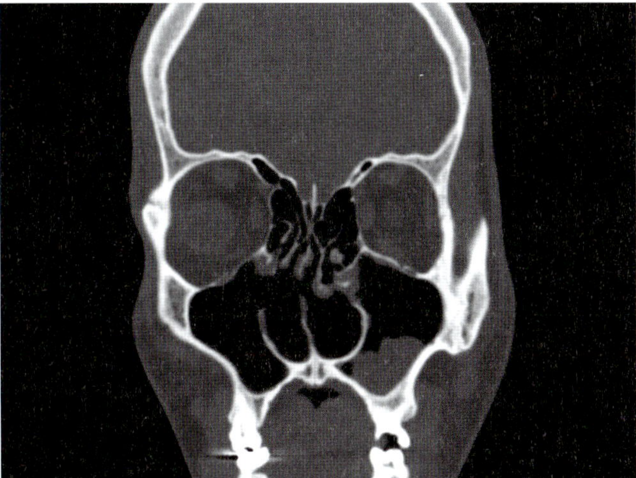

Fig. 7.4: Computed tomography scan of patient with empty nose syndrome. Both inferior turbinates and portions of the middle turbinates have been resected. A septal perforation is also present.

cleft. The ENS from superior turbinate resection alone has not been described, but a judicious approach to the superior turbinate is recommended due to its association with olfaction and proximity to the skull base.[36]

THE ROLE OF IMPLANT THERAPY FOR EMPTY NOSE SYNDROME

Although still somewhat controversial, there is evidence to suggest a physiologic relationship between the sensation of nasal airflow and the central respiratory center. Rhinomanometry, biomechanical, and physical resistance computational modeling have served to increase our understanding of the air passage through the nasal conduit. An appreciation of nasal airflow and how it relates to paradoxical obstruction is central to understanding the role of implant therapy for ENS.

A study of minimum air velocities required to produce subjective sensations at various nasal sites suggests that the nasal vestibule and anterior aspect of the lateral nasal walls are significantly more sensitive to airflow than the nasal cavum.[37] This may be due in part to the skin-lined nasal vestibule and the inferior meatus when compared with the mucosally lined nasal cavity or the middle meatus.[36,38] Physiologically, one may expect the greatest concentration of receptors to be present at the entrance to the nasal system, thereby allowing ample opportunity for the nasal-respiratory reflex arc to adjust accordingly in a dynamic flow system. However, the perplexing aspect of ENS is that patients have dramatically increased nasal airflow, especially at the nasal vestibule, yet they report a paradoxical obstruction. A possible explanation is that the loss of inferior turbinate tissue produces turbulent airflow, especially over the middle meatus. This may result in dryness and crusting along the lateral aspect of the middle turbinate and in the middle meatus where other airflow receptors exist, ultimately leading to a sensation of nasal obstruction.[39] Although these studies highlight the middle meatus as an important location of airflow sensation, it is still not known which area of the nose is most important for the subjective sensation of nasal patency and airflow.

The sensation of nasal airflow is of central importance for both the patient and the physician to assess clinical symptoms. Ultimately, it is the subjective sensation of nasal obstruction, rather than an objective change in nasal airway resistance, which causes symptoms and complaints. Objective values are much easier to quantify than subjective sensation though. This may explain why the literature focuses on objective measures of nasal airflow and yet has not yielded a strong correlation between turbinate resection and aberrant nasal sensation due to changes in airflow and resistance.

Nasal breathing is far more satisfying and effective than breathing through an open mouth. With a loss of turbinates as resistors of the nasal cavity, the patient suffers from derangements in nasal breathing. The majority of humans breathe primarily through their nose and switch to oral breathing only at high levels of physical strain.[40] The goal of surgical treatment for ENS is to improve nasal sensation, by redirecting airflow away from an insensate empty region toward an unoperated native region. Aggressive nasal hygiene and nasal moisturizers alone may be of limited efficacy. Surgical implantation to augment intranasal volume is the mainstay of operative treatment for the ENS patient. A recent systematic review of 128 patients across eight studies who underwent implantation demonstrated the most clinical improvement in the ENS *SNOT* subdomains and psychological issues.[41] The most common form of surgery is through a transnasal submucosal approach to augment the region of the absent turbinate tissue. Turbinate reconstruction, sometimes termed endonasal microplasty, utilizes various implant materials. Autografts such as temporalis fascia and cartilage have been described.[25,42] Additional options include silastic, acellular dermal matrix, hydroxyapetite cement, hyaluronic acid, beta-tricalcium phosphate, and porous polyethylene.[26,42,43] The desired implant should be weighed against clinical experience, composition, possible resorption or extrusion rates, and long-term efficacy.

The location of the implant will typically simulate the premorbid location of absent or resected turbinate tissue. The exact implant site and size is best identified through the in-office cotton test. In certain cases, such as with ENS–both patients, a large septal implant that bridges both the inferior and middle turbinates may be of benefit. The ENS-IT subtype presents the option of both sidewall and septal implantation, whereas ENS-MT repair is limited to the septal site. The ENS-type symptoms may be ameliorated through direct IT expansion. In all cases, the simple cotton test is useful to confirm ENS and aid in implant site selection.

OPERATIVE PROCEDURE FOR SURGICAL IMPLANTATION

While a multitude of grafts exist to surgically reconstruct the empty nose, Houser recommends acellular dermis as a reliable, predictable, and pliable choice for optimal rehabilitation. Examples include Alloderm (LifeCell, Bridgewater, NJ, USA), Allomax (Bard, Warwick RI, USA), FlexHD (MTF, Edison, NJ and Ethicon, Somerville, NJ), Graft Jacket (Wright Medical, Memphis, TN, USA) or SureDerm (HansBiomed, Seoul, South Korea). The implant is placed into a submucoperichondrial (smpc) or submucoperiosteal (smpo) plane, or directly beneath the mucosa. Preoperative evaluation with a thorough history and clinical examination, CT imaging, and the cotton test will help determine the ideal location for implant placement. Once the patient is deemed a satisfactory candidate for implantation, the goal is to create permanent tissue expansion that simulates the moistened cotton and will improve symptomatology.

Infection is a possible complication of any allogenic graft, and therefore, the patient is given a 1-g (or weight appropriate) dose of intravenous Cephazolin immediately preoperatively, and the perifacial and nose region is prepped with betadine paint and draped in the normal, sterile fashion. Hydrogen peroxide diluted to half-strength with normal saline is used to lavage the nasal cavity in an effort to sterilize the area. To date, the senior author has surgically implanted over 60 patients in 15 years without any graft infections.

To simulate the anatomic loss of inferior turbinate tissue, the implant is placed at the septum, floor, and/or the lateral nasal wall. For lateral wall implants, the incision is usually made anterior to the limen nasi or just posterior to it (Figs. 7.5A and B). An angled beaver blade or ophthalmologic knife is helpful for a lateral incision behind the nasal sill. As the inferior meatus slopes laterally, endoscopic assistance may be necessary to raise the flap and the *smpo* is then raised with the blunt end of a Cottle elevator or a Freer elevator. The pocket is created all along the length of the IT and from the floor to the IT

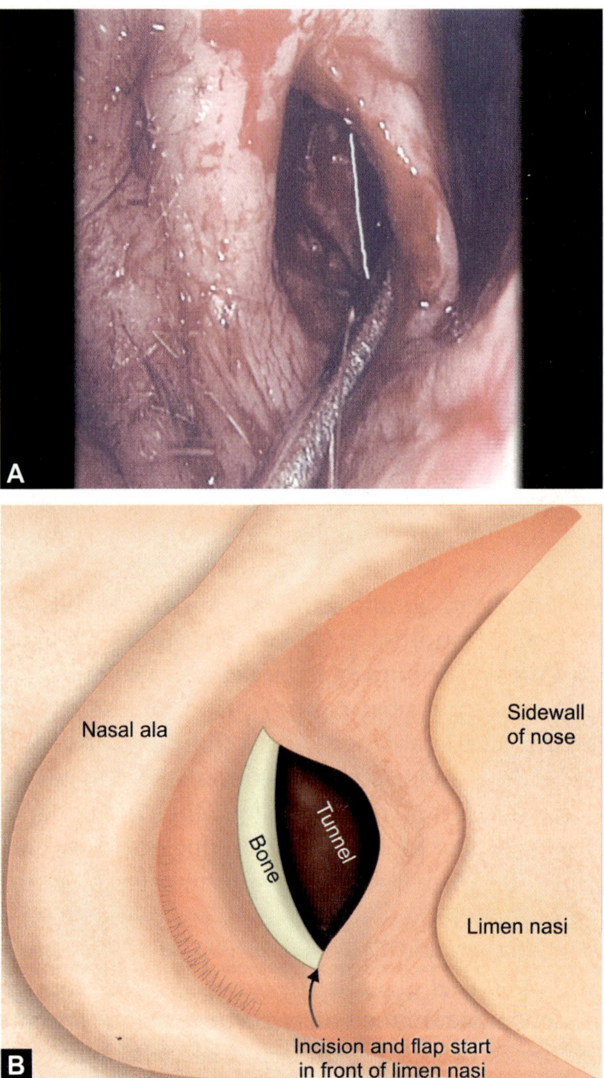

Figs. 7.5A and B: Incision (A) and schematic representation (B) of the placement for a lateral wall implant. The pocket is usually created just anterior to the limen nasi in the nasal vestibule.

remnant above. Dissection near the lacrimal duct orifice should be done with care as the tethered mucosa will often tear. Although nasolacrimal duct occlusion was initially feared with sidewall expansion, none has occurred. The mucosa of the *smpo* seems to provide excellent blood supply to the graft while the bone offers minimal blood vessel ingrowth. Two or three 2 × 4 cm acellular dermis sheets are cut into strips and packed loosely into the lateral wall pocket. The operator should expect some attenuation as the graft incorporates and the air pockets are ablated; therefore, it is recommended to overcorrect the site of implantation by at least 25%. The surgical pocket is closed deeply at the pyriform with a Vicryl suture, and chromic is used superficially in the vestibule. If a revision procedure or additional expansion is needed, the same approach can be readily used to lift the mucosa and the attached graft away from the underlying bone. Interestingly, the sharp pyriform bone will be found to be blunt or rounded after previous dissection in the area. Any revision operations should be deferred for at least 6 months to allow for adequate healing and graft integration (Figs. 7.6A and B).

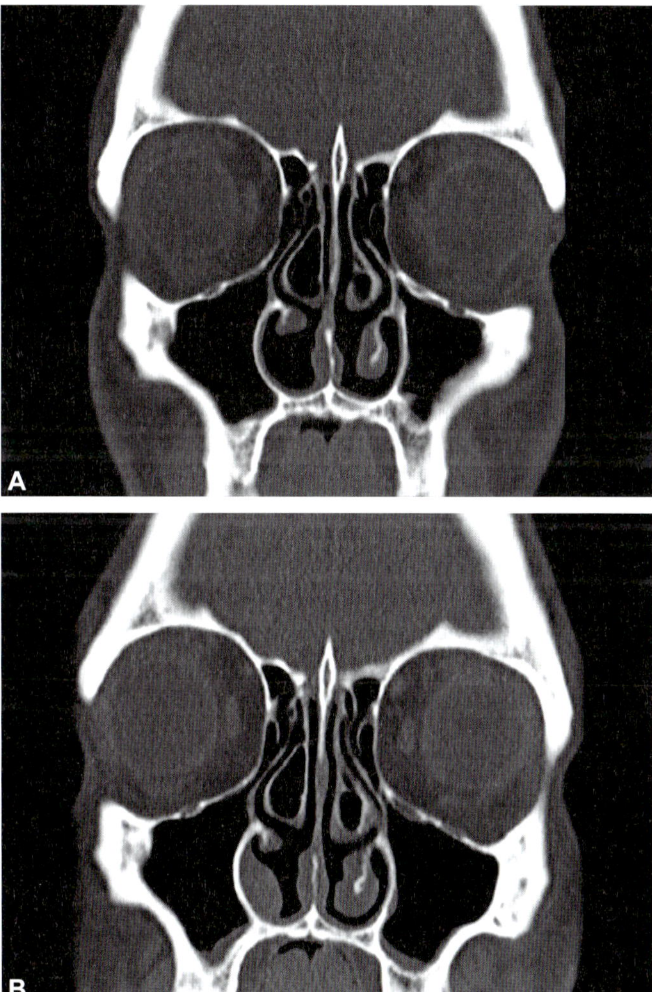

Figs. 7.6A and B: Preoperative (A) and 2-year postoperative (B) radiographic imaging of a right lateral wall implant. The graft has integrated well into the surrounding tissue and simulates the location of the resected inferior turbinate.

Medial or septal implantation via a septoplasty incision is challenging as most ENS patients have previously undergone septoplasty. Delicate and meticulous elevation will help preserve adequate mucosa underneath which the implant can be placed. The graft should be placed sufficiently anteriorly to be opposite the former head of the inferior turbinate. The septal incision and pocket usually extends onto the nasal floor. The acellular dermis can be fashioned through cutting, folding, and suturing with 4-0 chromic, often to resemble a teardrop with the narrowest portion positioned anteriorly and inferiorly. Two stitches (4-0 gut on baby Keith needles) are fixed to the graft prior to final placement, passed through the septum, and secured on the contralateral side. The hemitransfixion septal incision is closed in a standard fashion with several interrupted sutures. The senior author prefers chromic suture but larger grafts placed near the incision may swell postoperatively and result in suture dehiscence and graft exposure. Although these areas have healed by secondary intention without apparent consequence, Vicryl suture may provide more tensile strength if one fears the graft is in danger of exposure. Vicryl sutures may not fall away as easily as chromics; therefore, office removal may be necessary after several weeks. The volume of acellular dermis is individualized to the patient's needs but generally two 2 × 4-cm-thick sheets are sufficient.

A difficult subtype of ENS to surgically address is ENS-MT. The lateral nasal wall contains the drainage pathways for the paranasal sinuses, and implantation in this region may cause chronic or recurrent infections or disturb patent drainage pathways. In addition, the mucosa in the middle meatus and opposite the middle turbinate is exceedingly thin. For these reasons, lateral wall implants for ENS-MT are avoided in favor of implanting the septum, which simulates a "Bolgerized" or well-medialized middle turbinate.[4] A standard septal flap is elevated to the sphenoid rostrum. Acellular dermis is then positioned and its ideal location opposite the absent middle turbinate can be confirmed per endoscopic visualization. In ENS-MT, typically one thick 2 × 4 cm piece of acellular dermis is shaped per chromic sutures and anchored in position via 4-0 gut on baby Keith needles tied on the opposite side of the septal flap.

In a patient with ENS-both, the septum is also the optimal location for grafting a large implant to span the region of both the middle and inferior turbinates. A relatively large volume of acellular dermis is required, such as three or more 2 × 4-cm-thick sheets. The graft is anchored in position to the septal mucosa as described above.

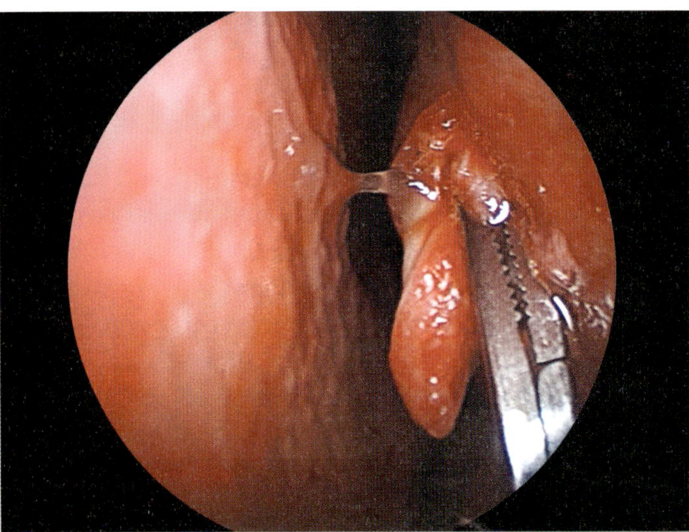

Fig. 7.7: Endoscopic view of the "spear technique". For empty nose syndrome-type patients, multiple strips of acellular dermis are placed submucosally with alligator forceps.

The inferior turbinates of ENS-type patients can be directly expanded in a submucosal fashion. A tunnel within the turbinate tissue is filled with strips cut from acellular dermis. This technique was dubbed the "spear technique" as extra thick sheets allowed for an only partially rehydrated segment to be passed into the tunnel like a spear. The name stuck, despite extra thick sheets no longer being made. Rehydrated segments are passed into the IT tunnel with the aid of small ear alligator forceps (Fig. 7.7). Multiple segments can be passed and may lay adjacent to one another. The anterior half to two-thirds of the inferior turbinate can be expanded. The tunnel is closed with a single chromic suture, and postoperative packing is generally not required.

Since the nasal mucosa is not as distensible as external skin, instillation of injectable fillers may serve only limited benefit. Excess injection may risk mucosal rupture and leakage of filler material into the nasal cavity. The adherence of mucosa to underlying periosteal and perichondrial attachments, namely the septum and nasal floor, make injection in these regions particularly difficult. The submucosal layer of the inferior turbinate, as opposed to the *smpo*, is more readily able to accept fillers; hence, ENS-type patients are the main candidates for injection therapy. There are a myriad of injectable products, which may be temporary or permanent; the senior author has found Acell™ (Acell Inc., Columbia, MD, USA), and Cymetra™ (Lifecell, Bridgewater, NJ) to be useful. Additional investigation into the realm of injectables for ENS treatment is needed to further elucidate their role and determine long-term efficacy.

CONCLUSION

Empty nose syndrome is a poorly understood and rare iatrogenic disorder that results from the destruction of normal nasal and turbinate tissue. It is important to understand the distinction between ENS and atrophic rhinitis as a lack of recognition can prolong patient complaints and symptoms. While further research is needed to better elucidate pathophysiologic mechanisms of ENS, an astute clinical suspicion coupled with the use of diagnostic tools such as the *SNOT-25* and cotton test will greatly benefit the otolaryngologist in clinical practice. In addition, a judicious and cautious approach to turbinate reduction is recommended to help prevent this rare but debilitating sequela of nasal surgery. The goal of surgical rehabilitation is to augment the nasal airway and help restore functional nasal anatomy toward the premorbid state, which will attain dramatic improvements in symptomatology and quality of life for patients afflicted with ENS.

REFERENCES

1. Moore EJ, Kern EB. Atrophic rhinitis: a review of 242 cases. Am J Rhinol. 2001; 15:355-61.
2. Goodman WS, De Souza FM. Atrophic rhinitis. Otolaryngol Clin North Am. 1973;6:773-82.
3. Cottle M. Nasal atrophy, atrophic rhinitis, ozena: medical and surgical treatment. J Int Coll Surg. 1958;29:472-84.
4. Houser SM. Empty nose syndrome associated with middle turbinate resection. Otolaryngol Head Neck Surg. 2006;135:972-73.
5. Clarke RW, Jones AS. Editorial: nasal airflow sensation. Clin Otolaryngol. 1995; 20:97-9.
6. Clarke RW, Jones AS, Charters P, et al. The role of mucosal receptors in the nasal sensation of airflow. Clin Otolaryngol. 1992;17:383-87.
7. Ramadan MF, Campbell IT, Linge K. The effect of nose breathing and mouth breathing on pulmonary ventilation. Clin Otolaryngol. 1984;9:136.
8. Young A. Closure of the nostrils in atrophic rhinitis. J Laryngol Otol. 1967;81: 515-24.
9. Chatterji P. Autogenous medullary (cancellous) bone graft in ozaena. J Laryngol Otol. 1980;94:737-49.
10. Shehata M, Dogheim Y. Surgical treatment of primary chronic atrophic rhinitis—an evaluation of silastic implants. J Laryngol Otol. 1986;100:803-07.
11. Wu X, Myers AC, Goldstone AC, et al. Localization of nerve growth factor and its receptors in the human nasal mucosa. J Allergy Clin Immunol. 2006;118(2): 428-33.

12. Mikkelsen T, Werner MU, Lassen B, et al. Pain and sensory dysfunction 6 to 12 months after inguinal herniotomy. Anesth Analg. 2004;99(1):146-51.

13. Frampton SJ, Pringle M. Cutaneous sensory deficit following post-auricular incision. J Laryngol Otol. 2011;125(10):1014-9.

14. Zhao K, Dalton P. The way the wind blows: implications of modeling nasal airflow. Curr Allergy Asthma Rep. 2007;7:117-25.

15. Sozansky J, Houser SM. Pathophysiology of empty nose syndrome. Laryngoscope. 2015;125(1):70-4.

16. Huizing EH, de Groot JAM. Functional Reconstructive Nasal Surgery. Stuttgart, Germany: Thieme; 2003. p. 48.

17. Swift AC, Campbell IT, McKown TM. Oronasal obstruction, lung volumes, and arterial oxygenation. Lancet. 1988;25(8600):1458-59.

18. Schelegl ES, Green JF. An overview of the anatomy and physiology of slow adapting pulmonary stretch receptors. Respir Physiol. 2001;125:17-31.

19. Elad D, Liebenthal R, Wenig BL, et al. Analysis of airflow patterns in the human nose. Med Biol Eng Comput. 1993;31:585-92.

20. Elad D, Naftali S, Rosenfeld M, et al. Physical stresses at the air-wall interface of the human nasal cavity during breathing. J Appl Physiol. 2006;100(3):1003-10.

21. Grützenmacher S, Lang C, Mlynski G. The combination of acoustic rhinometry, rhinoresistometry and flow simulation in noses before and after turbinate surgery: a model study. J Otorhinolaryngol Relat Spec. 2003;65(6):341-47.

22. Passàli D, Lauriello M, Anselmi M, et al. Treatment of the inferior turbinate: long-term results of 382 patients randomly assigned to therapy. Ann Otol Rhinol Laryngol. 1999;108:569-75.

23. Naftali S, Rosenfeld M, Wolf M, et al. Pathophysiology of nasal air conditioning. In: Proceedings of the Second Joint EMBS/BMES Conference, Houston, TX, USA, October 23–26, 2002. pp. 1523-24.

24. Elad D, Wolf M, Keck T. Air-conditioning in the human nasal cavity. Respir Physiol Neurobiol. 2008;163(1-3):121-7.

25. Houser SM. Surgical treatment for empty nose syndrome. Arch Otolaryngol Head Neck Surg. 2007;133:858-63.

26. Chhabra N, Houser SM. The diagnosis and management of empty nose syndrome. Otolaryngol Clin North Am. 2009;42(2):311-30.

27. Coste A, Dessi P, Serrano E. Empty nose syndrome. Eur Ann Otorhinolaryngol Head Neck Dis. 2012;129:93-7.

28. Jiang C, Wong F, Chen K, et al. Assessment of surgical results in patients with empty nose syndrome using the 25-item Sino-Nasal Outcome Test Evaluation. JAMA Otolaryngol Head Neck Surg. 2014;140(5):453-8.

29. Saafan ME. Acellular dermal (alloderm) grafts versus silastic sheets implants for management of empty nose syndrome. Eur Arch Otorhinolaryngol. 2013; 270(2):527-33.

30. Yaniv E, Hadar T, Shvero J, et al. Objective and subjective nasal airflow. Am J Otolaryngol. 1997;18(1):29-32.

31. Eccles R. Nasal airway resistance and nasal sensation of airflow. Rhinol Suppl. 1992;14:86-90.

32. Moore GF, Freeman TJ, Ogren FP, et al. Extended follow-up of total inferior turbinate resection for relief of chronic nasal obstruction. Laryngoscope. 1985; 95:1095-99.

33. Kennedy DW. Middle turbinate resection: evaluating the issues—should we resect normal middle turbinates? Arch Otolaryngol Head Neck Surg. 1998;124:107.
34. Houser SM. Empty nose syndrome associated with middle turbinate resection. Otolaryngol Head Neck Surg. 2006;135:972-3.
35. Cook PR, Begegni A, Bryant WC, et al. Effect of partial middle turbinectomy on nasal airflow and resistance. Otolaryngol Head Neck Surg. 1995;113:413-9.
36. Wrobel BB, Leopold DA. Olfactory and sensory attributes of the nose. Otolaryngol Clin North Am. 2005;38(6):1163-70.
37. Clarke RW, Jones AS, Charters P, et al. The role of mucosal receptors in the nasal sensation of airflow. Clin Otolaryngol. 1992;17:383-7.
38. Wrobel BB, Bien AG, Holbrook EH, et al. Decreased nasal mucosal sensitivity in older subjects. Am J Otolaryngol. 2006;20:364-8.
39. Wight RG, Jones AS, Beckingham E. Trimming of the inferior turbinates: a prospective long-term study. Clin Otolaryngol Allied Sci. 1990;15(4):347-50.
40. Niinimaa V, Cole P, Mintz S, et al. Oronasal distribution of respiratory airflow. Resp Physiol. 1981;43:69-75.
41. Leong SC. The clinical efficacy of surgical interventions for empty nose syndrome: a systematic review. Laryngoscope. 2015;125(7):1557-62.
42. Kuan EC, Suh JD, Wang MB. Empty nose syndrome. Curr Allergy Asthma Rep. 2015;15(1):493.
43. Bastier PL, Bennani-Baiti AA, Stoll D, et al. β-Tricalcium phosphate implant to repair empty nose syndrome: preliminary results. Otolaryngol Head Neck Surg. 2013;148(3):519-22.

Chapter 8

Acute Sinusitis

Rakesh K Chandra, Benjamin P Hull

INTRODUCTION

Rhinosinusitis, or "sinusitis" as it is often called, refers to inflammation of the paranasal sinuses. The paranasal sinuses are eight paired hollow cavities that are bordered by the orbits laterally, the skull base superiorly, the palate inferiorly, and the clivus posteriorly. They are lined with ciliated pseudostratified columnar epithelium. As the epithelium is affected by various inciting factors, inflammation can occur that results in symptoms that often cause patients to seek medical care. In fact, in 1996 rhinosinusitis was responsible for approximately 17 million ambulatory visits.[1] Currently, approximately one in eight adults in the United States is affected by sinusitis annually,[2,3] resulting in over 25–30 million annual diagnoses.[2,4] About 20 million cases of presumed bacterial acute rhinosinusitis (ARS) are diagnosed in the United States annually,[5] and based on population estimates in 2012, approximately 77,000 adults will suffer from recurrent acute rhinosinusitis (RARS) in a given year.[6]

Rhinosinusitis has a tremendous impact on current medical practice. It is the fifth most common diagnosis responsible for outpatient antibiotic therapy,[5] and more than one in five antibiotics prescribed for adults are for rhinosinusitis.[5] From 2006 to 2010, rhinosinusitis accounted for approximately 11% of all primary care antibiotic-related visits and ARS accounted for 3.9%.[7,8]

Rhinosinusitis is costly to society — the direct annual cost of managing acute and chronic sinusitis exceeds \$11 billion per year;[5] ARS-related health care expenditures total between \$3 and \$3.5 billion annually in the United States.[5] Bhattacharyya et al. elucidated that the average patient with RARS can expect to pay about \$1,100 per year in total direct health costs based on claims paid and third party reimbursements.[6] The indirect costs of rhinosinusitis are also substantial and include decreased productivity and lost workdays;[4,7] and the cost of antibiotic treatment failure includes additional prescriptions, outpatient visits, tests, and procedures.[9] Indeed, rhinosinusitis is common and expensive.

Sinusitis is classified into ARS, chronic rhinosinusitis (CRS), and RARS. Acute rhinosinusitis is defined as an infection of the paranasal sinuses with clinical symptoms lasting 4 weeks or less,[10] and patients with CRS are symptomatic for at least 12 weeks.[10] Recurrent acute rhinosinusitis is defined as four or more distinct episodes of ARS within 12 months time.[7] This chapter will focus on ARS.

PATHOPHYSIOLOGY OF ARS

Most ARS begins with a viral upper respiratory infection that extends into the paranasal sinuses, which may be followed by a bacterial infection.[7] The average adult will experience two to five episodes of viral ARS a year.[11] The viral infection promotes growth of bacteria that colonize the nose and nasal cavities.[12] As patients with upper respiratory infections blow their nose, bacteria are deposited into the paranasal sinuses.[7] Additionally, inflammation associated with the viral infection can obstruct the natural drainage pathways during the nasal cycle, the natural cycle in which the nasal mucosa swell and decongest intermittently throughout the day. This can further predispose the patient to a bacterial infection.[13] Certain anatomic variations, like nasal septal deviation, concha bullosa, or infraorbital ethmoid cells, can predispose to the development of obstructive rhinosinusitis.[14] The obstruction of the natural sinus outflow tracts can result in hypoxia, which leads to subatmospheric pressure that in turn causes the release of vascular-endothelial growth factors and increases the release of inflammatory and fibrotic factors in the affected paranasal sinuses.[15] Fortunately, viral upper respiratory tract infections are complicated by bacterial ARS in only 0.5–2% of cases.[11,12]

With the widespread prevalence of bacterial resistance to antibiotics, it is imperative that clinicians distinguish accurately between viral processes and those that are bacterial.[7] Viral ARS is a self-limited disease characterized by cough, sneezing, rhinorrhea, sore throat, and nasal congestion.[16] It promotes a vigorous inflammatory response causing epithelial disruption, edema, and excessive mucous production, which further impairs normal ciliary function.[17] But the symptoms typically peak in 2–3 days, then gradually decline, and usually resolve by 14 days after onset.[16,18] Therefore, attention to the duration, illness pattern, and severity of symptoms can help differentiate viral ARS from bacterial.[7]

MICROBIOLOGY OF ARS

In patients without ARS, the mucous is sterile.[19] Bacterial ARS is most often caused by *Streptococcus pneumoniae*, *Hemophilus influenzae*,

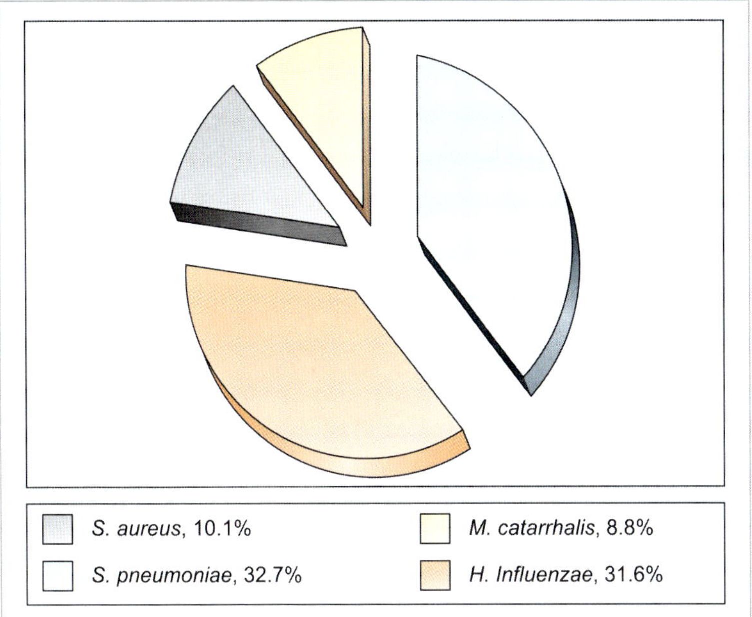

Fig. 8.1: Bacterial causes of acute rhinosinusitis.[20]

Moraxella catarrhalis, and *Staphylococcus aureus*[5] (*see* Fig. 8.1). Aspiration studies have demonstrated that *S. pneumoniae* makes up approximately 20–43% of bacterial ARS.[19-21] As many as 35% of pneumococcal strains have been noted to demonstrate antibiotic resistance with some geographic variation.[5] *H. influenzae* has been noted in 22–35% of aspiration studies.[19-21] Importantly, b-lactamase producing *H. influenzae* has a national prevalence of 27–43%.[22] *M. catarrhalis* makes up about 2–10% of bacterial ARS.[19-21] It is more common in children with bacterial ARS than *S. pneumoniae* and *H. influenzae*[7] and most strains of *M. catarrhalis* produce b-lactamase and are resistant to penicillins.[23] *S. aureus* has also been found in up to 10.1% of bacterial ARS specimens[20] and a significant number of specimens are methicillin-resistant.[24] Another variant of bacterial ARS is odontogenic sinusitis with historical prevalence estimates ranging 10–12% of maxillary sinusitis.[25] These cases are typically polymicrobial with a large portion of their flora represented by anaerobes.[26] Odontogenic sinusitis classically has a severe radiologic appearance,[25] and definitive treatment is incomplete without addressing the dental source.

Historically, sinus cultures have been obtained using a sinus puncture technique. Now, middle meatal swabs or aspirates are performed because they are much less uncomfortable and demonstrate a high degree of diagnostic accuracy when purulence is present in the middle meatus.[27] Endoscopically directed middle meatal cultures have demonstrated a sensitivity of 81%, specificity of 91%, positive predictive value of 83%, negative predictive value of 89%, and overall accuracy of 87% when compared with direct sinus aspiration.[28] While routine culture of uncomplicated ARS is not always indicated,[28] it can help guide subsequent antibiotic therapy.[7] Certainly complicated ARS warrants endoscopically directed culture.

DIAGNOSIS

The diagnosis of ARS is typically made based on clinical evaluation. Patients with ARS describe purulent rhinorrhea, nasal obstruction and, or, facial pain or pressure[7] for at least 10 days beyond the onset of symptoms.[7,18,29] Sometimes symptoms worsen within 10 days of onset after an initial improvement.[7,29] This pattern of initial improvement followed by worsening, or "double worsening", is consistent with bacterial ARS.[30,31] Purulent rhinorrhea is a strong predictor of sinusitis,[32] although the coloration of nasal discharge does not enable one to predict the bacterial flora of the nose.[33-35] The combination of rhinorrhea, nasal congestion, and facial pain or pressure has a high sensitivity and relatively high specificity for bacterial ARS.[36-38] It is important to note that facial pain is often the reason that patients with bacterial ARS seek medical care.[36,38] In addition to the common symptoms of ARS, patients can also present with fever, cough, fatigue, malaise, hyposmia or anosmia, maxillary dental pain, or halitosis.[7,10]

Imaging studies are not indicated for uncomplicated bacterial ARS but may be appropriate in cases refractory to medical therapy when an alternative diagnosis is suspected.[7,39] Imaging may also be obtained when patients have modifying factors or comorbidities that predispose to complications like diabetes mellitus, immunocompromised state, or a history of facial trauma or surgery.[7] In those cases noncontrast computed tomography (CT) scans may be obtained as plain films of the sinuses are inaccurate in a high percentage of patients.[40] If CT scans are obtained, they must be interpreted in conjunction with clinical and endoscopic findings[40] as it is impossible to distinguish viral ARS from ARS based solely on imaging.[7] Moreover, abnormalities on CT typically accompany viral ARS and sinus involvement is common in documented upper respiratory tract infections.[41] In the proper clinical context, CT findings suggestive of bacterial ARS include sinus opacification, air-fluid levels, and moderate-to-severe mucosal thickening[7] — *see* Figure 8.2. The positive predictive value for a sinus CT showing an air-fluid level and total opacification for the diagnosis of ARS is 90%.[31]

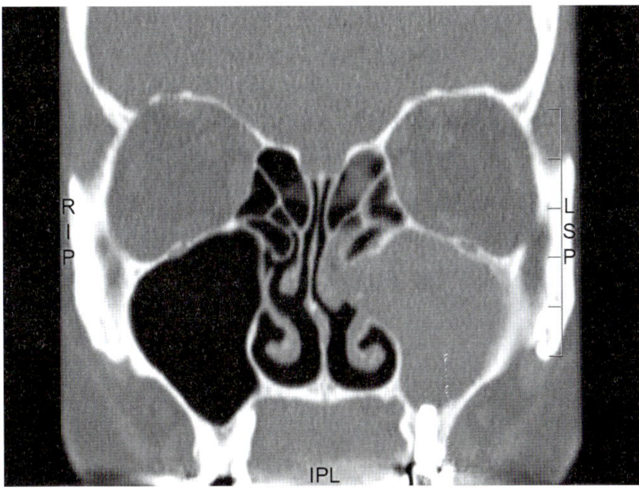

Fig. 8.2: Coronal computed tomography scan of acute rhinosinusitis. This patient developed rapidly progressive severe left facial pain 3 weeks status postdental implantation. Note the complete maxillary sinus opacification and the post from the maxillary implant, which has penetrated the sinus floor.

One special case in which imaging is indicated for ARS is if intracranial or intraorbital complications are suspected.[7,39,40] In those cases, unless patients have contraindications clinicians should obtain an iodine contrast-enhanced CT scan or a gadolinium-based magnetic resonance image (MRI) to characterize extra-sinus extension or involvement.[39,42-44] In the setting of bacterial ARS, suspected complications are the only indication for MRI of the paranasal sinuses.[7,40]

Differential Diagnosis

When considering the diagnosis of ARS, it is imperative to consider all potential causes for the patient's presentation. As previously stated, one of the most common reasons patients with ARS present for medical care is due to facial pain or pressure.[36,38] Other disease processes can cause facial pain similar to that seen in ARS. For example, tension headaches can mimic ARS, as can cluster headaches.[7] The latter are often accompanied by unilateral epiphora with or without nasal congestion. Temporomandibular joint dysfunction should also be considered,[7] and clinicians should focus their physical exams to evaluate the joint. Another common cause of facial pain that can mimic ARS is migraine.[7] In fact, up to 88% of patients with a history of "sinus headaches" have been shown to have migraine headaches.[45] Patients with recurrent facial pain or pressure without fever or purulent rhinorrhea often have symptoms related to migraines and may warrant an empiric diagnostic and therapeutic trial of triptan therapy.[45,46] Similarly, patients with a presenting symptom of rhinorrhea or nasal congestion should be evaluated for nasal septal deviation and nasal valve collapse, and the diagnoses of allergic rhinitis and vasomotor rhinitis should also be considered.[7]

COMPLICATIONS

The complications of ARS occur more frequently in children or immunocompromised adults, and can be life threatening and sight-threatening. They may also occur in patients who have been treated with antibiotic therapy who develop pronounced worsening of symptoms.[7] Complicated ARS occurs when a sinonasal infection spreads into the orbit or the cranium.[7] It may present with periorbital cellulitis and develop into an orbital infection that can spread intracranially.[7,47,48] These patients will have impressive periorbital erythema and edema, and may have restriction of eye movement and proptosis.[7] Paranasal sinus infections may also bypass the orbit and spread directly into the cranium causing meningitis or intracranial abscesses.[47,48] If diagnosed early, these patients will have high fevers and neck stiffness.[7] Often they are diagnosed late and can have neurologic changes.

One unique complication of sinusitis has been termed Pott's puffy tumor — *see* Figures 8.3A to C. First described by Sir Percivall Pott in 1768,[49] Pott's puffy tumor consists of a subperiosteal abscess with associated frontal osteomyelitis. Up to 60% of cases demonstrate intracranial spread of infection. With the widespread use of antibiotics for sinusitis, it has become a rare occurrence.[49]

Complicated ARS can be challenging to treat. Patients require hospitalization, intravenous antibiotics, steroids, and sometimes operative intervention. Consultation with either ophthalmology or neurosurgery is often warranted.

MANAGEMENT

Although related, the treatment for viral ARS and bacterial ARS has important differences. In either case, clinicians should provide patients with clear information on management options including symptomatic relief.[7]

As previously stated, viral ARS is characterized by 2–3 days of progressive rhinorrhea, nasal congestion, and facial pain or pressure that resolves over the next 1–2 weeks. Most infections are self-limited, and as such, treatment should be directed toward relief of the presenting symptoms.[7] Treatment options include analgesics, anti-inflammatory

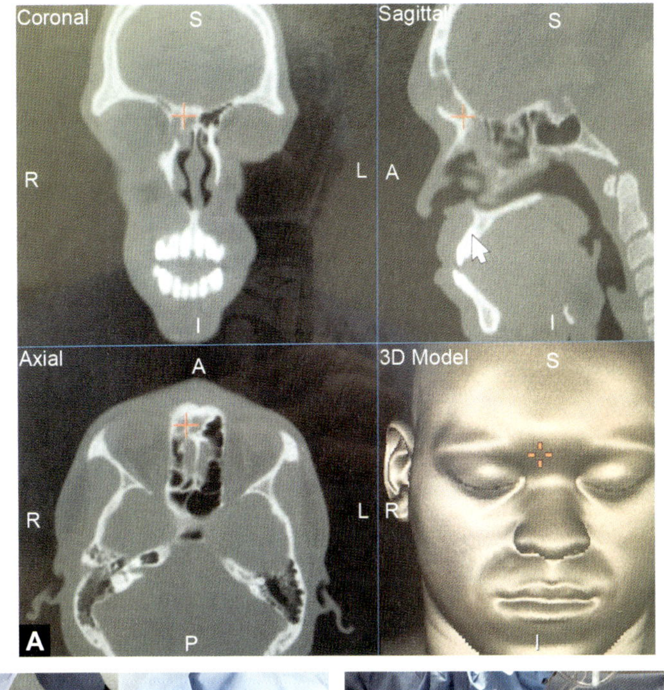

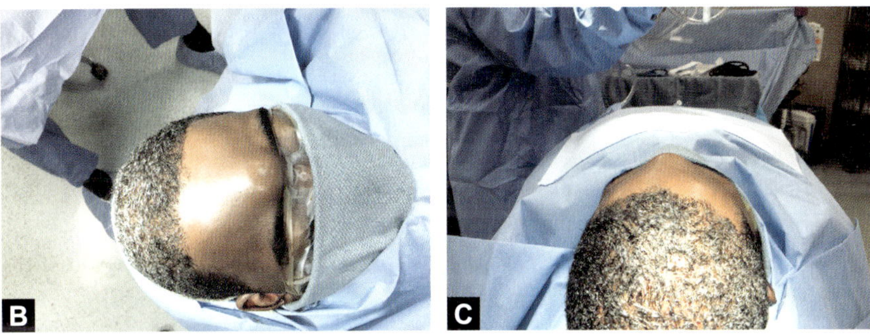

Figs. 8.3A to C: Pott's puffy tumor. (A) Computed tomography scan revealing frontal sinusitis complicated by frontal bone osteomyelitis and erosion of the anterior table with abscess formation extending to the frontal soft tissues. (B) Frontal view of patient depicted prior to surgical incision and drainage. (C) Top down view of patient depicted prior to surgical incision and drainage.

medications, nasal saline sprays and rinses, decongestant medications, and in some cases topical corticosteroids.[50] Antibiotics should not be prescribed for cases of viral ARS.

Bacterial ARS occurs when sinonasal symptoms persist or worsen 10 days after the onset of symptoms.[7,29] Pain relief is a major goal for management of bacterial ARS[7] and unless contraindicated, nonsteroidal anti-inflammatory drugs (NSAIDS) may be recommended to provide needed relief. Narcotic pain medications are rarely necessary and their use for the treatment of ARS should be discontinued due to potential adverse effects.[7] If patients describe pain that is only adequately managed by narcotic analgesia, an alternate diagnosis should be considered, as should complicated ARS.

Antibiotics have traditionally been the mainstay of treatment for bacterial ARS. In fact, they are prescribed in up to 85% of ambulatory care visits for ARS.[8] Some data suggest that antibiotic therapy for uncomplicated ARS do not significantly affect clinical cure rates, but do aid in the relief of symptoms.[51] Current recommendations no longer mandate the use of antibiotics. In fact, for uncomplicated bacterial ARS, clinicians should solicit patient preferences.[7] The use of antibiotics favors a small clinical benefit but also slightly increases the chance of adverse events.[7] Specifically, when compared to patients who were not treated with antibiotics, those who used them more frequently described nausea, vomiting, diarrhea, abdominal pain, headache, skin rashes, photosensitivity, and vaginal moniliasis.[7] Furthermore, there was no difference in clinical success for antibiotics given for 3–7 days when compared to a 6–10 days course.[52,53] Therefore, current recommendations for uncomplicated bacterial ARS are to solicit patient preferences, and treat accordingly. Patients may elect to undergo a short course of antibiotic therapy, or they may undergo watchful waiting with the assurance of follow-up and subsequent antibiotic therapy if symptoms worsen or fail to improve in 7 days.[7] Clinicians may allow patients to call in during the next 7 days for a prescription, or they may elect to give patients a safety-net antibiotic prescription.[7] In either case, patients should be re-evaluated if symptoms persist or worsen.[7]

When patients elect to undergo antibiotic therapy for uncomplicated bacterial ARS, first-line therapy should include amoxicillin with or without clavulanic acid because it is safe, effective, inexpensive, and amoxicillin has a narrow microbial spectrum.[7] Patients who are allergic to penicillins should be offered doxycycline, levofloxacin, or moxifloxacin.[7] Macrolides and trimethoprim-sulfa are not recommended as first-line treatment because of antibiotic resistance. While there is considerable geographic variability among resistance patterns,[54] macrolide resistance has been identified in up to 30–40% of *S. pneumoniae* in the United States, and resistance to trimethoprim-sulfa has been identified in up to 50% of *S. pneumoniae* and up to 27% of *H. influenzae*.[54,55] If patients fail initial empiric treatment, combination therapy with clindamycin and a third generation cephalosporin is recommended in adults without a history of type-1 hypersensitivity to penicillins.[7] Intravenous antibiotics are rarely required and their use is typically more a function of a patient's overall health and medical comorbidities than of the disease process itself.[56] But they may be considered for a patient who is unable to take oral preparations, an immunocompromised patient, or those with poor bowel absorption.[56] Cultures may also be used to guide antibiotic selection for treatment failures and for all cases of complicated ARS.

Other medications may also be beneficial for the treatment of bacterial ARS. Saline irrigation may be safely recommended to all patients.[29] When used alone or in conjunction with other adjunctive measures, saline irrigation may improve quality of life, decrease symptoms, and decrease medication use for bacterial ARS.[7,57] Some studies have suggested that hypertonic saline may have a mildly improved ability to transiently thin mucous than isotonic saline,[58,59] but others conclude that there is no difference in patient outcomes for hypertonic saline compared to isotonic saline or observation.[60] Still, nasal saline irrigation poses no risk to patients and may safely be recommended to help alleviate patient symptoms.

Antihistamines and steroids have a limited role in the treatment of ARS. Antihistamines provide no relief to nonatopic patients and should not be encouraged unless patients have symptoms supportive of allergy.[7,11,61] The use of topical intranasal steroids should be left largely to patient preference.[7] Topical intranasal steroids may have a small but statistically significant effect in the relief of facial pain and nasal congestion in patients with ARS,[62,63] and clinicians and patients should weigh the modest but clinically important benefits of nasal steroid treatment against their associated costs and the risk of minor adverse events.[7] Oral steroids provide no benefit when compared with placebo when used as monotherapy for the treatment of bacterial ARS,[64] and data to support their routine use for treatment of bacterial ARS is currently lacking.[7]

Decongestants may be used to alleviate symptoms associated with ARS. Oral decongestants may be recommended in patients without any medical contraindications, such as hypertension.[7] Topical decongestants like xylometazoline may safely be recommended to patients so long as their continuous use does not exceed 3–5 days.[7,65] Xylometazoline nasal spray has been shown to reduce congestion of the turbinates and nasal mucosa on imaging studies,[13,66] but its prolonged use can cause rhinitis medicamentosa.[65]

PEDIATRIC ACUTE SINUSITIS

A complete discussion of pediatric ARS is beyond the scope of this chapter. Still, clinicians should familiarize themselves with some basic facts regarding this disease process. Similar to adults, pediatric bacterial ARS is typically secondary to a viral upper respiratory infection.[67]

In fact, up to 10% of viral ARS in children may develop into bacterial ARS.[12] Clinicians should suspect bacterial ARS in children with a history of an acute upper respiratory tract infection with persistent rhinorrhea or daytime cough that has been present for over 10 days.[68] Additionally, children with a history of an acute upper respiratory infection with a worsening clinical course, or those with a severe onset, defined as a temperature >39°F and rhinorrhea for at least 3 days meet diagnostic criteria for bacterial ARS.[68] Imaging should always be obtained if there is any suspicion of orbital or central nervous system involvement,[68] as complications more commonly present in the pediatric population.

Treatment for uncomplicated pediatric ARS is similar to adults in that antibiotic treatment is not always required initially. The decision on whether to treat with antibiotics empirically depends on patient and caregiver preference, as well as the reliability of the caregiver. If the child has a reliable caregiver, observation may be offered as long as the caregiver is taught to look for progression of symptoms or new clinical signs.[68] Children who are observed should be reassessed in 48–72 hours.[68] If empiric antibiotics are prescribed, amoxicillin with or without clavulanic acid is recommended for first-line therapy, and the child should be reassessed in 3 days to evaluate treatment efficacy.[68]

SUMMARY

Acute rhinosinusitis may be viral or bacterial. Viral ARS is a self-limited disease process and treatment should be aimed at palliation. Antibiotics should not be prescribed for viral ARS. Bacterial ARS is diagnosed clinically, and initial management may include a period of observation in uncomplicated patients or empiric antibiotic therapy. Treatment is also directed at symptom control, and many adjunctive options are available. Clinicians should have a low index of suspicion for complications of ARS.

REFERENCES

1. Schappert SM. Ambulatory care visits to physician offices, hospital outpatient departments, and emergency departments: United States, 1996. Vital Health Stat 13. 1998:1-37.
2. Lethbridge-Çejku M, Rose D, Vickerie J. Summary health statistics for U.S. adults: national health interview survey, 2004. Vital Health Stat 10. 2006:1-164.
3. Blackwell DL, Lucas JW, Clarke TC. Summary health statistics for U.S. adults: national health interview survey, 2012. Vital Health Stat 10. 2014:1-161.
4. Anand VK. Epidemiology and economic impact of rhinosinusitis. Ann Otol Rhinol Laryngol Suppl. 2004;193:3-5.
5. Anon JB, Jacobs MR, Poole MD, et al. Antimicrobial treatment guidelines for acute bacterial rhinosinusitis. Otolaryngol Head Neck Surg. 2004;130:1-45.

6. Bhattacharyya N, Grebner J, Martinson NG. Recurrent acute rhinosinusitis: epidemiology and health care cost burden. Otolaryngol Head Neck Surg. 2012; 146:307-12.

7. Rosenfeld RM, Piccirillo JF, Chandrasekhar SS, et al. Clinical practice guideline (update): adult sinusitis. Otolaryngol Head Neck Surg. 2015;152:S1-S39.

8. Smith SS, Evans CT, Tan BK, et al. National burden of antibiotic use for adult rhinosinusitis. J Allergy Clin Immunol. 2013;132:1230-2.

9. Wu JH, Howard DH, McGowan JE, et al. Patterns of health care resource utilization after macrolide treatment failure: results from a large, population-based cohort with acute sinusitis, acute bronchitis, and community-acquired pneumonia. Clin Ther. 2004;26:2153-62.

10. Lanza DC, Kennedy DW. Adult rhinosinusitis defined. Otolaryngol Head Neck Surg. 1997;117:S1-7.

11. Fokkens WJ, Lund VJ, Mullol J, et al. European position paper on rhinosinusitis and nasal polyps 2012. Rhinol Suppl. 2012;3p preceding table of contents, 1-298.

12. Gwaltney JM. Acute community-acquired sinusitis. Clin Infect Dis. 1996;23: 1209-23; quiz 24-5.

13. Stringer SP, Mancuso AA, Avino AJ. Effect of a topical vasoconstrictor on computed tomography of paranasal sinus disease. Laryngoscope. 1993;103:6-9.

14. Caughey RJ, Jameson MJ, Gross CW, et al. Anatomic risk factors for sinus disease: fact or fiction? Am J Rhinol. 2005;19:334-9.

15. Early SB, Hise K, Han JK, et al. Hypoxia stimulates inflammatory and fibrotic responses from nasal-polyp derived fibroblasts. Laryngoscope. 2007;117:511-5.

16. Gwaltney JM, Hendley JO, Simon G, et al. Rhinovirus infections in an industrial population. II. Characteristics of illness and antibody response. JAMA. 1967; 202:494-500.

17. Lund VJ. Therapeutic targets in rhinosinusitis: infection or inflammation? Medscape J Med. 2008;10:105.

18. Rosenfeld RM, Andes D, Bhattacharyya N, et al. Clinical practice guideline: adult sinusitis. Otolaryngol Head Neck Surg. 2007;137:S1-31.

19. Gwaltney JM, Scheld WM, Sande MA, et al. The microbial etiology and antimicrobial therapy of adults with acute community-acquired sinusitis: a fifteen-year experience at the University of Virginia and review of other selected studies. J Allergy Clin Immunol. 1992;90:457-61; discussion 62.

20. Payne SC, Benninger MS. *Staphylococcus aureus* is a major pathogen in acute bacterial rhinosinusitis: a meta-analysis. Clin Infect Dis. 2007;45:e121-7.

21. Low DE, Desrosiers M, McSherry J, et al. A practical guide for the diagnosis and treatment of acute sinusitis. CMAJ. 1997;156(Suppl 6):S1-14.

22. Sahm DF, Brown NP, Draghi DC, et al. Tracking resistance among bacterial respiratory tract pathogens: summary of findings of the TRUST Surveillance Initiative, 2001–2005. Postgrad Med. 2008;120:8-15.

23. Murphy TF, Parameswaran GI. *Moraxella catarrhalis,* a human respiratory tract pathogen. Clin Infect Dis. 2009;49:124-31.

24. McCoul ED, Jourdy DN, Schaberg MR, et al. Methicillin-resistant *Staphylococcus aureus* sinusitis in nonhospitalized patients: a systematic review of prevalence and treatment outcomes. Laryngoscope. 2012;122:2125-31.

25. Bomeli SR, Branstetter BF, Ferguson BJ. Frequency of a dental source for acute maxillary sinusitis. Laryngoscope. 2009;119:580-4.

26. Brook I. Microbiology of acute and chronic maxillary sinusitis associated with an odontogenic origin. Laryngoscope. 2005;115:823-5.

27. Dubin MG, Ebert CS, Coffey CS, et al. Concordance of middle meatal swab and maxillary sinus aspirate in acute and chronic sinusitis: a meta-analysis. Am J Rhinol. 2005;19:462-70.

28. Benninger MS, Appelbaum PC, Denneny JC, et al. Maxillary sinus puncture and culture in the diagnosis of acute rhinosinusitis: the case for pursuing alternative culture methods. Otolaryngol Head Neck Surg. 2002;127:7-12.

29. Chow AW, Benninger MS, Brook I, et al. IDSA clinical practice guideline for acute bacterial rhinosinusitis in children and adults. Clin Infect Dis. 2012;54:e72-e112.

30. Meltzer EO, Hamilos DL, Hadley JA, et al. Rhinosinusitis: establishing definitions for clinical research and patient care. J Allergy Clin Immunol. 2004;114:155-212.

31. Lindbaek M, Hjortdahl P, Johnsen UL. Use of symptoms, signs, and blood tests to diagnose acute sinus infections in primary care: comparison with computed tomography. Fam Med. 1996;28:183-8.

32. Lindbaek M, Hjortdahl P. The clinical diagnosis of acute purulent sinusitis in general practice—a review. Br J Gen Pract. 2002;52:491-5.

33. Hays GC, Mullard JE. Can nasal bacterial flora be predicted from clinical findings? Pediatrics. 1972;49:596-9.

34. Winther B. Effects on the nasal mucosa of upper respiratory viruses (common cold). Dan Med Bull. 1994;41:193-204.

35. Winther B, Brofeldt S, Grønborg H, et al. Study of bacteria in the nasal cavity and nasopharynx during naturally acquired common colds. Acta Otolaryngol. 1984;98:315-20.

36. Axelsson A, Runze U. Symptoms and signs of acute maxillary sinusitis. ORL J Otorhinolaryngol Relat Spec. 1976;38:298-308.

37. Axelsson A, Runze U. Comparison of subjective and radiological findings during the course of acute maxillary sinusitis. Ann Otol Rhinol Laryngol. 1983;92:75-7.

38. Williams JW, Simel DL, Roberts L, et al. Clinical evaluation for sinusitis. Making the diagnosis by history and physical examination. Ann Intern Med. 1992;117:705-10.

39. Setzen G, Ferguson BJ, Han JK, et al. Clinical consensus statement: appropriate use of computed tomography for paranasal sinus disease. Otolaryngol Head Neck Surg. 2012;147:808-16.

40. Cornelius RS, Martin J, Wippold FJ, et al. ACR appropriateness criteria sinonasal disease. J Am Coll Radiol. 2013;10:241-6.

41. Gwaltney JM, Phillips CD, Miller RD, et al. Computed tomographic study of the common cold. N Engl J Med. 1994;330:25-30.

42. Younis RT, Anand VK, Davidson B. The role of computed tomography and magnetic resonance imaging in patients with sinusitis with complications. Laryngoscope. 2002;112:224-9.

43. Mafee MF, Tran BH, Chapa AR. Imaging of rhinosinusitis and its complications: plain film, CT, and MRI. Clin Rev Allergy Immunol. 2006;30:165-86.

44. Hoxworth JM, Glastonbury CM. Orbital and intracranial complications of acute sinusitis. Neuroimaging Clin N Am. 2010;20:511-26.

45. Schreiber CP, Hutchinson S, Webster CJ, et al. Prevalence of migraine in patients with a history of self-reported or physician-diagnosed "sinus" headache. Arch Intern Med. 2004;164:1769-72.

46. Kari E, DelGaudio JM. Treatment of sinus headache as migraine: the diagnostic utility of triptans. Laryngoscope. 2008;118:2235-9.

47. Clayman GL, Adams GL, Paugh DR, et al. Intracranial complications of paranasal sinusitis: a combined institutional review. Laryngoscope. 1991;101:234-9.

48. Brook I. Acute sinusitis in children. Pediatr Clin North Am. 2013;60:409-24.

49. Karaman E, Hacizade Y, Isildak H, et al. Pott's puffy tumor. J Craniofac Surg. 2008; 19:1694-7.

50. Desrosiers M, Evans GA, Keith PK, et al. Canadian clinical practice guidelines for acute and chronic rhinosinusitis. Allergy Asthma Clin Immunol. 2011;7:2.

51. Williams JW, Aguilar C, Cornell J, et al. Antibiotics for acute maxillary sinusitis. Cochrane Database Syst Rev. 2003;2:CD000243.

52. Falagas ME, Karageorgopoulos DE, Grammatikos AP, et al. Effectiveness and safety of short vs. long duration of antibiotic therapy for acute bacterial sinusitis: a meta-analysis of randomized trials. Br J Clin Pharmacol. 2009;67:161-71.

53. Ip S, Fu L, Balk E, et al. Update on acute bacterial rhinosinusitis. Evid Rep Technol Assess (Summ). 2005:1-3.

54. Jenkins SG, Farrell DJ, Patel M, et al. Trends in anti-bacterial resistance among *Streptococcus pneumoniae* isolated in the USA, 2000-2003: PROTEKT US years 1-3. J Infect 2005;51:355-63.

55. Harrison CJ, Woods C, Stout G, et al. Susceptibilities of *Hemophilus influenzae, Streptococcus pneumoniae*, including serotype 19A, and *Moraxella catarrhalis* paediatric isolates from 2005 to 2007 to commonly used antibiotics. J Antimicrob Chemother. 2009;63:511-9.

56. Han J, Wold S. Acute rhinosinusitis. In: Rhinology—Diseases of the Nose, Sinuses, and Skull Base. New York, NY: Thieme Medical Publishers, Inc; 2012.

57. Kassel JC, King D, Spurling GK. Saline nasal irrigation for acute upper respiratory tract infections. Cochrane Database Syst Rev. 2010;3:CD006821.

58. Keojampa BK, Nguyen MH, Ryan MW. Effects of buffered saline solution on nasal mucociliary clearance and nasal airway patency. Otolaryngol Head Neck Surg. 2004;131:679-82.

59. Wabnitz DA, Wormald PJ. A blinded, randomized, controlled study on the effect of buffered 0.9% and 3% sodium chloride intranasal sprays on ciliary beat frequency. Laryngoscope. 2005;115:803-5.

60. Adam P, Stiffman M, Blake RL. A clinical trial of hypertonic saline nasal spray in subjects with the common cold or rhinosinusitis. Arch Fam Med. 1998;7:39-43.

61. Slavin RG, Spector SL, Bernstein IL, et al. The diagnosis and management of sinusitis: a practice parameter update. J Allergy Clin Immunol. 2005;116:S13-47.

62. Hayward G, Heneghan C, Perera R, et al. Intranasal corticosteroids in management of acute sinusitis: a systematic review and meta-analysis. Ann Fam Med. 2012;10:241-9.

63. Zalmanovici A, Yaphe J. Intranasal steroids for acute sinusitis. Cochrane Database Syst Rev. 2009;4:CD005149.

64. Venekamp RP, Thompson MJ, Hayward G, et al. Systemic corticosteroids for acute sinusitis. Cochrane Database Syst Rev. 2014;3:CD008115.

65. Mortuaire G, de Gabory L, François M, et al. Rebound congestion and rhinitis medicamentosa: nasal decongestants in clinical practice. Critical review of the literature by a medical panel. Eur Ann Otorhinolaryngol Head Neck Dis. 2013; 130:137-44.

66. Caenen M, Hamels K, Deron P, et al. Comparison of decongestive capacity of xylometazoline and pseudoephedrine with rhinomanometry and MRI. Rhinology. 2005;43:205-9.

67. Fireman P. Diagnosis of sinusitis in children: emphasis on the history and physical examination. J Allergy Clin Immunol. 1992;90:433-6.

68. Wald ER, Applegate KE, Bordley C, et al. Clinical practice guideline for the diagnosis and management of acute bacterial sinusitis in children aged 1 to 18 years. Pediatrics. 2013;132:e262-80.

Chapter 9

Contemporary Management of Paraganglioma: Jugulare and Tympanicum

Jennifer Alyono, Carleton Eduardo Corrales

INTRODUCTION

Paragangliomas are rare, vascular tumors of the paraganglion system. Over 90% are found in the adrenal gland and are termed pheochromocytomas. The remaining 10% are found in extra-adrenal sites including the abdomen and thorax, with 3% found in the head and neck.[1] The most common paraganglioma in the head and neck is the carotid body tumor, followed by paraganglioma of the jugular bulb (jugulare), middle ear (tympanicum), and finally vagal paragangliomas.[2] This chapter will focus on paraganglioma jugulare and tympanicum, which are the most common primary neoplasms of the jugular foramen and middle ear, respectively.[3,4]

HISTORY AND TERMINOLOGY

In 1840, Valentin was the first to describe the tympanic ganglion to Jacobsen's nerve in the middle ear.[5] William Wilde then described in 1853 a pulsation of the tympanic membrane that was synchronous with the heartbeat that was associated with a small posterior tympanic membrane perforation.[6] More than two decades later, Robert Weir described two cases of intratympanic vascular tumors with a pulsating intact tympanic membrane in 1879.[7,8] The histology of glomus tumors was characterized by Stacy Guild in 1941 when he described glomus jugulare as small formations in the adventitia of the dome of the jugular bulb along the tympanic branch (Jacobsen's nerve) of the glossopharyngeal nerve and the auricular branch (Arnold's nerve) of the vagus nerve.[9] Alford and Guilford more formally classified these lesions in 1960 into *glomus tympanicum* (tumors located within the middle ear) and *glomus jugulare* (tumors involving the jugular bulb and foramen with extension into the middle ear).

Historically, many terms have been used to describe paragangliomas including glomus tumors, nonchromaffin paraganglioma, and chemodectoma.[10] Originally, paragangliomas were termed "glomus" tumors because of the belief that the chief cells were derived from specialized pericytes, similar to true cutaneous arteriovenous (glomus) anastomosis tumors (glomangiomas). However, these cutaneous tumors are unrelated to paragangliomas both developmentally and functionally.[11,12] The term "nonchromaffin" paraganglioma derives from the histologic examination of adrenal autonomic paraganglia using chromium salts (staining used to determine the presence or absence of catecholamines). Extra-adrenal paraganglia do not stain with chromium salts, hence the term "nonchromaffin" paragangliomas.[10] A "chemodectoma" inaccurately describes paragangliomas of the temporal bone, as the only paraganglion in the head and neck region known to act as a chemoreceptor is the carotid body.[10]

HISTOPATHOLOGY

Paraganglia are cells derived from the neural crest that are associated with the autonomic nervous system. Within the adrenal gland, they are found within the adrenal medulla. Extra-adrenal paraganglia are then classified by the system to which they are related: parasympathetic or sympathetic.[13] Extra-adrenal abdominal and thoracic paraganglia are typically associated with the sympathetic nervous system. Those in the head and neck are more closely associated with the parasympathetic nervous system, with the largest paraganglia represented by the carotid body.[14] Temporal bone paraganglia are distributed along the auricular branch of the vagus nerve (Arnold's nerve), and the tympanic branch of the glossopharyngeal nerve (Jacobson's nerve).[15] Approximately 70% of paraganglia related to the vagus nerve occur at the jugular bulb. Paraganglia along the glossopharyngeal nerve occur anywhere from the origin of the nerve at the petrosal ganglion (10%) to the jugular bulb (28%), tympanic canaliculus (40%), promontory of the middle ear (20%), and beyond (2%).[11] Paragangliomas of the jugular bulb may thus arise along either the vagus or glossopharyngeal nerves, with the former being more common. Paraganglioma tympanicums are most typically associated with Jacobson's nerve, and only rarely with Arnold's nerve.

Histologically, all paragangliomas are characterized by polygonal-shaped chief (type I) cells surrounded by spindle-shaped sustentacular (type II) cells, in defined nests, which are termed cells of "Zellballen" (Figs. 9.1A and B). Type I cells often have enlarged hyperchromatic nuclei with an abundant granular eosinophilic cytoplasm, and stain positive for synaptophysin. Type II cells are basophilic and stain S-100 protein positive.[13] Of note, no histologic or immunohistochemical

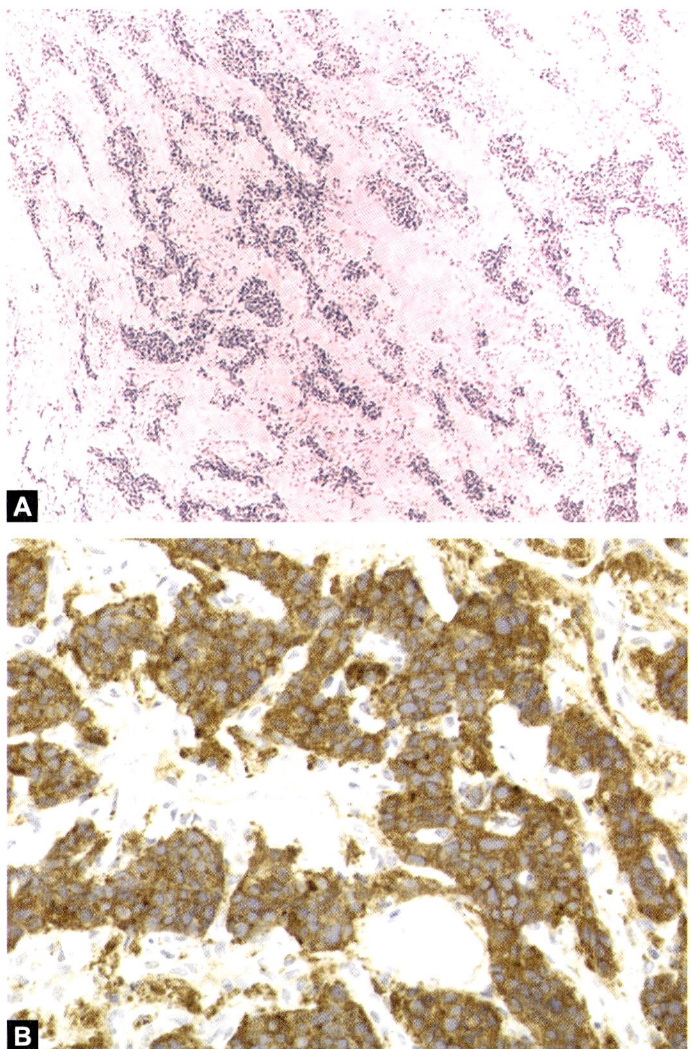

Figs. 9.1A and B: Histology (A) Low magnification hematoxylin and eosin stained paraganglioma demonstrating nests of cells (Zellballen) with prominent vascular network. (B) Synaptophysin stain (brown immunohistochemistry stain) demonstrates the neuroendocrine origin, suggestive of paraganglioma.

markers exist to distinguish malignant from benign paraganglioma. Rather, the diagnosis of malignancy is based on the clinical presence metastasis to non-neuroendocrine tissue.[16,17]

EPIDEMIOLOGY AND PATHOGENESIS

Of all head and neck tumors, 1 in 30,000–100,000 is a paraganglioma.[14,18] Paragangliomas may occur at any age, though most patients present between the 4th and 5th decades of life.[16,17,19] Females are affected

3–4 times more commonly than males.[4,17] The majority of paragangliomas are solitary, with multiple or synchronous tumors occurring in 3–10% of patients.[10, 20, 21] The most common multifocal combination is a carotid body tumor with an ipsilateral tympanic paraganglioma.[21]

Functional catecholamine secretion from paragangliomas of the head and neck region is reported to be 1–3%.[10,22] All paragangliomas have neurosecretory granules that contain catecholamines, though few tumors clinically manifest with symptoms. Norepinephrine is the most commonly secreted catecholamine, though dopamine secretion has also been reported.[22]

While most are thought to arise sporadically, up to 40% of paragangliomas have been found to arise due to heritable genetic mutations.[23-27] Heritable forms can be further classified into paraganglioma syndromes 1-4 (PGL1-4, attributable to mutations in *SDHx* or associated cofactors), familial pheochromocytoma (associated with *TMEM127* and *MAX* mutations), and those associated with other neuroendocrine syndromes including multiple endocrine neoplasia type 2 (MEN2, from mutations in *RET*), neurofibromatosis 1 (NF1, caused by mutations in *NF1*), and von Hippel-Lindau disease (from mutations in *VHL*) (Table 9.1).

Compared to patients with sporadic paragangliomas of the head and neck, patients with PGL syndromes develop paragangliomas earlier in life and demonstrate a higher propensity toward multifocal paraganglial tumors. Burnichon et al. found that patients with PGL syndromes presented at an average age of 36 compared to 50.2 years in patients with sporadic tumors.[28] Furthermore, patients with PGL syndromes have a higher risk of malignant paragangliomas, though this difference can largely be attributed to those patients with PGL4, who have a higher propensity to develop malignant paragangliomas compared to patients with sporadic or other PGL syndromes.[17,28] Over a third of all malignant tumors and >80% of familial paraganglioma and pheochromocytoma are attributable to PGL syndromes.[29]

Baysal et al. was the first to identify germline mutations of the succinate dehydrogenase subunit *D* gene (*SDHD* gene) as the underlying cause of paraganglioma syndrome 1 (PGL1) in the year 2000.[30] Since then other mutations in the SDH complex have been discovered: Niemann et al.[31] described mutations in *SDHC* causing PGL3, and Astuti et al.[32] described PGL4 as a mutation in the *SDHB* gene. Mutations in SDH complex assembly factor 2 gene (*SDHAF2*, also known as *SDH5*) were then found to cause PGL2.[33-35] Mutations of *SDHA* are most commonly associated with Leigh's disease, a familial neurologic disorder encephalopathy.[33] However, in 2011, Korepershoek reported

Table 9.1: Genetics of hereditary paraganglioma.

Syndrome	Gene (chromosome)	Features
Paraganglioma syndrome 1	SDHD (chr 11)	Most common gene mutation. Head and neck paragangliomas > pheochromocytomas. Moderate malignant potential.
Paraganglioma syndrome 2	SDHAF2 (chr 11)	Least common PGL syndrome.
Paraganglioma syndrome 3	SDHC (chr 1)	Less common than PGL 1 and 4. Twenty percent develop multiple tumors. Rare malignant potential.
Paraganglioma syndrome 4	SDHB (chr 1)	Pheochromocytomas > head and neck paragangliomas. High risk of malignancy
Neurofibromatosis type 1	NF1 (chr 17)	Pheochromocytomas > head and neck paragangliomas. Café-au-lait spots, neurofibromas, optic gliomas, axillary, and inguinal freckling.
Multiple endocrine neoplasia type 2	RET (chr 10)	Type 2A: Pheochromocytomas, parathyroid neoplasia, and medullary thyroid carcinoma Type 2B: Pheochromocytomas, medullary thyroid carcinomas, neuromas, marfanoid habitus. Both have sporadic associations with head and neck paraganglioma.
Von Hippel-Lindau	VHL (chr 3)	Pheochromocytomas > head and neck paragangliomas. Hemangioblastomas, renal cell carcinoma, endolymphatic sac tumors, renal and pancreatic cysts.
Familial pheochromocytoma	TMEM127 (chr 2) MAX (chr 14)	Pheochromocytomas > head and neck paragangliomas.

(SDHD: Succinate dehydrogenase subunit D; SDHAF2: Succinate dehydrogenase complex assembly factor 2; SDHC: Succinate dehydrogenase subunit C; SDHB: Succinate dehydrogenase subunit B; NF1: Neurofibromin 1; RET: Ret proto-oncogene; VHL: Von Hippel-Lindau tumor suppressor; TMEM127: Transmembrane protein 127; MAX: MYC-associated factor X).

that 3% of patients in a series of 316 patients with apparently sporadic paragangliomas and pheochromocytomas demonstrated germline mutations in *SHDA*.[36]

Each of these genes encodes subunits or cofactors of SDH, which is critical to mitochondrial function.[34] Mutations of the SDH complex result in a pseudohypoxic state and activation of hypoxic-inducible factor pathways.[37]

The majority of these hereditary paragangliomas are due to PGL1, 3, and 4. Important for molecular screening, a study by Neumann et al. found that no patients in a pool of 598 demonstrated *multiple* mutations when screened for SDHB, SDHC, and SDHD.[24]

Paraganglioma Syndromes

Paraganglioma Syndrome 1

Paraganglioma syndrome 1 was the first hereditary paraganglioma syndrome to be associated with a germline mutation, and is also the most common PGL syndrome. In 2000, Baysal et al. identified a mutation in *SDHD* on chromosome 11 to be the molecular genetic basis.[30] Although the mutation can be inherited either maternally or paternally, those inherited maternally only rarely develop paragangliomas, while those inherited paternally follow an autosomal dominant pattern. Paraganglioma syndrome 1 may appear to skip generations, as maternally inherited carriers still pass on the mutation to 50% of offspring. Paraganglioma syndrome 1 patients are more likely than other PGL syndrome and sporadic paraganglioma patients to have multifocal disease, with Neumann et al. reporting 74% of tumor patients who were *SDHD* carriers to have metachronous or synchronous tumors.[25] Though more frequent in carriers of *SDHB* mutations, malignancy has also been reported *SDHD* mutation carriers.[24]

Paraganglioma Syndrome 2

In 2009, Hao et al. described SDH5 as a mitochondrial protein interacting with the SDH complex, and linked its loss of function to a family with hereditary paraganglioma.[35] Later known as *SDHAF2* and found on chromosome 11, mutations in this gene linked to paraganglioma/ pheochromocytoma have only been described in two families, and another isolated case.[33,35,38] Patients with an isolated head and neck paraganglioma who do not have gene mutations in *SDHD, SDHC,* or *SDHB,* should be analyzed for an *SDHAF2* gene mutation.[33]

Paraganglioma Syndrome 3

Paraganglioma syndrome 3 is caused by a mutation in the *SDHC* gene, located on chromosome 1.[31] Less common than PGL1 or PGL4, Neumann et al.[24] found that 4.3% of a pooled cohort of 598 patients with paraganglioma/pheochromocytoma had a mutation in *SDHC*. Patients with *SDHC* mutations are more likely to present with carotid body tumors, and have a lower incidence of multifocal tumors.[24,26] Malignant paragangliomas have been described but are rare, and have not been associated with jugular or tympanic paragangliomas.[39]

Paraganglioma Syndrome 4

Astuti et al. first linked paraganglioma syndrome 4 (PGL4) to a mutation in the *SDHB* gene, found on chromosome 1.[32] Compared to other PGL syndromes, patients with *SDHB* mutations are more likely to have pheochromocytomas and also to develop malignant disease, with rates of 20–41% malignancy.[24,25,29] Additionally, patients with PGL4 have an increased risk of developing renal cell and thyroid carcinomas.[25,37,40]

Familial Pheochromocytoma Syndrome

Familial pheochromocytoma syndromes have been linked to tumor suppressor genes *TMEM127* (transmembrane protein 127, chromosome 2) and *MAX* (MYC-associated factor X, chromosome 14). While mutations are most frequently associated with pheochromocytomas, mutations in TMEM127 have also been linked to head and neck paragangliomas.[27,34,41,42]

Neurofibromatosis 1

Neurofibromatosis 1, previously known as von Recklinghausen disease, is associated with mutations in the *NF1* gene on chromosome 17, which encodes neurofibromin, a tumor suppressor. Pheochromocytomas and paragangliomas have only rarely been associated, reported in 0.1–5.7% of patients.[43-45] Similar to those with PGL syndromes, these patients have presented at an earlier age compared to those with sporadic disease, in the third decade.[27]

Multiple Endocrine Neoplasia 2

Multiple endocrine neoplasia 2 is associated with mutations in the *RET* proto-oncogene, and divided into two subtypes: MEN2A and MEN2B. Multiple endocrine neoplasia 2 is characterized by development of pheochromocytomas, parathyroid neoplasia, and medullary thyroid carcinoma, while MEN2B patients develop medullary thyroid carcinomas, neuromas, and pheochromocytomas, and present with a marfanoid habitus. In contrast to the high prevalence of pheochromocytomas (adrenal paragangliomas) in patients with MEN2 syndromes, only sporadic cases of associations with head and neck paragangliomas have been described.[46] Boedeker et al.[46] studied a registry of 809 registered with head and neck paraganglioma. Of these, only one patient had a *RET* mutation.

Von Hippel-Lindau Disease

Von Hippel-Lindau disease is an autosomal dominant disorder associated with a mutation in the *VHL* tumor suppressor gene on chromosome 3. It is characterized by the formation of multiple hemangioblastomas, cysts of the kidney and pancreas, and endolymphatic sac adenomas. Pheochromocytomas are more common in this population than are head and neck paragangliomas.[47] In the Boedeker et al. study referenced above, 11 patients had a *VHL* mutation. The authors suggest that molecular genetic testing for *RET* or *VHL* in patients with head and neck paraganglioma should only be performed if personal or family history are suggestive.[46]

MALIGNANCY AND OCCULT PARAGANGLIOMA

Metastasis to non-neuroendocrine tissues is the sole criterion defining a malignant paraganglioma. There are no histologic changes or immunohistochemical markers yet available that determine malignancy.[16,17,48] Traditional markers of malignancy, such as central necrosis, vascular invasion, mitotic figures, and nuclear atypia have not been correlated with metastasis.

Less than 10% of paragangliomas in the head and neck region are malignant.[16,17,49] The most common of these are thought to arise from vagal tumors with a 16–19% malignancy rate, followed by a 6% malignancy rate for carotid body tumors. Only 2–4% of jugulotympanic paragangliomas are thought to be malignant.[16,50]

Malignancy is more commonly identified in those with *SDHx*-related mutations.[50] Furthermore, asymptomatic *SDHx* mutation carriers have a higher prevalence of occult paraganglioma. Heesterman et al.[51] screened 294 asymptomatic relatives for mutations in *SDHD* and *SDHB*, and found 64 mutation carriers. In those with *SDHD* mutations, paragangliomas were detected in 59.6%. In the *SDHB* cohort, 11.8% were found to have a paraganglioma.

A survey of the National Cancer Database found that metastases for head and neck paragangliomas are most often confined to regional cervical lymph nodes. Accordingly, most malignant paragangliomas were treated with surgery, including neck dissection, with or without adjuvant radiation. In this study, 5-year survival was 76.8% for regional confined lesions, and 11.8% for those with distant metastases.[16]

As radiotherapy is increasingly being used for tumors of the temporal bone including jugular paragangliomas, and patients are living longer, radiation-induced malignancies are being reported.[52] Though rare, these tumors have poor prognosis.[10]

CLINICAL PRESENTATION AND GROWTH PATTERNS

Jugular and tympanic paragangliomas demonstrate slow and insidious growth, with patients most commonly presenting with otologic disturbances. The three most common symptoms for both jugular and tympanic paragangliomas are pulsatile tinnitus, hearing loss and otalgia.[4,53-56] Tympanic paragangliomas typically present at a younger age than jugular paragangliomas due to their closer proximity to and earlier involvement of the tympanic membrane and ossicles, with resultant pulsation transmission and conductive hearing loss.

Tympanic Paraganglioma

A pulsatile, reddish-blue mass emanating from the hypotympanum is characteristic on physical examination. Brown's sign, which is pneumotoscopy-induced blanching of the retrotympanic vascular mass, is rarely present.[4,57] Apparent blanching of the lesion might not occur because as the tympanic membrane medializes with positive pressure, the contact area with the tumor increases, making it appear larger. In the rare case that all borders of the tumor are visible through physical examination, the lesion may be limited to only the middle ear. However, the majority of tympanic paragangliomas include the hypotympanum producing a "setting sun" appearance, thus necessitating further diagnostic imaging to determine any extent beyond the middle ear.[4,10,58] Another phenomenon that can also present as a vascular mass emanating from the hypotympanum is a high riding jugular bulb, and should always be considered in the differential diagnosis.

While tympanic paragangliomas may be confined to the cochlear promontory with clearly visible borders, they can also present after extension inferiorly into the hypotympanum, posteriorly into retrofacial air cells and the mastoid, superiorly into the epitympanum and middle cranial fossa and to the protympanum adjacent to carotid, jugular bulb and Eustachian tube. They can also grow laterally and erode through the tympanic membrane, into the external auditory canal (Fig. 9.2).

Jugular Paraganglioma

In addition to otologic symptoms such as pulsatile tinnitus, hearing loss and otalgia, jugular paragangliomas often also present with neurologic

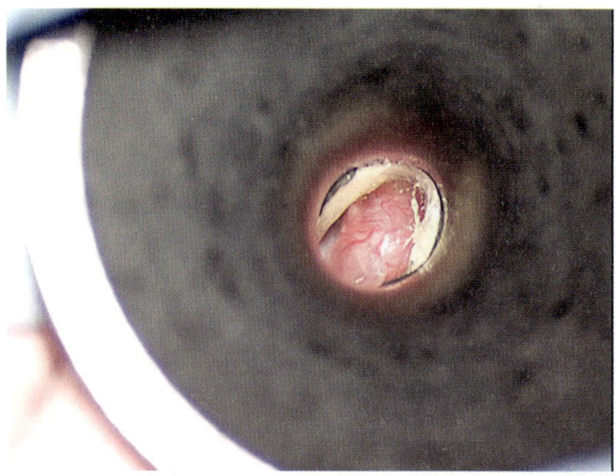

Fig. 9.2: *Otoscopic view.* Paraganglioma tympanicum eroding through the tympanic membrane into the external auditory canal.

deficits. Cranial nerve deficits are found in 39–46% of patients with jugular paragangliomas.[59-62] When the facial nerve is involved, it is generally affected at the mastoid segment as tumor growth proceeds laterally.[63] As the paraganglioma extends to and potentially through the jugular foramen, compression of cranial nerves IX, X, XI, and XII is possible, leading to hoarseness, dysphagia or arm weakness. The vagus nerve is most commonly affected, followed by cranial nerves IX > XI > XII.[64] Patients with preoperative cranial nerve deficits have a higher risk of intracranial tumor extension, with an overall prevalence of approximately 15%.[59,61,65,66] Extension into the cavernous sinus may compromise cranial nerves III, IV, V, and VI, and a Horner's syndrome may develop should the sympathetic plexus be compressed at the internal carotid artery.[65]

As jugular paragangliomas enlarge, they tend to grow along paths of least resistance through vascular channels, fissures, and foramina of the temporal bone.[54,67] Jugular paragangliomas have the potential to grow through the Eustachian tube to the nasopharynx, invade the petrous apex through peritubal air cells, or track through the petrous portion of the carotid artery to reach the middle cranial fossa and cavernous sinus. Superior extension into the hypotympanum is common, and the tumor can extend proximally within the lumen of the sigmoid sinus and distally into the jugular vein. Similar to tympanic paragangliomas, jugular paragangliomas can also erode laterally through the tympanic membrane into the external auditory canal.

DIFFERENTIAL DIAGNOSIS

The differential diagnosis of jugulotympanic paragangliomas includes vascular anomalies and both benign and malignant masses of the temporal bone (Table 9.2). The most common vascular anomaly of the

Table 9.2: Differential diagnoses of temporal bone paragangliomas.

Tympanic paraganglioma	*Jugular paraganglioma*
Primary masses/neoplasms • Jugular paraganglioma • Cholesteatoma • Cholesterol granuloma • Hemangioma • Hemangioendothelioma • Meningioma	Primary neoplasms • Schwannoma of the 9th, 10th, 11th, and 12th cranial nerves • Meningioma • Chordoma • Chondrosarcoma
Vascular anomalies • Aberrant or laterally displaced internal carotid artery • Congenital or acquired internal carotid artery aneurysm • Dehiscent or high-riding jugular bulb • Jugular bulb diverticulum • Persistent stapedial artery • Arteriovenous malformation	Vascular anomalies • Aberrant or laterally displaced internal carotid artery • Congenital or acquired internal carotid artery aneurysm • Dehiscent or high-riding jugular bulb • Arteriovenous malformation • Thrombosis of the jugular bulb, sigmoid sinus, internal jugular vein
	Metastatic neoplasms • Squamous cell carcinoma • Plasmacytoma

middle ear is the high-riding jugular bulb, found in approximately 6–34% of patients, and is defined as a jugular bulb with superior extension above the tympanic annulus or at the level of or above the basal turn of the cochlea.[68,69] When dehiscent, a high-riding jugular bulb or jugular bulb diverticulum, which is an abnormal extraluminal outpouching of the jugular bulb, can similarly present with conductive hearing loss, pulsatile tinnitus and a red pulsatile mass emanating from the hypotympanum. Aberrations of the internal carotid artery are also of consideration, including laterally displaced or intratympanic carotid artery aneurysms, which can be congenital or acquired.[70-72] Aberrant internal carotid arteries are more frequently diagnosed in female patients (90%) and in the right ear (75%).[10,73,74] Other lesions to include in the differential diagnosis of vascular lesions of the middle ear include arteriovenous malformations, persistent stapedial artery, cholesterol granuloma, cholesteatoma, and neoplasms such as hemangioma, hemangioendothelioma, and meningioma.[69]

Additional considerations in the differential diagnosis for jugular foramen masses include schwannomas of cranial nerves IX, X, XI, and XII, carotid artery aneurysms, thrombosis of the great vessels, or metastatic disease to the neck.[75] Because the differential for middle ear paragangliomas includes aberrations of the great vessels, biopsy of any vascular mass in the middle ear, or suspected paraganglioma is highly discouraged prior to imaging. Of note, several systemic conditions can also cause pulsatile tinnitus, including hyperthyroidism, anemia, pregnancy, and cardiac murmurs.[17]

WORKUP

Evaluation of paragangliomas includes a full history and physical, audiometry, imaging, and depending on the patient, possibly vestibular testing, endocrinologic screening, and genetic testing.

Audiometry and Vestibular Testing

Complete audiometric testing should be performed, including air and bone conduction pure tone audiometry. Depression of stapedial reflexes may reflect proximity to the ossicular chain. Should the patient history reveal disequilibrium or vertigo, formal videonystagmography is recommended.

Imaging

Radiographic imaging of paragangliomas at the skull base is critical as part of a comprehensive workup. High resolution computed tomography (CT) is the preferred imaging choice for middle ear vascular masses and magnetic resonance imaging (MRI) for tumors located at the jugular foramen. Formal angiography is typically performed when surgical treatment is being considered, and functional nuclear imaging performed when multifocal or metastatic disease is of consideration.

Computed Tomography

High resolution, thin-section CT scan (<1 mm) in both axial and coronal planes is the imaging modality of choice to determine the extent of the lesion, and involvement of surrounding bony structures. It is useful in discerning paragangliomas isolated to the middle ear from larger ones arising from the jugular bulb. This imaging modality delineates tumor extension beyond the tympanic annulus and illustrates any bony erosion of the temporal bone. Paragangliomas enhance intensely with contrast, allowing for the differentiation of paragangliomas from most but not all benign and malignant tumors of the skull base, as well as from aberrant vasculature such as an aberrant internal carotid artery or dehiscent jugular bulb.[76,77] Arteriovenous fistulas can appear similar to paragangliomas on CT. Finally, CT may allow for the identification of synchronous or multifocal tumors of the temporal bone and upper neck.

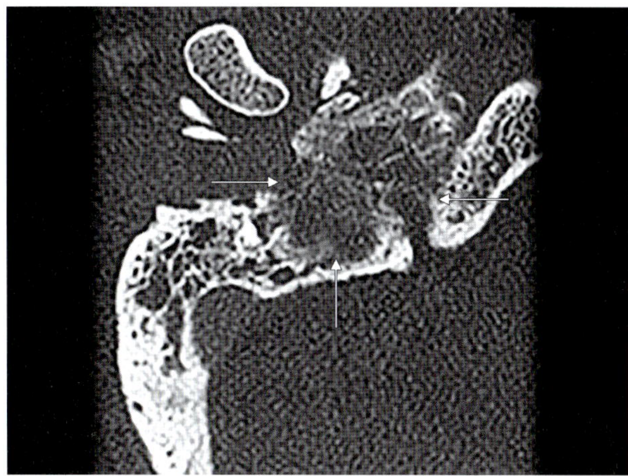

Fig. 9.3: *Computed tomography (CT) scan.* Axial high-resolution CT scan of the right jugular foramen showing a paraganglioma with the classical "moth-eaten" appearance secondary to bony erosion.

Tympanic Paragangliomas

These appear as well-circumscribed masses in the middle ear of soft tissue density. They are typically located at the cochlear promontory, with bony erosion uncommon.

Jugular Paragangliomas

These involve the hypotympanum. Due to bony destruction, these lesions demonstrate an irregular or "moth-eaten" appearance at the jugulocarotid spine, jugular foramen, or hypoglossal canal (Fig. 9.3).[10,78,79] Particular attention must be paid to the jugular plate, which is the bony covering of the jugular bulb. Erosion of the jugular plate suggests a jugular paraganglioma.

Magnetic Resonance Imaging

Magnetic resonance imaging performed with and without gadolinium contrast provides exquisite soft tissue detail, and is superior to CT in its ability to characterize the vascular nature of tumors involving the jugular bulb and skull base.[80] Paragangliomas typically are of intermediate intensity on T1-weighted images, and are hyperintense on T2-weighted images, with strong contrast enhancement, often allowing for differentiation from less vascular tumors such as neuro-fibromas, schwannomas or carcinomas (Figs. 9.4A and B). In both T1- and T2-weighted images, the characteristic "salt and pepper" appearance of paragangliomas corresponds to macroscopic flow voids, though this phenomenon can be present in other highly vascular tumors

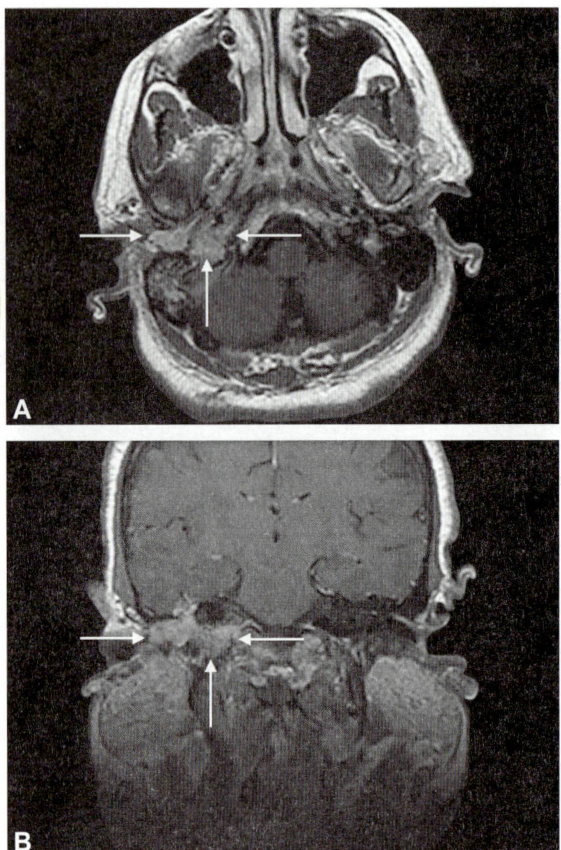

Figs. 9.4A and B: *Magnetic resonance imaging (MRI).* Gadolinium-enhanced T1-weighted axial (A) and coronal (B) MRI showing tumor involvement (arrows) of the right jugular foramen extending laterally into the external auditory canal.

such as metastatic thyroid carcinoma.[81] In addition to helping narrow one's differential diagnosis, MRI is useful to identify the presence and extent of intracranial tumor involvement. Magnetic resonance angiography (MRA) and magnetic resonance venography (MRV) provide information on the relationship of the tumor to the great vessels. Compression of the internal carotid artery can be evaluated with MRA, while MRV is useful to evaluate for collateral circulation within the dural sinuses of the skull, which may indicate occlusion of the jugular bulb and sigmoid sinus by tumor.

Angiography and Embolization

Conventional angiography serves multiple purposes, as an adjunct to other imaging modalities in diagnosis, and allowing for preoperative planning and intervention. Although angiography is not recommended simply for diagnostic purposes, it complements other imaging

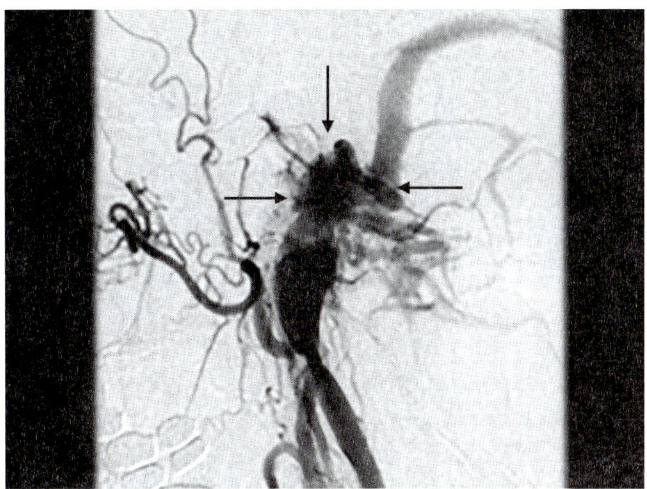

Fig. 9.5: *Angiography.* Angiography showing prominent tumor vasculature at the jugular foramen before embolization.

modalities in the diagnosis of paraganglioma, demonstrating these tumors' highly vascular nature, with shorter blush times than other tumors due to rapidly draining veins.[81] Angiography also allows identification of dominant feeding vessels that can then be embolized to reduce blood loss during surgical removal (Fig. 9.5). The most common feeding vessel in jugular paraganglioma is the ascending pharyngeal artery. Collateral vessels associated with the carotid and vertebral arteries that must be spared during surgery may be identified, and the patency of the contralateral venous system assessed. Multifocal tumors, as well as the presence of major venous sinus occlusion by tumor can also be identified.

Studies have demonstrated decreased operative time and intraoperative blood loss with preoperative embolization of jugular paragangliomas, thereby potentially facilitating more complete resection.[82,83] Angiography with embolization is typically performed 1–2 days before surgical excision because a longer interval between embolization and surgery may result in revascularization of the tumor, which may, paradoxically, increase intraoperative blood loss.[82] Due to their small size and easy accessibility, embolization for tympanic paragangliomas is not usually performed.

Nuclear Medicine Imaging

Numerous functional imaging modalities have been developed for detection of head and neck paragangliomas, the most common of which uses molecular tracers specific to catecholamine synthesis, storage and secretion. These agents include ^{123}I-Metaiodobenzylguanidin

(MIBG), ^{18}F-fluorodopamine (FDA), ^{18}F-fluorodihydroxyphenylalanine (^{18}F-FDOPA), and ^{18}F-fluorodopa (DOPA).[84] Radiolabelled octreotide is a somatostatin analogue that is used in defining neuroendocrine tumors that express somatostatin type 2 receptors.[85] Octreotide scintigraphy imaging for head and neck paragangliomas has been reported to have a sensitivity of 97% and specificity of 82%.[86,87] ^{123}I-Metaiodobenzylguanidin scintigraphy has the disadvantage of requiring two patient visits since the images are captured 2 and 24 hours after tracer injection. Furthermore, because the tracer also accumulates at salivary glands, this may obscure lesions.[88] If treatment with ^{131}I-MIBG is planned however, imaging with ^{123}I-MIBG is prudent.

A recent systematic review of the incremental benefit of functional imaging over CT and MRI found that functional imaging aided in localization of 1.4% of cases of catecholamine-producing tumors. In patients with metastasis, DOPA and FDA were the most successful in identifying disease missed by CT/MRI, with additional lesions identified in 10% and 6.4% of cases, respectively.[84] In patients with *SDHB*-associated tumors, one study showed ^{18}F-fluoro-2-deoxy-d-glucose (FDG) positron emission tomography (PET) to have a sensitivity approaching 100%.[89] While cell turnover is not high in these tumors, as found in most FDG-avid lesions, it is hypothesized that high FDG uptake in these tumors is due to SDH dysfunction leading to stabilization of hypoxia-inducible factor a protein, leading to an increase in glucose transporters and hexokinase activity.[90] In 2014, a Task Force of the Endocrine Society, European Society of Endocrinology, and American Association for Clinical Chemistry released a clinical practice guideline recommending ^{18}F-FDG PET/CT as the preferred imaging modality over ^{123}I-MIBG scintigraphy in patients with known metastatic disease.[91]

Endocrinologic Testing

Patients should specifically be screened for signs and symptoms of catecholamine secretion such as excessive sweating, palpitations, hypertension, tachycardia, irritability, anxiety, unexplained weight loss, severe headaches, nausea, pallor, or flushing. Because catecholamine release may be variable, symptoms are often intermittent. Patients who endorse the above signs and symptoms should be evaluated with a plasma metanephrine level or a 24-hour urine collection measuring levels of norepinephrine and its metabolites including metanephrine and vanillylmandelic acid (VMA). Of note, paragangliomas of the temporal bone are unable to convert norepinephrine to epinephrine due to lack of the enzyme phenylethanolamine-N-methyltransferase.

Thus, if high levels of epinephrine or metanephrine are found, this should prompt workup for a concomitant adrenal pheochromocytoma with an abdominal CT scan.[21] In general, preoperative screening for urinary metanephrines and VMA and serum catecholamines is indicated for glomus jugulare, carotid body tumors, multiple glomus tumors, and familial paragangliomas. For glomus tympanicum tumors, there is little evidence to recommend ordering preoperative tests for detecting neurosecretory activity.[4]

Genetic Testing

Historically, molecular genetic analysis for patients with head and neck paraganglioma or pheochromocytoma was recommended only for those patients with a positive family history or multifocal disease.[92] However, even in patients with apparently sporadic head and neck paragangliomas, germline mutations have been found in 25–56%.[27,34] Several authors, including the Endocrine Society Task Force consensus, agree that genetic testing should at least be offered to all patients.[17,27,91] Identification of particular genetic mutations may be useful in prognosis, predicting risk of malignancy, in screening asymptomatic family members with the potential for earlier identification of disease, and in genetic counseling for prospective parents.[91] Advantageous to molecular screening is the fact that no patients have been found to have more than one mutation when tested for *SDHB, SDHC,* and *SDHD.*[24]

Recommendations on the best testing strategies are evolving as new technologies emerge. For patients presenting with syndromic features, testing for the corresponding genetic association (e.g. NF1, RET, and VHL) is appropriate. For nonsyndromic patients, "next-generation sequencing" also known as "massively parallel sequencing" is an option whereby mutations in numerous genes are screened at once in a single assay.[27,93,94] For sequential testing, clinical features can help guide the most efficient testing order. Forehead and neck paragangliomas in particular, Boedeker[17] has proposed the following algorithm:

- *Multiple paragangliomas:* (1) SDHD (2) SDHB (3) SDHC
- *Solitary paraganglioma, positive family history:* (1) SDHD (2) SDHB (3) SDHC
- *Paraganglioma(s) and pheochromocytoma(s):* (1) SDHD (2) SDHB (3) SDHC
- *Solitary paraganglioma, negative family history:* (1) SDHB (2) SDHD (3) SDHC
- *Malignant paraganglioma(s):* (1) SDHB (2) SDHD (3) SDHC

In carriers of PGL syndrome mutations, screening recommendations include an annual history and physical examination, blood pressure monitoring, annual levels of urinary cathecholamines and metanephrines, and an MRI with contrast of the head and neck, the thorax, and the abdomen every 1–3 years.[17,27,95]

TUMOR CLASSIFICATION

Several classification schemas have been developed to describe the growth patterns of temporal bone paraganglioma:

1. *Fisch and Mattox classification:*[96] This system delineates four types based on the extent of the lesion and structures involved:
   a. *Type A (glomus tympanicum):* Tumor is limited to the middle ear cleft.
   b. *Type B (glomus hypotympanicum):* Tumor originates in the canalis tympanicus of the hypotympanum and invades the middle ear and mastoid. Jugular bulb plate is intact.
   c. *Type C:* Tumor originates at the dome of the jugular bulb and erodes the overlying plate. Further classification denotes the degree of carotid canal erosion (C1–C4). C1: Erosion of the carotid foramen with limited involvement of the vertical carotid canal. C2: Erosion of the vertical carotid canal. C3: Erosion of the horizontal carotid canal, not reaching the foramen lacerum. C4: Erosion into the foramen lacerum and along the carotid artery to the cavernous sinus.
   d. *Type De (extradural):* Intracranial extension of tumor, displacing the posterior fossa dura. De1: <1 cm and De2: >2 cm.
   e. *Type Di (intracranial):* Tumor with intracranial extension. Di1: <2 cm and Di2: >2 cm.
2. *Glasscock-Jackson classification:*[97] This system classifies lesions based on their origin, tympanic or jugular, then based on the tumor extent:
   a. Tympanic paragangliomas:
      i. *Type I:* Small mass limited to the promontory.
      ii. *Type II:* Tumor filling the middle ear space.
      iii. *Type III:* Tumor filling the middle ear, extending into the mastoid.
      iv. *Type IV:* Tumor filling the middle ear, extending into the mastoid and through the tympanic membrane to fill the external auditory canal; may also extend anterior to the internal carotid artery.
   b. Jugular paragangliomas:
      i. *Type I:* Small mass involving the jugular bulb, middle ear, and mastoid.
      ii. *Type II:* Tumor extending beneath the internal auditory canal; may have intracranial extension.
      iii. *Type III:* Tumor extending into the petrous apex; may have intracranial extension.

    iv. *Type IV*: Tumor extending beyond the petrous apex into the clivus or infratemporal fossa; may have intracranial extension.

3. *De la Cruz classification*:[10] This system pairs a surgical approach with the type of tumor:
   a. *Tympanic*: Transcanal
   b. *Tympanomastoid*: Mastoid-extended facial recess
   c. *Jugular bulb*: Transmastoid-transcervical (possible limited facial nerve rerouting)
   d. *Carotid artery*: Infratemporal fossa ± subtemporal
   e. *Transdural*: Infratemporal fossa/Intracranial
   f. *Craniocervical*: Transcondylar
   g. *Vagal*: Cervical

TREATMENT

Observation

Given the slow growth and benign nature of the majority of paragangliomas, a watchful waiting, or observational approach may be considered for select patients. Such an approach may be especially prudent for elderly patients, those with small tumors, or those who have multiple comorbidities that might increase perioperative risk. Follow-up imaging is typically performed 6 months, then at intervals of 12 months thereafter. At any point, should the patient become increasingly symptomatic or the tumor demonstrate growth, alternatives such as surgery or radiotherapy may be pursued. In young, otherwise healthy patients, an interventional rather than observational approach is preferred, as tumor growth is more likely to occur during their lifetimes.

Radiation

Radiotherapy may be considered as a primary treatment option, as adjunctive to subtotal resection, or as salvage therapy following surgical recurrence. Because isolated tympanic paragangliomas can typically be resected with minimal risk to hearing and facial nerve function, radiation has not been considered a primary treatment modality.

For jugular bulb paragangliomas, conventional external beam, conformal radiotherapy, and stereotactic radiotherapy have all been used for local tumor control. Because of the increased risk of temporal osteoradionecrosis, cranial nerve palsy, or secondary malignancy, conventional external beam therapy has fallen to the wayside, and conformal radiotherapy with or without intensity modulation and stereotactic radiation (Cyberknife, Gamma Knife, or LINAC) have become more common due to their more precise delivery adapted to the tumor shape and size. For conformal radiotherapy typical doses range from 40 to 50 Gy over the course of 4–5 weeks. Stereotactic radiotherapy is performed with both CT and MRI image fusion guidance. Although historically, delivered doses were as high as 50 Gy, more contemporary treatment has decreased to 12–14 Gy, which can be delivered in a single session or with dose fractionation.

The efficacy of radiotherapy, as defined by stabilization of growth and lack of symptom progression, has ranged from 71% to 100% in series with follow-up ranging from 1 to 12 years.[98-101] Transient acute toxicity such as nausea, mucositis, or weight loss may interrupt or preclude completion of therapy. Longer-term complications include skull base osteomyelitis, temporal bone osteoradionecrosis, brain abscess, pituitary gland insufficiency, and radiation-induced malignancies.[52,102] Less serious complications include chronic otitis media, TMJ disorder, and stenosis of the external auditory canal.[103,104]

Systemic Therapy

Systemic therapy is reserved for those patients with malignant paraganglioma, largely as palliative therapy to reduce or stop the rate of growth. In such cases, overall 5-year survival has been reported to be <50%. Current systemic therapies include traditional chemotherapy with combination of cyclophosphamide, vincristine and dacarbazine and radionuclide ^{131}I-MIBG therapy.[105,106] Investigational therapies include radionuclide therapy with radiolabelled somatostatin analogues, and sunitinib, an oral tyrosine kinase inhibitor that prevents angiogenesis.[105,107]

Surgery

For patients with secreting tumors, special antihypertensive management is indicated pre-procedurally, as manipulation of the tumor can induce sudden release of catecholamines. Alpha-blockade should always be performed before β-blockade, as unopposed α-adrenoreceptor stimulation can result in hypertensive crisis. Combined α- and β-blockers such as labetalol should also be avoided as solo agents, as the β-blockade outweighs the α effect. Adrenoreceptor blockade, which has been shown to significantly decrease perioperative risk of complications, should be initiated at least 2 weeks prior to surgery.[107]

The surgical approach to resection of paragangliomas of the temporal bone depends on the location and extent of the tumor. Patients with paragangliomas isolated to the middle ear or should be counseled of the routine risks of tympanomastoidectomy. For jugular paragangliomas, a larger surgical approach is required with inherently more risks to local structures, including facial nerve palsy, lower cranial nerve deficits, vascular injury, and hearing loss. Neck dissection should be performed if clinical examination or preoperative imaging suggests metastasis.[16,17]

Tympanic Paragangliomas

For tumors limited to the middle ear, a transcanal exploration may allow adequate access. A tympanomeatal flap is raised tailored to the tumor location. The tumor can then be removed with cupped forceps, which typically leads to brisk bleeding. Hemostasis can be achieved using the bipolar cautery or an absorbable hemostatic agent such as oxidized regenerated cellulose (Surgicel). As with other middle ear surgery, attention to preservation of the ossicular chain during tumor removal and hemostasis is important. Monopolar cautery should be avoided to prevent conduction to the cochlea or facial nerve, leading to potential hearing loss or facial paresis, respectively. Tympanomastoidectomy (with an extended facial recess approach) may be required if the tumor extends into the mastoid and hypotympanum.

Jugular Paragangliomas

Cranial nerve monitoring: Continuous intraoperative cranial nerve monitoring allows for earlier identification of the lower cranial nerves in a distorted operative field. Electrodes are placed in the pharyngeal plexus (IX), larynx (X), trapezius muscle (XI), and tongue (XII). The relative incidence of new nerve deficits after surgery is IX>X + XI> XII.[60,64] Though variable, observations of up to 45% of patients having postoperative hearing loss have been reported.[62,108-111] Overall, 59–72% of patients have one or more new cranial nerve deficits detected after surgery.[17,59-61,64,112]

Approaches

Transmastoid-transcervical: Smaller jugular paragangliomas that do not involve the carotid artery or posterior cranial fossa are removed via a transmastoid-transcervical approach. The cervical portion of the procedure is necessary for distal jugular vein control and ligation. Mastoidectomy with extended facial recess approach is performed, and the skin incision is carried inferiorly to the neck along a natural skin crease. A Fallopian bridge technique is performed, preserving a thin covering of bone surrounding the facial nerve circumferentially and drilling the air cells medial to the nerve.[112,113] The sternocleidomastoid and digastric muscles are amputated at the mastoid tip, and the mastoid tip is removed. The internal jugular vein and internal carotid artery are dissected superiorly to skull base. The sigmoid sinus and jugular bulb are exposed using diamond burrs. The proximal sigmoid sinus is occluded with extraluminal packing within the mastoid. Distal control of the internal jugular vein is then achieved by ligation in the superior neck. This is performed immediately prior to tumor resection to prevent tumor emboli, air emboli, and to reduce back-bleeding. As the sigmoid sinus and jugular bulb are opened for tumor removal, brisk bleeding may occur from the inferior petrosal sinus and condylar vein. Hemostasis can be achieved with gentle application of absorbable hemostatic agents. Cautery of the medial jugular bulb should not be performed to avoid injury to the lower cranial nerves.

Infratemporal fossa: Larger jugular paragangliomas with significant carotid artery involvement may benefit from a wider infratemporal fossa approach. This allows dissection of tumor from the internal carotid artery into the petrous apex. Transposition of the facial nerve is usually not required, though an option. To minimize intracranial hemorrhage, resection of any intracranial components should be performed after tumor at the jugular bulb has been removed and hemostasis achieved. Ear canal closure and packing of the Eustachian tube is indicated in cases of extensive erosion of the ear canal, deaf ear, and tumor extension anterior to cochlea and encasing carotid.

Outcomes

Recurrence rates

Tympanic paragangliomas have low recurrence rates with most published series reporting rates <1%.[4,17,55,114-116] Recurrence may occur when residual tumor is present within infracochlear cells between the cochlea and carotid artery. Jugular paragangliomas have higher rates of recurrence of approximately 5–10% in the setting of subtotal resections. In cases of cavernous sinus extension, central nervous system invasion, or involvement of the lower clivus marrow, total excision may not be possible.[59-62,116,117]

Complications

A systematic review of treatment of jugular paragangliomas identified cerebrospinal fluid leak, aspiration/pneumonia, wound infection, meningitis, and stroke as the most common life-threatening postoperative complications.[62] An increase in impairment was also observed for cranial nerves VII, IX, X, XI, and XII following surgery.[62] Because of their less extensive involvement, surgery for tympanic paragangliomas is associated with lower rates of complications. Risks include hearing loss, facial weakness, and rarely, vascular injury.[118]

REFERENCES

1. Sykes JM, Ossoff RH. Paragangliomas of the head and neck. Otolaryngol Clin North Am. 1986;19:755-67.
2. Wenig BM. Atlas of Head and Neck Pathology, 2nd edition. Philadelphia, PA: Saunders/Elsevier; 2008. pp. xvi, 1139.
3. Jackler RK, Brackmann DE. Neurotology, 2nd edition. Philadelphia, PA: Elsevier Mosby; 2005. pp. xxiii, 1411.
4. O'Leary MJ, Shelton C, Giddings NA, et al. Glomus tympanicum tumors: a clinical perspective. Laryngoscope. 1991;101:1038-43.
5. Valentin G. Über eine gangliose Anschwellung in der Jacobsonchen Anastomose des Menschen. Arch Anat Physiolog Lpz. 1840;16:287-90.
6. Wilde WR. Practical observations on aural surgery and the nature and treatment of diseases of the ear, with illustrations. London: John Churchill;1853.
7. Weir RF. Two cases of intratympanic vascular tumor, with a pulsating intact drum-membrane. Am J Otol. 1979;1:129-31.
8. Jackler RK. A century ago in the American Journal of Otology. Am J Otol. 1995;16:823-6.
9. Guild SR. A hitherto unrecognized structure, the glomus jugularis in man. Anat Rec. 1941;79:28.
10. Jackler RK, Driscoll CLW. Tumors of the Ear and Temporal Bone. Philadelphia: Lippincott Williams & Wilkins; 2000. pp. xvi, 494.
11. Mills SE. Histology for Pathologists, 4th edition. Philadelphia: Wolters Kluwer/ Lippincott Williams & Wilkins Health; 2012.
12. Winship T, Klopp CT, Jenkins WH. Giomus-jugularis tumors. Cancer. 1948;1: 441-8.
13. Rosai J, Ackerman LV, Rosai J. Rosai and Ackerman's surgical Pathology, 10th edition. Edinburgh; New York: Mosby; 2011.
14. Fletcher CDM. Diagnostic Histopathology of Tumors, 4th edition. Philadelphia, PA: Elsevier/Saunders; 2013.
15. Guild SR. The glomus jugulare, a nonchromaffin paraganglion, in man. Ann Otol Rhinol Laryngol. 1953;62:1045-71.
16. Lee JH, Barich F, Karnell LH, et al. National Cancer Data Base report on malignant paragangliomas of the head and neck. Cancer. 2002;94:730-7.
17. Boedeker CC. Paragangliomas and paraganglioma syndromes. GMS Curr Top Otorhinolaryngol Head Neck Surg. 2011;10:Doc03.
18. Wasserman PG, Savargaonkar P. Paragangliomas: classification, pathology, and differential diagnosis. Otolaryngol Clin North Am. 2001;34:v-vi, 845-62.
19. Destito D, Bucolo S, Florio A, et al. Management of head and neck paragangliomas: a series of 9 cases and review of the literature. Ear Nose Throat J. 2012;91:366-75.
20. Sillars HA, Fagan PA. The management of multiple paraganglioma of the head and neck. J Laryngol Otol. 1993;107:538-42.
21. Spector GJ, Ciralsky R, Maisel RH, et al. Multiple glomus tumors in the head and neck. Laryngoscope. 1975;85:1066-75.
22. Schwaber MK, Glasscock ME, Nissen AJ, et al. Diagnosis and management of catecholamine secreting glomus tumors. Laryngoscope. 1984;94:1008-15.
23. Neumann HP, Bausch B, McWhinney SR, et al. Germ-line mutations in nonsyndromic pheochromocytoma. N Engl J Med. 2002;346:1459-66.

24. Neumann HP, Erlic Z, Boedeker CC, et al. Clinical predictors for germline mutations in head and neck paraganglioma patients: cost reduction strategy in genetic diagnostic process as fall-out. Cancer Res. 2009;69:3650-6.

25. Neumann HP, Pawlu C, Peczkowska M, et al. Distinct clinical features of paraganglioma syndromes associated with SDHB and SDHD gene mutations. JAMA. 2004;292:943-51.

26. Schiavi F, Boedeker CC, Bausch B, et al. Predictors and prevalence of paraganglioma syndrome associated with mutations of the SDHC gene. JAMA. 2005;294:2057-63.

27. Favier J, Amar L, Gimenez-Roqueplo AP. Paraganglioma and phaeochromocytoma: from genetics to personalized medicine. Nat Rev Endocrinol. 2015;11: 101-11.

28. Burnichon N, Rohmer V, Amar L, et al. The succinate dehydrogenase genetic testing in a large prospective series of patients with paragangliomas. J Clin Endocrinol Metab. 2009;94:2817-27.

29. Pasini B, Stratakis CA. SDH mutations in tumorigenesis and inherited endocrine tumours: lesson from the phaeochromocytoma-paraganglioma syndromes. J Intern Med. 2009;266:19-42.

30. Baysal BE, Ferrell RE, Willett-Brozick JE, et al. Mutations in SDHD, a mitochondrial complex II gene, in hereditary paraganglioma. Science. 2000;287:848-51.

31. Niemann S, Muller U. Mutations in SDHC cause autosomal dominant paraganglioma, type 3. Nat Genet. 2000;26:268-70.

32. Astuti D, Latif F, Dallol A, et al. Gene mutations in the succinate dehydrogenase subunit SDHB cause susceptibility to familial pheochromocytoma and to familial paraganglioma. Am J Hum Genet. 2001;69:49-54.

33. Bayley JP, Kunst HP, Cascon A, et al. SDHAF2 mutations in familial and sporadic paraganglioma and phaeochromocytoma. Lancet Oncol. 2010;11:366-72.

34. Boedeker CC, Hensen EF, Neumann HP, et al. Genetics of hereditary head and neck paragangliomas. Head Neck. 2014;36:907-16.

35. Hao HX, Khalimonchuk O, Schraders M, et al. SDH5, a gene required for flavination of succinate dehydrogenase, is mutated in paraganglioma. Science. 2009;325:1139-42.

36. Korpershoek E, Favier J, Gaal J, et al. SDHA immunohistochemistry detects germline SDHA gene mutations in apparently sporadic paragangliomas and pheochromocytomas. J Clin Endocrinol Metab. 2011;96:E1472-6.

37. Ricketts CJ, Forman JR, Rattenberry E, et al. Tumor risks and genotype-phenotype-proteotype analysis in 358 patients with germline mutations in SDHB and SDHD. Hum Mutat. 2010;31:41-51.

38. Zhu WD, Wang ZY, Chai YC, et al. Germline mutations and genotype-phenotype associations in head and neck paraganglioma patients with negative family history in China. Eur J Med Genet. 2015;58:433-8.

39. Niemann S, Muller U, Engelhardt D, et al. Autosomal dominant malignant and catecholamine-producing paraganglioma caused by a splice donor site mutation in SDHC. Hum Genet. 2003;113:92-4.

40. Vanharanta S, Buchta M, McWhinney SR, et al. Early-onset renal cell carcinoma as a novel extraparaganglial component of SDHB-associated heritable paraganglioma. Am J Hum Genet. 2004;74:153-9.

41. Neumann HP, Sullivan M, Winter A, et al. Germline mutations of the TMEM127 gene in patients with paraganglioma of head and neck and extraadrenal abdominal sites. J Clin Endocrinol Metab. 2011;96:E1279-82.

42. Rattenberry E, Vialard L, Yeung A, et al. A comprehensive next generation sequencing-based genetic testing strategy to improve diagnosis of inherited pheochromocytoma and paraganglioma. J Clin Endocrinol Metab. 2013;98:E1248-56.

43. Bausch B, Borozdin W, Neumann HP, European-American Pheochromocytoma Study G. Clinical and genetic characteristics of patients with neurofibromatosis type 1 and pheochromocytoma. N Engl J Med. 2006;354:2729-31.

44. Bausch B, Koschker AC, Fassnacht M, et al. Comprehensive mutation scanning of NF1 in apparently sporadic cases of pheochromocytoma. J Clin Endocrinol Metab. 2006;91:3478-81.

45. Walther MM, Herring J, Enquist E, et al. von Recklinghausen's disease and pheochromocytomas. J Urol. 1999;162:1582-6.

46. Boedeker CC, Erlic Z, Richard S, et al. Head and neck paragangliomas in von Hippel-Lindau disease and multiple endocrine neoplasia type 2. J Clin Endocrinol Metab. 2009;94:1938-44.

47. Cassol C, Mete O. Endocrine manifestations of von Hippel-Lindau disease. Arch Pathol Lab Med. 2015;139:263-8.

48. Offergeld C, Brase C, Yaremchuk S, et al. Head and neck paragangliomas: clinical and molecular genetic classification. Clinics (Sao Paulo). 2012;67(Suppl 1):19-28.

49. Batsakis JG. Tumors of the Head and Neck. Clinical and Pathological Considerations. Baltimore: Williams & Wilkins; 1974. pp. x, 388.

50. Boedeker CC, Neumann HP, Maier W, et al. Malignant head and neck paragangliomas in SDHB mutation carriers. Otolaryngol Head Neck Surg. 2007;137:126-9.

51. Heesterman BL, Bayley JP, Tops CM, et al. High prevalence of occult paragangliomas in asymptomatic carriers of SDHD and SDHB gene mutations. Eur J Hum Genet. 2013;21:469-70.

52. Lustig LR, Jackler RK, Lanser MJ. Radiation-induced tumors of the temporal bone. Am J Otol. 1997;18:230-5.

53. Green JD, Jr, Brackmann DE, Nguyen CD, et al. Surgical management of previously untreated glomus jugulare tumors. Laryngoscope. 1994;104:917-21.

54. House WF, Glasscock ME, 3rd. Glomus tympanicum tumors. Arch Otolaryngol. 1968;87:550-4.

55. Jackson CG, Welling DB, Chironis P, et al. Glomus tympanicum tumors: contemporary concepts in conservation surgery. Laryngoscope. 1989;99:875-84.

56. Larson TC, 3rd, Reese DF, Baker HL, Jr, et al. Glomus tympanicum chemodectomas: radiographic and clinical characteristics. Radiology. 1987;163:801-6.

57. Brown LA. Glomus jugulare tumor of the middle ear; clinical aspects. Laryngoscope. 1953;63:281-92.

58. Jackson CG, Glasscock ME, 3rd, Nissen AJ, et al. Glomus tumor surgery: the approach, results, and problems. Otolaryngol Clin North Am. 1982;15:897-916.

59. Jackson CG, McGrew BM, Forest JA, et al. Lateral skull base surgery for glomus tumors: long-term control. Otol Neurotol. 2001;22:377-82.

60. Lope Ahmad RA, Sivalingam S, Konishi M, et al. Oncologic outcome in surgical management of jugular paraganglioma and factors influencing outcomes. Head Neck. 2013;35:527-34.

61. Neskey DM, Hatoum G, Modh R, et al. Outcomes after surgical resection of head and neck paragangliomas: a review of 61 patients. Skull Base.2011;21:171-6.

62. Suarez C, Rodrigo JP, Bodeker CC, et al. Jugular and vagal paragangliomas: systematic study of management with surgery and radiotherapy. Head Neck. 2012;35:1195-204.

63. Makek M, Franklin DJ, Zhao JC, et al. Neural infiltration of glomus temporale tumors. Am J Otol. 1990;11:1-5.

64. Lustig LR, Jackler RK. The variable relationship between the lower cranial nerves and jugular foramen tumors: implications for neural preservation. Am J Otol. 1996;17:658-68.

65. Spector GJ, Gado M, Ciralsky R, et al. Neurologic implications of glomus tumors in the head and neck. Laryngoscope. 1975;85:1387-95.

66. Pellitteri PK, Rinaldo A, Myssiorek D, et al. Paragangliomas of the head and neck. Oral Oncol. 2004;40:563-75.

67. Spector GJ, Sobol S, Thawley SE, et al. Panel discussion: glomus jugulare tumors of the temporal bone. Patterns of invasion in the temporal bone. Laryngoscope. 1979;89:1628-39.

68. Glasscock ME, 3rd, Dickins JR, Jackson CG, et al. Vascular anomalies of the middle ear. Laryngoscope. 1980;90:77-88.

69. Kuhn MA, Friedmann DR, Winata LS, et al. Large jugular bulb abnormalities involving the middle ear. Otol Neurotol. 2012;33:1201-6.

70. Conley J, Hildyard V. Aneurysm of the internal carotid artery presenting in the middle ear. Arch Otolaryngol. 1969;90:35-8.

71. Sinnreich AI, Parisier SC, Cohen NL, et al. Arterial malformations of the middle ear. Otolaryngol Head Neck Surg. 1984;92:194-206.

72. Stallings JO, McCabe BF. Congenital middle ear aneurysm of internal carotid. Arch Otolaryngol. 1969;90:39-43.

73. Lo WW, Solti-Bohman LG, McElveen JT, Jr. Aberrant carotid artery: radiologic diagnosis with emphasis on high-resolution computed tomography. Radiographics. 1985;5:985-93.

74. McElveen JT, Jr, Lo WW, el Gabri TH, et al. Aberrant internal carotid artery: classic findings on computed tomography. Otolaryngol Head Neck Surg. 1986;94:616-21.

75. Nanda A, Murray RD. Diverse pathologies of the jugular foramen. World Neurosurg. 2015;83:164-6.

76. Arriaga MA, Brackmann DE. Differential diagnosis of primary petrous apex lesions. Am J Otol. 1991;12:470-4.

77. Swartz JD, Bazarnic ML, Naidich TP, et al. Aberrant internal carotid artery lying within the middle ear. High resolution CT diagnosis and differential diagnosis. Neuroradiology. 1985;27:322-6.

78. Lo WW, Solti-Bohman LG, Lambert PR. High-resolution CT in the evaluation of glomus tumors of the temporal bone. Radiology. 1984;150:737-42.

79. Som PM, Reede DL, Bergeron RT, et al. Computed tomography of glomus tympanicum tumors. J Comput Assist Tomogr. 1983;7:14-7.

80. Olsen WL, Dillon WP, Kelly WM, et al. MR imaging of paragangliomas. AJR Am J Roentgenol. 1987;148:201-4.

81. Vogl TJ, Bisdas S. Differential diagnosis of jugular foramen lesions. Skull Base. 2009;19:3-16.

82. Murphy TP, Brackmann DE. Effects of preoperative embolization on glomus jugulare tumors. Laryngoscope. 1989;99:1244-7.

83. Tasar M, Yetiser S. Glomus tumors: therapeutic role of selective embolization. J Craniofac Surg. 2004;15:497-505.

84. Brito JP, Asi N, Gionfriddo MR, et al. The incremental benefit of functional imaging in pheochromocytoma/paraganglioma: a systematic review. Endocrine. 2015;50:176-86.

85. Telischi FF, Bustillo A, Whiteman ML, et al. Octreotide scintigraphy for the detection of paragangliomas. Otolaryngol Head Neck Surg. 2000;122:358-62.

86. Bustillo A, Telischi F, Weed D, et al. Octreotide scintigraphy in the head and neck. Laryngoscope. 2004;114:434-40.

87. Bustillo A, Telischi FF. Octreotide scintigraphy in the detection of recurrent paragangliomas. Otolaryngol Head Neck Surg. 2004;130:479-82.

88. Hoegerle S, Ghanem N, Altehoefer C, et al. 18F-DOPA positron emission tomography for the detection of glomus tumours. Eur J Nucl Med Mol Imaging. 2003;30:689-94.

89. Timmers HJ, Kozupa A, Chen CC, et al. Superiority of fluorodeoxyglucose positron emission tomography to other functional imaging techniques in the evaluation of metastatic SDHB-associated pheochromocytoma and paraganglioma. J Clin Oncol. 2007;25:2262-9.

90. Taieb D, Timmers HJ, Shulkin BL, et al. Renaissance of (18)F-FDG positron emission tomography in the imaging of pheochromocytoma/paraganglioma. J Clin Endocrinol Metab. 2014;99:2337-9.

91. Lenders JW, Duh QY, Eisenhofer G, et al. Pheochromocytoma and paraganglioma: an endocrine society clinical practice guideline. J Clin Endocrinol Metab. 2014;99:1915-42.

92. Young AL, Baysal BE, Deb A, et al. Familial malignant catecholamine-secreting paraganglioma with prolonged survival associated with mutation in the succinate dehydrogenase B gene. J Clin Endocrinol Metab. 2002;87:4101-5.

93. Luchetti A, Walsh D, Rodger F, et al. Profiling of somatic mutations in phaeochromocytoma and paraganglioma by targeted next generation sequencing analysis. Int J Endocrinol. 2015;2015:138573.

94. Toledo RA, Dahia PL. Next-generation sequencing for the diagnosis of hereditary pheochromocytoma and paraganglioma syndromes. Curr Opin Endocrinol Diabetes Obes. 2015;22:169-79.

95. Drucker AM, Houlden RL. A case of familial paraganglioma syndrome type 4 caused by a mutation in the SDHB gene. Nat Clin Pract Endocrinol Metab. 2006;2:702-6; quiz following 6.

96. Brackmann DE. Ear Research Foundation of Florida, House Ear Institute. Neurological Surgery of the Ear and Skull Base. New York: Raven Press; 1982. pp. xviii, 408.

97. Jackson CG, Glasscock ME, 3rd, Harris PF. Glomus tumors. Diagnosis, classification, and management of large lesions. Arch Otolaryngol. 1982;108:401-10.

98. Powell S, Peters N, Harmer C. Chemodectoma of the head and neck: results of treatment in 84 patients. Int J Radiat Oncol Biol Phys. 1992;22:919-24.

99. Chino JP, Sampson JH, Tucci DL, et al. Paraganglioma of the head and neck: long-term local control with radiotherapy. Am J Clin Oncol. 2009;32:304-7.

100. Boyle JO, Shimm DS, Coulthard SW. Radiation therapy for paragangliomas of the temporal bone. Laryngoscope. 1990;100:896-901.

101. Tran Ba Huy P. Radiotherapy for glomus jugulare paraganglioma. Eur Ann Otorhinolaryngol Head Neck Dis. 2014;131:223-6.

102. Lalwani AK, Jackler RK, Gutin PH. Lethal fibrosarcoma complicating radiation therapy for benign glomus jugulare tumor. Am J Otol. 1993;14:398-402.

103. Hinerman RW, Mendenhall WM, Amdur RJ, et al. Definitive radiotherapy in the management of chemodectomas arising in the temporal bone, carotid body, and glomus vagale. Head Neck. 2001;23:363-71.

104. Gabriel EM, Sampson JH, Dodd LG, et al. Glomus jugulare tumor metastatic to the sacrum after high-dose radiation therapy: case report. Neurosurgery. 1995;37:1001-5.

105. Niemeijer ND, Alblas G, van Hulsteijn LT, et al. Chemotherapy with cyclophosphamide, vincristine and dacarbazine for malignant paraganglioma and pheochromocytoma: systematic review and meta-analysis. Clin Endocrinol. 2014;81:642-51.

106. van Hulsteijn LT, Niemeijer ND, Dekkers OM, et al. (131)I-MIBG therapy for malignant paraganglioma and phaeochromocytoma: systematic review and meta-analysis. Clin Endocrinol. 2014;80:487-501.

107. Martucci VL, Pacak K. Pheochromocytoma and paraganglioma: diagnosis, genetics, management, and treatment. Curr Probl Cancer. 2014;38:7-41.

108. Moe KS, Li D, Linder TE, et al. An update on the surgical treatment of temporal bone paraganglioma. Skull Base Surg. 1999;9:185-94.

109. Poe DS, Jackson G, Glasscock ME, et al. Long-term results after lateral cranial base surgery. Laryngoscope. 1991;101:372-8.

110. Pareschi R, Righini S, Destito D, et al. Surgery of glomus jugulare Tumors. Skull Base. 2003;13:149-57.

111. Fayad JN, Keles B, Brackmann DE. Jugular foramen tumors: clinical characteristics and treatment outcomes. Otology Neurotol. 2010;31:299-305.

112. Pensak ML, Jackler RK. Removal of jugular foramen tumors: the fallopian bridge technique. Otolaryngol Head Neck Surg. 1997;117:586-91.

113. Oghalai JS, Leung MK, Jackler RK, et al. Transjugular craniotomy for the management of jugular foramen tumors with intracranial extension. Otol Neurotol. 2004;25:570-9; discussion 9.

114. Sanna M, Fois P, Pasanisi E, et al. Middle ear and mastoid glomus tumors (glomus tympanicum): an algorithm for the surgical management. Auris Nasus Larynx. 2010;37:661-8.

115. Schick B, Draf W, Kahle G. Jugulotympanic paraganglioma: therapy concepts under development. Laryngorhinootologie. 1998;77:434-43.

116. Gstoettner W, Matula C, Hamzavi J, et al. Long-term results of different treatment modalities in 37 patients with glomus jugulare tumors. Eur Arch Otorhinolaryngol. 1999;256:351-5.

117. Woods CI, Strasnick B, Jackson CG. Surgery for glomus tumors: the Otology Group experience. Laryngoscope. 1993;103:65-70.

118. Carlson ML, Sweeney AD, Pelosi S, et al. Glomus tympanicum: a review of 115 cases over 4 decades. Otolaryngol Head Neck Surg. 2015;152:136-42.

Chapter 10

Music Perception and Enjoyment with Cochlear Implants

Brianna M Griffin, Anil K Lalwani

INTRODUCTION

The cochlear implant (CI) is a prosthetic device that restores auditory function to individuals with sensorineural hearing loss. It does so by bypassing inner hair cells and directly stimulating the auditory nerve. Over the past several decades, advances in CI hardware, software, and surgical techniques have led to significant improvement in speech perception to a level where many CI recipients are able to use the telephone. Following implantation, children and adults with CIs also function at high levels in everyday life and report a greater degree of self-esteem.[1] Despite the remarkable advances in speech perception with newer hardware and software, music perception remains difficult for most CI recipients.[2-4] This chapter reviews various topics concerning music and CIs, including coding strategies, music perception and enjoyment, rehabilitation, and future strategies for improving music listening.

Music is an integral component of human well-being and social interaction, and it is present among myriad societies and cultures.[5] In her review on CIs and both music appreciation and training, Looi describes music as:

an emotionally expressive and a culturally significant acoustic phenomenon that helps regulate mood, connects us with important memories, and fosters social cohesiveness throughout the life span. In daily life, we hear music on the television and radio, in places of business, at worship, at sporting events, concerts, and dances, and at home … As music is such a pervasive acoustic phenomenon, CI recipients are likely to be exposed to music on a regular basis.[6]

Considering music's sociocultural and psychological significance, this is an aspect of CI users' quality of life worth restoring and improving. Recognizing this role that music plays in their quality of life, all three CI manufacturers—Cochlear, Advanced Bionics, and Med-El—address how to best appreciate music with their devices, and some have even developed music-specific coding programs for CI users to turn on when listening to music. For example, Cochlear released its Music Program for its Nucleus 6 processor specifically designed for music listening experiences.

MUSIC PERCEPTION IN NORMAL-HEARING LISTENERS

The basic psychological attributes of musical sound are timbre, pitch duration, and loudness. The combinations and interactions between those attributes create the music with which normal-hearing (NH) listeners are familiar. Music and speech share similar qualities; they both rely on frequency, timbral, temporal, and intensity components presented systematically to convey meaning, whether concrete (speech) or abstract (music).[7] However, though they both share qualities, music is abstract and its interpretation is highly subjective. This and other differences effect the perceptual challenges of CI users for both speech and music.[8,9]

The fundamental frequency (f0) is the primary determinant of pitch perception. Moreover, the harmonic content determines the strength of pitch perception; the low harmonics are most important since they are resolvable by a normal auditory system.[10] For pure-tones, both the peak of the traveling wave on the basilar membrane and the temporal pattern of neural firing affect their perception. Complex tones are likely perceived by a combination of these.[11-13] The lower resolved harmonics of a complex tone or temporal cues from unresolved harmonics can determine pitch information.[14-16] The unresolved harmonics vibrate along the basilar membrane with specific spots excited by multiple harmonics simultaneously, and this complex vibration pattern repeats at a rate equal to f0.

Timbre is the quality that allows one to distinguish between two instruments playing the same pitch at the same loudness level, and it is an encompassing quality related to differences in sound spectra. Part of every musical instrument's unique timbre originates from its harmonic structure, specifically the number and spacing of harmonics.[17] The three spectral dimensions of timbre are rise time (or attack time), spectral centroid (the center of the spectrum, affecting the perception of a "bright" or "dull" sound), and spectral flux (the number and spread of components in the spectrum) (Fig. 10.1).[18]

MUSIC PERCEPTION AND CI CODING

Normal hearing and hearing aid (HA) use are both types of acoustic hearing. In contrast, CIs utilize electrical hearing, directly and electronically stimulating the cochlea. Despite this fundamental difference in

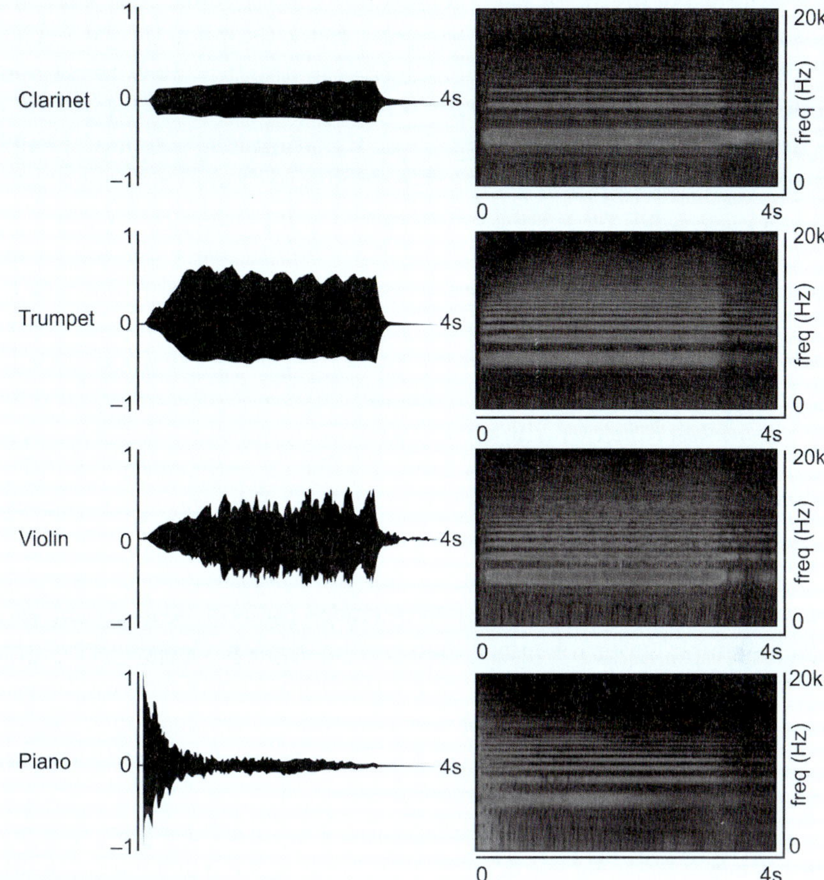

Fig. 10.1: Comparison of middle C (261.6 Hz) played by instruments of different instrument families (woodwind, brass, strings, and percussion). The left column graphs show the acoustic waveforms of each instrument. The *y*-axis is the amplitude proportional to the voltage level of the resulting audio output. Differences in rise time among instruments can be appreciated from these graphs. The right column graphs show log-based spectrograms of the waveforms, and differences in spectral flux among instruments can be appreciated from these graphs. The timbral elements of rise time and spectral flux, exhibited in this figure, contribute to the timbral fingerprints of these instruments, helping listeners to distinguish them from one another.
Source: Adapted from Donnelly PJ, Limb CJ, Niparko JK. Music perception in cochlear implant users. Cochlear implants: Principles and practices. 2009:223-8.

hearing modality, temporal resolution skills in CI users equal those of NH listeners. However, frequency-resolution skills are significantly worse for CI users, which contribute to their difficulties perceiving music.

For pitch perception among CI users, there are two schools of thought: The place or rate-place theory and the temporal theory. In the rate-place theory, pitches are encoded by the location of the peak of the traveling wave on the basilar membrane of the cochlea, which has the greatest excitation or neuronal firing rate. In the temporal theory, pitches are encoded based on temporal pattern of neural firing; neurons fire in time with the pitch heard, and the intervals between those subsequent action potentials equal the period of the stimulus.[19] Temporal pitch cues are affected by modulating the amplitude or changing the stimulating pulse train rate. Most speech-processing strategies do not alter the stimulation rate, keeping it at a constant, relatively high rate. Thus, temporal pitch cues are mostly driven by pulse amplitude. However, CI users reliably receive pitch cues from modulations of pulse amplitude in only the low frequency region, up to about 300 Hz. Therefore, CI users would only reliably be able to use temporal pitch cues to identify pitches with an f0 below about middle-C.[20-23] This upper limit of rate pitch also limits how closely spaced action potentials can be—the backbone of the temporal theory, and above which there is not a distinguishable change in pitch.

As mentioned previously, the ability to perceive f0 is integral to pitch perception. The range of frequencies for both f0 and loudness level is much wider for music than it is for speech. Consequently, this wider frequency range affects CI users' difficulties perceiving f0 and, subsequently, pitches in music. For perceiving complex tones, consistent rate-place and temporal pitch information are needed. Varying the rate-place information stymies accurate pitch perception.[24]

Other factors besides rate-place and temporal cues hamper pitch perception among CI users as well. Inhibitors such as factors related to the electrode (e.g. insertion depth and placement), the sound processor (e.g. processing strategy specifications and stimulation mode), interaction with other stimuli features (e.g. loudness level and pulse duration), and patient factors (e.g. pathology and tissue impedance surrounding array) affect pitch perception.[25-27] Specifically, rate-place cues are limited by both number of electrodes and depth of electrode insertion.[28] Having a limited number of electrodes in an array causes ranges of frequencies to be assigned to single electrodes, which impede a robust frequency resolution. Shallow electrode insertion results in low-frequency content loss (speech included) since the apical regions of the cochlea that encode those frequencies are not sufficiently stimulated by the electrode.

Melody perception relates to pitch perception since melody involves a series of pitch intervals. However, melody also involves rhythm, lyrics, musical style, and other musical elements. Thus, it merits evaluation separate from pitch. Temporal pitch cues are sufficient for CI users to discern pitch intervals as small as one semitone (a half-step in music) at stimulation rates (<200 Hz) applied to one electrode.[28] For rate-place cues, distortion refers to large frequency ranges assigned to single electrodes. Rate-place cues may not adequately transmit low pitch stimuli (<500 Hz) because of increased distortion that occurs in the lower registers.[29] However, rate-place cues do transmit sufficient information to discern pitch directions with intervals also as small as one semitone, though perhaps at higher registers where there is less distortion.[30]

Factors contributing to impaired pitch perception also contribute to impaired timbre perception. Accurate timbral perception requires perception of both the temporal envelope and the spectral shape.[31] Among CI listeners, and even bimodal users (CI with a contralateral HA), attack time is the salient cue that helps them identify musical instruments.[32] Instruments with a sharp attack time—e.g. guitar or piano—are better recognized than other instruments.[33] Multichannel CIs seek to restore part of the spectral flux aspect of timbre by electrically stimulating different sites along the cochlea. Unfortunately, existing CI processors conduct a crude spectral analysis of the input signal, and spectral selectivity is quite important for listening to musical stimuli.[34] Moreover, the presence of spectral smearing—arising from current spread around the electrode, neural survival characteristics, or channel interactions—for many CI users may also affect timbre perception.[35,36]

CI USERS AND MUSIC PERCEPTUAL PERFORMANCE

The CI currently faces numerous challenges translating the complex acoustic information in a music signal into electrical information that is perceived as music. These challenges effect the difficulties experienced by CI users in both perceiving music and performing musical tasks.

Considering the difficulties CIs encounter encoding pitch information, CI users accordingly perform much worse on pitch-related tasks than their NH counterparts.[37,38] Upon completing tasks identifying six semitone and one semitone intervals, CI users performed significantly worse than NH listeners.[39] Furthermore, CI users also perform worse than HA users on pitch-related tasks. When compared against HA users—with similar levels of hearing loss—on their ability to perceive intervals sung an octave, half-octave, and quarter-octave apart, CI users performed much worse on this task than HA users. For the quarter-octave interval, CI users performed near chance level.[40] Thus, CI users perform worse on pitch-related tasks than both NH listeners and HA users with similar levels of hearing loss, likely impacting their music perception as well.

Timbre perception, across numerous studies, is typically assessed via instrument identification. As discussed previously, CIs have difficulty in processing timbral information. Therefore, it is not surprising that CI users also perform significantly worse than NH listeners at perceiving musical instruments.[41-45] In a study asking CI users and NH listeners to identify seven instruments each playing the same melody, NH individuals were almost perfect (91% correct), while CI users exhibited greater difficulty with the task (47% correct). Despite maintaining the timbral perceptual advantage of acoustic hearing, however, HA users also appear to have difficulties identifying instruments. When asked to identify single instruments, solo instruments with background accompaniment, and musical ensembles, not only did both CI and HA users fare similarly, but they also both exhibited decreasing performance as timbral complexity increased.[47] Thus, deviating a bit from pitch perceptual tasks, CI users perform worse on tasks of timbral perception than NH listeners, but perform equal to HA users. Moreover, timbral perception decreases as the timbral complexity of the music increases.

For melody perception, CI users rely more heavily on rhythm and lyrical cues to glean melodic perceptual information, though they still perform worse than NH listeners on melodic tasks. Upon evaluating melody recognition across pop, country and western, and classical genres, CI users performed generally worse than NH listeners for all three genres. However, they performed significantly worse than NH listeners for identifying melodies in the classical genre, which further supports the notion that CI users utilize lyrical and rhythm information to discern melodies.[47-53] A similar trend exists between CI and HA users; in the above study, CI users exhibited much more difficultly identifying melodies than HA users.[54] In a study investigating the smallest identifiable pitch interval (ranging from two octaves to one semitone) within a single piano melody, CI users performed much worse than NH participants, and there was no correlation between melody discrimination and pitch discrimination for the same instrument and key. Considering that likely a combination of temporal and rate-place cues contribute to pitch perception among NH listeners, the lack of both reliable temporal cues in higher registers and reliable rate-place cues at lower registers also likely contribute to decreased melody perception overall.[55]

Unlike pitch, timbre, and melody, rhythm is perceived quite well by CI users, performing similarly to NH adults as well as HA users on tasks of rhythmic or temporal discrimination.[56-66] The temporal cues perceived in rhythm occur on a more macrotemporal scale, different than the microtemporal ones perceived in pitch. The temporal frameworks that influence the rhythm of music are on the order of 0.2–20 Hz, while much higher-frequency temporal components comprise the acoustic signal to convey pitch information.[61]

Music perception correlates with age and postimplant listening habits, but does not correlate with speech processing strategy, device manufacturer, or insertion depth of the electrode.[62-72] Speech perception scores do predict music perception, but only for tests with music samples that included lyrics. Conversely, formal music training predicted performance on tests without lyrics. Specifically, CI users with formal music training at the high school level or above did significantly better on tests without lyrics.[73] For speech perception, duration of implant use is a strong predictor of speech performance. However, despite this correlation, duration of implant use impacts upon neither music perception nor music enjoyment.[74] In fact, for pitch discrimination, duration of implant use is negatively correlated.[75] Therefore, correlations between duration of implant use and performance for music do not mirror those for speech.

MUSIC PERCEPTION IN ELECTROACOUSTIC HEARING

Due to the limitations of current strategies to simulate acoustic hearing, pure electric hearing does not transmit pitch and timbre information incredibly well. However, electroacoustic hearing may enhance perception of these musical elements. Electroacoustic hearing takes advantage of residual acoustic hearing in CI users by either using an HA in the contralateral ear (referred to as bimodal stimulation [BMS]) or implanting the implant device with a modified surgical technique and/or a shorter electrode array to preserve residual acoustic hearing (Figs. 10.2A and B). Since acoustic hearing provides more accurate f0 information—specifically at lower frequencies, electroacoustic hearing may improve aspects of music perception for those users.[76-83]

On pitch-ranking tasks among NH listeners, conventional CI users, and "hybrid" CI users with a shorter electrode array to preserve low-frequency hearing, NH listeners performed better than both CI groups. However, the "hybrid" CI user group performed better than the conventional CI user group and more similarly to the NH listener group. Furthermore, the lower the f0 of the first pitch, the more accurate the responses among the "hybrid" CI users, suggesting that preserving lower frequency hearing enhances pitch perception.[84]

"Hybrid" CI users exhibit improved timbral perception compared to conventional CI users as well. In another study investigating tasks

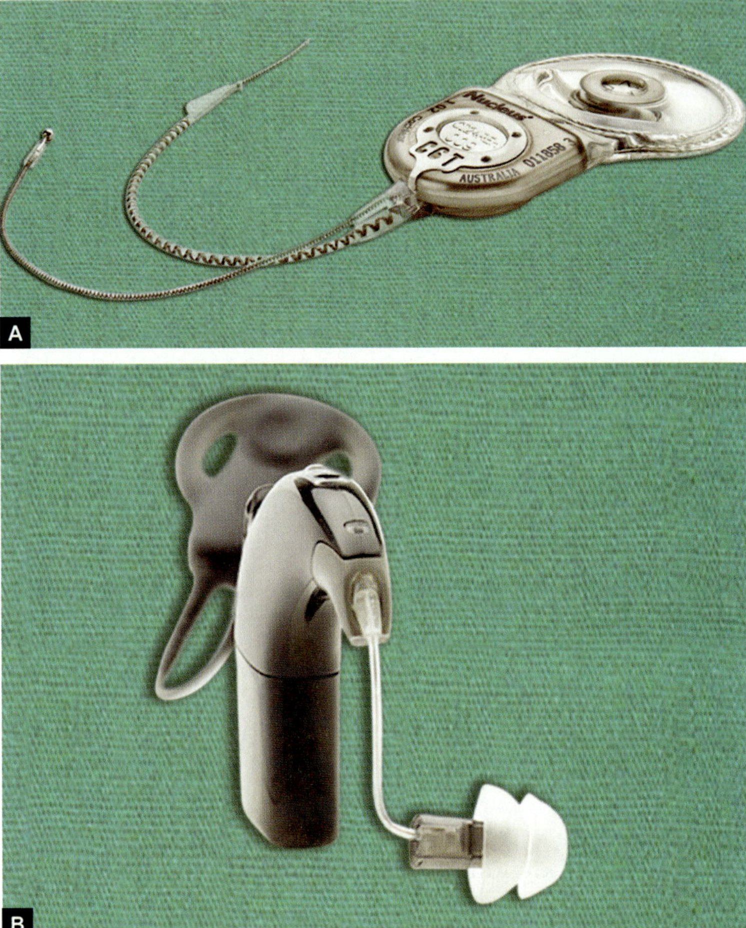

Figs. 10.2A and B: (A) A cochlear implant with a shorter electrode to preserve residual low-frequency hearing. (B) Cochlear Hybrid Hearing™ device, a type of electroacoustic hearing device. This is a hybrid device from the CI company Cochlear that combines both a shorter-electrode CI and hearing aid into one device. The cochlear implant component electrically stimulates the cochlea, and the hearing aid component amplifies acoustic sound and transmits it via the normal pathway of hearing through the external auditory canal.
Courtesy: Cochlear.

of song recognition without lyrics, NH listeners performed better than conventional CI users, as one may expect, but "hybrid" CI users also performed better than conventional CI users. On tasks of instrument identification among three frequency ranges, "hybrid" CI users performed better than conventional CI users for both low and high frequency ranges. Moreover, for instrument identification at low frequencies, "hybrid" CI users performed similarly to NH listeners, suggesting that the lower-frequency hearing preservation among these users enhances timbral perception as well.[85]

For melody recognition tasks among HA users, CI users, and BMS users, HA and BMS users both scored similarly and better than CI users, further exhibiting the impact of residual acoustic hearing on music perception.[86]

For the above studies, the "hybrid" CI users using the short-electrode array performed more similarly to NH listeners than to conventional CI users. However, though the prospects for music perception among electroacoustic hearing users appear promising, only a fraction of CI candidates qualify for utilizing an electroacoustic hearing modality. Thus, only a small portion of CI users would benefit. Furthermore, the degree of residual acoustic hearing likely contributes more significantly to the improved performance among "hybrid" users than shorter electrode arrays.[87]

It is interesting to note, however, that the perceptual advantage "hybrid" users have over conventional CI users—most of whom are postlingually deafened adults—disappears among prelingually deafened children. In a study involving prelingually deafened children that investigated pitch-ranking tasks among NH listeners, HA users, conventional CI users, and BMS users, both the NH and HA user groups performed better than conventional CI and BMS users, and the BMS and conventional CI users performed similarly to each other. Thus, for this study of NH and prelingually deafened children, those using electrical hearing of any kind performed worse than those using acoustic hearing only.[88] This suggests that in these tests largely developed by NH individuals, the prior history of musical interaction as an NH individual among postlingually deaf CI users affords a perceptual advantage over prelingually deafened CI users whose musical interactions have likely differed significantly.

CI USERS AND MUSIC ENJOYMENT

Except rhythm, we have established that CI users have difficulty perceiving timbre, pitch, and melody, performing worse on related tasks compared to NH listeners for all three attributes. However, music perception is a separate entity from music appraisal, or enjoyment, and the difficulties CI users encounter perceiving music may not necessarily impact upon their subsequent music enjoyment. Music listening habits among CI users do decline after implantation, but they do not disappear.[89] Thus, CI users still glean something from listening to music despite their perceptual relationship to music radically changing.

In a study investigating appraisal of the piano, clarinet, trumpet, and violin among CI and NH listeners, appraisal among CI users was lower than that for NH listeners. Furthermore, the amount of time CI users spent listening to music postimplantation and music background scores significantly correlated with appraisal, while speech perception and music perception scores did not.[90,91]

Similar to timbral complexity negatively affecting its perception, complexity of musical genre influences its preference. In a study investigating musical preferences differing in musical genre, CI users preferred country and western music to both pop and classical music. Furthermore, CI users preferred classical music the least of the three musical genres. The authors attributed the preference of country and western music to its decreased complexity and heavy reliance on lyrics, which also explains classical music's lack of appraisal by CI users.[92] Looi et al. evaluated appraisal of single and multiple instrument music samples among CI and HA users. The authors found that both users rated samples with multiple instruments to sound less pleasant, hinting that perhaps more complex musical stimuli decreases its quality among these two groups.[93] Concerning musical genres, Gfeller and colleagues found that CI users' appraisal ratings did not differ significantly among various genres. However, users did exhibit a strong preference for music perceived to be more "simple," supporting the complexity argument. In contrast, NH listeners not only exhibited musical preferences by genre, but also far preferred music perceived to be more complex.[94]

Reverberation time adds another type of complexity to music by increasing the echo of sounds in a musical piece. In a study evaluating the effect of reverberation time (or echo) on music enjoyment among NH listeners and CI-simulated music samples, the CI-simulated samples with greater amounts of reverberation time had lower appraisal ratings.[95] These results further buttress the argument that increased musical complexity—greater number of musical instruments, more reverberation—decreases its enjoyment.

For "hybrid" CI users, the trends for music appraisal follow those of music perception. When comparing CI users and BMS users, significantly more BMS users describe instruments to sound more pleasant and natural, musical styles to sound more "normal" and easier to identify, and melody as easier to follow.[96]

Complexity of musical stimuli, whether timbral, genre-related, or melodic, is a major factor in music appraisal, which is understandable considering the processing issues related to complex pitch and timbre perception. However, though one may anticipate an association between music perception and music enjoyment, no correlation actually exists between the two. In a large study by Drennan et al., the authors describe a weak correlation between timbral perception and music enjoyment, but found all other correlations between perception and appraisal to be insignificant.[97] Not only does this make a case for separating both the clinical evaluation and research investigation of perception and enjoyment, but it is also encouraging because the poor perceptual abilities of CI users do not stymie their enjoyment of music. However, though there are not correlations between perception and enjoyment, attenuating the difficulties CI users experience perceiving music can enhance subsequent music enjoyment. Selecting familiar music, less complex music, music with a strong rhythm, or music with lyrics improves the experience of enjoying music among CI users.[98] Furthermore, similar to communication tactics given to CI users to improve speech perception, controlling the music listening environment (quiet room, good quality of sound) and using visual cues (watching a performer, following lyrics) can improve music enjoyment.[99-101] These are all salient principles discussed with CI users when counseling them on how to rehabilitate their music-listening habits postimplantation.

REHABILITATION OF MUSIC PERCEPTION AND ENJOYMENT

The music listening experience changes dramatically postimplantation. Despite this, however, there is potential for postimplantation music rehabilitation. Duration of implant use is a strong predictor of speech performance as speech perception is constantly rehabilitated through conversations in everyday life. Similarly, music-specific rehabilitation may be able to improve both music perception and enjoyment. After computer-based, direct instruction that trained CI users to evaluate computer-generated melodies and real world melodies over the course of 12 weeks, both recognition and appraisal of real-world melodies improved. No improvement was noted for the computer-generated melodies, likely due to the lack of other cues (rhythmic, etc.) available to aid CI users in these melodies. It is important to note that appraisal for real world melodies also improved, which is encouraging for the potential of music enjoyment rehabilitation.[102] Cochlear implant users also improved in recognition and appraisal of musical instruments.[103] Remediation results are also promising for shorter training intervals. In training involving either direct instruction or repeated exposure with feedback, CI users exhibited improvement in instrument recognition in as little as 3 weeks of training, with improved benefit with longer training.[104]

A different angle to this topic is music habilitation among prelingually deafened children. Though this population lacks the music listening experiences of NH children, pediatric CI users are involved in various music activities at school and at home, and many do enjoy music, despite their less accurate perception of both pitch and timbre.[105-108] In a study involving a 2-year music-training program for pediatric CI users, after the first year, children exhibited greater interest in music exposure in daily life and awareness of musical elements. After the second year, children were rated by their parents to be more attentive to music, be more willing to voluntarily participate in music outside of training exercises, perform better on discrimination and identification of pitch and rhythm patterns, and have improved emotional responses to music.[109]

There is promise for both rehabilitation and habilitation of music in postlingual adult CI users and prelingual pediatric users, respectively. Furthermore, at least among adult CI users, they desire music rehabilitation. In a survey, over half of adult CI users expressed interest in a music training program, noting recognizing previously known tunes, appreciating musical instruments and pitch changes, and performing tasks related to enhancing pitch or timbre perception as skills they considered most important.[110] These findings pose a compelling argument for future incorporation of music into current clinical postimplantation rehabilitation or habilitation.

CONCLUSION

Music is an integral aspect of human quality of life that unfortunately eludes many CI users. These implant devices face engineering challenges hindering them from simulating the acoustic hearing of salient musical elements, and these challenges, in turn, effect subpar musical perception among its users. However, the fraction of users lucky enough to preserve a portion of acoustic hearing postimplantation retain some musical perceptual ability at low frequencies. Though not correlated with perception, music enjoyment is similarly challenging, but is more generally influenced by musical complexity than by individual pitches, melodies, or instruments. Furthermore, both music perception and enjoyment can be rehabilitated through directed training.

So, how does the horizon look for the future of music in the lives of CI users? Much emphasis and inquiry has been directed toward improving CI processing strategies to improve perception and enjoyment. The thought is that by improving the CI technology, perception and enjoyment also improve. However, as evidenced by the progress in music rehabilitation, perception and enjoyment can also be improved despite current CI technology challenges.

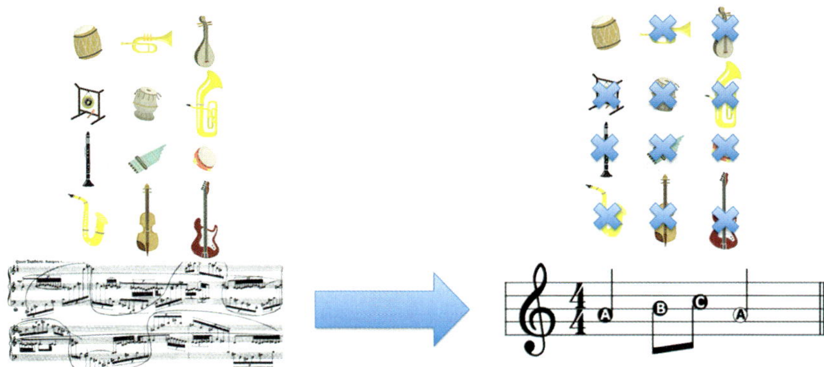

Fig. 10.3: Music Engineering. A proposed strategy for augmenting music enjoyment is re-engineering music to decrease its complexity. Kohlberg et al. had positive results upon reducing the number of instruments in a piece of music. Simplifying the melody in a piece of music is another possible strategy for music re-engineering.
Courtesy: www.dreamstime.com.

Recently, researchers have begun to focus on music engineering as a strategy to improve enjoyment. Moreover, modifying existing music to underscore its more enjoyable aspects based on appraisal ratings may be a novel way to restore this facet of quality of life. In a study modifying the number of instruments used in a country and Western song, CI users preferred versions of the song that used one to three instruments rather than versions using the full musical set (Fig. 10.3).[111]

After implantation, general attitudes toward music improve compared to those experienced while hearing-impaired preimplantation. However, attitudes postimplantation are still less positive than those prior to hearing impairment. Thus, in the postlingual, hearing-impaired CI users, musical experiences worsen over the course of progressive hearing impairment preimplant, improve postimplant, but still greatly fall short of musical experiences prior to onset of hearing impairment.[112,113] This is likely due to comparisons of current musical appreciation to those experienced prior to hearing loss, and these findings have implications for how to manage expectations for music enjoyment with the implant when counseling CI users in the clinical setting.

Through these endeavors, there is potential for restoration of enjoyable music listening experiences within the CI population. As CI technologies continue to slowly improve, music rehabilitation and habilitation, along with music engineering and proper music counseling, are strategies for improving music enjoyment and perception.

REFERENCES

1. Lassaletta L, Castro A, Bastarrica M, et al. Quality of life in postlingually deaf patients following cochlear implantation. Eur Arch Otorhinolaryngol. 2006; 263:267-70.
2. Gfeller K, Lansing CR. Melodic, rhythmic, and timbral perception of adult cochlear implant users. J Speech Hear Res. 1991;34:916-20.
3. Leal MC, Shin YJ, Laborde M, et al. Music perception in adult cochlear implant recipients. Acta Otolaryngol. 2003;123:826-35.
4. Kong YY, Cruz R, Jones JA, et al. Music perception with temporal cues in acoustic and electric hearing. Ear Hear. 2004;25:173-85.
5. Gfeller K, Christ A, Knutson JF, et al. Musical backgrounds, listening habits, and aesthetic enjoyment of adult cochlear implant recipients. J Am Acad Audiol. 2000;11:390406.
6. Looi V, Gfeller K, Driscoll V. Music appreciation and training for cochlear implant recipients: a review. Semin Hear. 2012;33:307-34.
7. Donnelly PJ, Limb CJ, Niparko JK. Music perception in cochlear implant users. Cochlear implants: Principles and Practices. 2009:223-8.
8. Looi V, Gfeller K, Driscoll V. Music appreciation and training for cochlear implant recipients: a review. Semin Hear. 2012;33:307-34.
9. Donnelly PJ, Limb CJ, Niparko JK. Music perception in cochlear implant users. Cochlear implants. Principles and Practices. 2009:223-8.
10. Rasch RA, Plomp R. The perception of musical tones. In: Deutsch D (Eds). The Psychology of Music. New York: Academic Press; 1982. pp. 1-22.
11. Moore BCJ. An Introduction to the Psychology of Hearing, 5th edition. San Diego: Academic Press; 2003.
12. Goldstein JL. An optimum processor theory for the central formation of the pitch of complex tones. J Acoust Soc Am. 1973;54:1496-516.
13. Meddis R, O'Mard L. A unitary model of pitch perception. J Acoust Soc Am. 1997;102:1811-20.
14. Moore BCJ. Coding of sounds in the auditory system and its relevance to signal processing and coding in cochlear implants. Otol Neurotol. 2003;24: 243-54.
15. Plomp R. Pitch of complex tones. J Acoust Soc Am. 1967;41:1526-33.
16. Ritsma RJ. Frequencies dominant in the perception of the pitch of complex sounds. J Acoust Soc Am. 1967;42:191-8.
17. Looi V, Gfeller K, Driscoll V. Music appreciation and training for cochlear implant recipients: a review. Semin Hear. 2012;33: 307-34.
18. Grey JM. Multidimensional scaling of musical timbres. J Acoust Soc Am. 1977; 61:1270-7.
19. Erfanian Saeedi N, Blamey PJ, Burkitt AN, et al. Application of a pitch perception model to investigate the effect of stimulation field spread on the pitch ranking abilities of cochlear implant recipients. Hear Res. 2014;316:129-37.
20. Shannon RV, Fu QJ, Galvin JJ, et al. Speech perception with cochlear implants. In: Zeng FG, Popper AN, Fay RR (Eds). Cochlear Implants: Auditory Prostheses and Electric Hearing. New York: Springer; 2004. pp. 334-76.
21. McKay CM. Psychophysics and electrical stimulation. In: Zeng FG, Popper AN, Fay RR (Eds). Cochlear Implants: Auditory Prostheses and Electric Hearing. New York: Springer; 2004. pp. 286-333.

22. Zeng FG. Temporal pitch in electric hearing. Hear Res. 2002;174:101-6.

23. Pijl S, Schwarz DW. Melody recognition and musical interval perception by deaf subjects stimulated with electrical pulse trains through single cochlear implant electrodes. J Acoust Soc Am. 1995;98:886–95.

24. Oxenham AJ, Bernstein JG, Penagos H. Correct tonotopic representation is necessary for complex pitch perception. Proc Natl Acad Sci USA. 2004;101: 1421-5.

25. Busby PA, Whitford LA, Blamey PJ, et al. Pitch perception for different modes of stimulation using the cochlear multiple-electrode prosthesis. J Acoust Soc Am. 1994;95:2658-69.

26. McDermott HJ. Music perception with cochlear implants: a review. Trends Amplif. 2004;8:49- 82.

27. McKay CM. Psychophysics and electrical stimulation. In: Zeng FG, Popper AN, Fay RR (Eds). Cochlear Implants: Auditory Prostheses and Electric Hearing. New York: Springer; 2004. pp. 286-333.

28. Blamey PJ, Dooley GJ, Parisi ES, et al. Pitch comparisons of acoustically and electrically evoked auditory sensations. Hear Res. 1996;99:139-50.

29. Schatzer R, Vermeire K, Visser D, et al. Electric-acoustic pitch comparisons in single-sided-deaf cochlear implant users: frequency-place functions and rate pitch. Hear Res. 2014;309:26-35.

30. Maarefvand M, Marozeau J, Blamey PJ. A cochlear implant user with exceptional musical hearing ability. Int J Audiol. 2013;52:424-32.

31. Looi V, Gfeller K, Driscoll V. Music appreciation and training for cochlear implant recipients: a review. Semin Hear. 2012;33:307-34.

32. Kong YY, Mullangi A, Marozeau J. Timbre and speech perception in bimodal and bilateral cochlear-implant users. Ear Hear. 2012;33:645-59.

33. Macherey O, Delpierre A. Perception of musical timbre by cochlear implant listeners: a multidimensional scaling study. Ear Hear. 2013;34:426-36.

34. Shannon RV, Fu QJ, Galvin JJ, et al. Speech perception with cochlear implants. In: Zeng FG, Popper AN, Fay RR (Eds). Cochlear Implants: Auditory Prostheses and Electric Hearing. New York: Springer; 2004. pp. 334-76.

35. McDermott HJ. Music perception with cochlear implants: a review. Trends Amplif. 2004;8:49-82.

36. McKay CM. Psychophysics and electrical stimulation. In: Zeng FG, Popper AN, Fay RR (Eds). Cochlear Implants: Auditory Prostheses and Electric Hearing. New York: Springer; 2004. pp. 286-333.

37. McDermott HJ. Music perception with cochlear implants: a review. Trends Amplif. 2004;8:49-82.

38. Looi V. The effect of cochlear implantation of music: a review. Otorinolaringologia. 2008;58:169-90.

39. Sucher CM, McDermott HJ. Pitch ranking of complex tones by normally hearing subjects and cochlear implant users. Hear Res. 2007;230:80-7.

40. Looi V, McDermott H, McKay C, et al. Music perception of cochlear implant users compared with that of hearing aid users. Ear Hear. 2008;29:421-34.

41. McDermott HJ. Music perception with cochlear implants: a review. Trends Amplif. 2004;8:49-82.

42. Looi V. The effect of cochlear implantation of music: a review. Otorrinolaringologia. 2008;58:169-90.

43. Gfeller K, Knutson JF, Woodworth G, et al. Timbral recognition and appraisal by adult cochlear implant users and normal-hearing adults. J Am Acad Audiol. 1998;9:1-19.

44. Leal MC, Shin YJ, Laborde ML, et al. Music perception in adult cochlear implant recipients. Acta Otolaryngol. 2003;123:826-35.

45. Gfeller K, Witt S, Woodworth G, et al. Effects of frequency, instrumental family, and cochlear implant type on timbre recognition and appraisal. Ann Otol Rhinol Laryngol. 2002;111:349-56.

46. Looi V, McDermott H, McKay C, et al. Music perception of cochlear implant users compared with that of hearing aid users. Ear Hear. 2008;29:421-34.

47. Leal MC, Shin YJ, Laborde ML, et al. Music perception in adult cochlear implant recipients. Acta Otolaryngol. 2003;123:826-35.

48. Vongpaisal T, Trehub SE, Schellenberg EG, et al. Music recognition by children with cochlear implants. In: Miyamoto RT (Eds). The VIII International Cochlear Implant Conference. Indianapolis, Indiana USA: Elsevier; 2004. pp. 193-6.

49. Gfeller K, Turner C, Mehr M, et al. Recognition of familiar melodies by adult cochlear implant recipients and normal-hearing adults. Cochlear Implants Int. 2002;3:29-53.

50. Fujita S, Ito J. Ability of nucleus cochlear implantees to recognize music. Ann Otol Rhinol Laryngol. 1999;108:634-40.

51. Gfeller K, Olszewski C, Rychener M, et al. Recognition of "real-world" musical excerpts by cochlear implant recipients and normal-hearing adults. Ear Hear. 2005;26:237-50.

52. Gfeller K, Witt S, Stordahl J, et al. The effects of training on melody recognition and appraisal by adult cochlear implant recipients. J Acad Rehabil Audiol. 2000;33:115-38.

53. Kong YY, Cruz R, Jones JA, et al. Music perception with temporal cues in acoustic and electric hearing. Ear Hear. 2004;25:173-85.

54. Gfeller K, Olszewski C, Rychener M, et al. Recognition of "real-world" musical excerpts by cochlear implant recipients and normal-hearing adults. Ear Hear. 2005;26:237-50.

55. Brockmeier SJ, Fitzgerald D, Searle O, et al. The music perception test: a novel battery for testing music perception of cochlear implant users. Cochlear Implants Int. 2011;12:10-20.

56. Gfeller K, Woodworth G, Robin DA, et al. Perception of rhythmic and sequential pitch patterns by normally hearing adults and adult cochlear implant users. Ear Hear. 1997;18:252-60.

57. Gfeller K, Christ A, Knutson JF, et al. Musical backgrounds, listening habits, and aesthetic enjoyment of adult cochlear implant recipients. J Am Acad Audiol. 2000;11:390-406.

58. Gfeller K, Lansing C. Musical perception of cochlear implant users as measured by the primary measures of music audiation: an item analysis. J Music Ther. 1992;29:18-39.

59. Gfeller K, Lansing CR. Melodic, rhythmic, and timbral perception of adult cochlear implant users. J Speech Hear Res. 1991;34:916-20.

60. Schulz E, Kerber M. Music perception with the MED-EL implants. In: Hochmair-Desoyer IJ, Hochmair ES (Eds). Advances in Cochlear Implants. Vienna: Datenkonvertierung, Reproduktion und Druck; 1994. pp. 326-32.

61. McDermott HJ. Music perception with cochlear implants: a review. Trends Amplif. 2004;8:49-82.

62. Gfeller K, Woodworth G, Robin DA, et al. Perception of rhythmic and sequential pitch patterns by normally hearing adults and adult cochlear implant users. Ear Hear. 1997;18:252-60.

63. Gfeller K, Christ A, Knutson JF, et al. Musical backgrounds, listening habits, and aesthetic enjoyment of adult cochlear implant recipients. J Am Acad Audiol. 2000;11:390-406.

64. Gfeller K, Lansing C. Musical perception of cochlear implant users as measured by the primary measures of music audiation: an item analysis. J Music Ther. 1992;29:18-39.

65. Gfeller K, Knutson JF, Woodworth G, et al. Timbral recognition and appraisal by adult cochlear implant users and normal-hearing adults. J Am Acad Audiol. 1998;9:1-19.

66. Gfeller K, Turner C, Mehr M, et al. Recognition of familiar melodies by adult cochlear implant recipients and normal-hearing adults. Cochlear Implants Int. 2002;3:29-53.

67. Gfeller K, Olszewski C, Rychener M, et al. Recognition of "real-world" musical excerpts by cochlear implant recipients and normal-hearing adults. Ear Hear. 2005;26:237-50.

68. Looi V, She JHK. Music perception of cochlear implant users: a questionnaire, and its implications for a music training program. Int J Audiol. 2010;49:116-28.

69. Gfeller K, Oleson J, Knutson JF, et al. Multivariate predictors of music perception and appraisal by adult cochlear implant users. J Am Acad Audiol. 2008;19: 120-34.

70. Gfeller K, Jiang D, Oleson J, et al. Temporal stability of music perception and appraisal scores of adult cochlear implant recipients. J Am Acad Audiol. 2010; 21:28-34.

71. Gfeller K, Witt S, Stordahl J, et al. The effects of training on melody recognition and appraisal by adult cochlear implant recipients. J Acad Rehabil Audiol. 2000;33:115-38.

72. Lassaletta L, Castro A, Bastarrica M, et al. Musical perception and enjoyment in post-lingual patients with cochlear implants. Acta Otorrinolaringol Esp. 2008; 59:228-34.

73. Gfeller K, Oleson J, Knutson JF, et al. Multivariate predictors of music perception and appraisal by adult cochlear implant users. J Am Acad Audiol. 2008;19: 120-34.

74. Gfeller K, Jiang D, Oleson J, et al. Temporal stability of music perception and appraisal scores of adult cochlear implant recipients. J Am Acad Audiol. 2010; 21:28-34.

75. Gfeller K, Turner C, Oleson J, et al. Accuracy of cochlear implant recipients on pitch perception, melody recognition, and speech reception in noise. Ear Hear. 2007;28:412-23.

76. Looi V, McDermott H, McKay C, et al. Comparisons of quality ratings for music by cochlear implant and hearing aid users. Ear Hear. 2007;28:59S-61S.

77. Tyler RS, Parkinson AJ, Wilson BS, et al. Patients utilizing a hearing aid and a cochlear implant: speech perception and localization. Ear Hear. 2002;23: 98-105.

78. Kiefer J, von Ilberg C, Reimer B, et al. Results of cochlear implantation in patients with severe to profound hearing loss—implications for patient selection. Audiology. 1998;37:382-95.

79. Gantz BJ, Turner C. Combining acoustic and electrical speech processing: Iowa/Nucleus hybrid implant. Acta Otolaryngol. 2004;124:344-7.

80. Gantz BJ, Turner C, Gfeller KE, et al. Preservation of hearing in cochlear implant surgery: advantages of combined electrical and acoustical speech processing. Laryngoscope. 2005;115:796-802.

81. Kong YY, Stickney GS, Zeng FG. Speech and melody recognition in binaurally combined acoustic and electric hearing. J Acoust Soc Am. 2005;117:1351-61.

82. Gfeller K, Turner C, Oleson J, et al. Accuracy of cochlear implant recipients on pitch perception, melody recognition, and speech reception in noise. Ear Hear. 2007;28:412-23.

83. Gfeller KE, Olszewski C, Turner C, et al. Music perception with cochlear implants and residual hearing. Audiol Neurootol. 2006;11:12-5.

84. Gfeller K, Turner C, Oleson J, et al. Accuracy of cochlear implant recipients on pitch perception, melody recognition, and speech reception in noise. Ear Hear. 2007;28:412-23.

85. Gfeller KE, Olszewski C, Turner C, et al. Music perception with cochlear implants and residual hearing. Audiol Neurootol. 2006;11:12-5.

86. Kong YY, Stickney GS, Zeng FG. Speech and melody recognition in binaurally combined acoustic and electric hearing. J Acoust Soc Am. 2005;117:1351-61.

87. Looi V, Gfeller K, Driscoll V. Music appreciation and training for cochlear implant recipients: a review. Semin Hear. 2012;33:307-34.

88. Looi V, Radford CJ. A comparison of the speech recognition and pitch ranking abilities of children using a unilateral cochlear implant, bimodal stimulation or bilateral hearing aids. Int J Ped Otorhinolaryngol. 2011;74:472-82.

89. Leal MC, Shin YJ, Ladorde ML, et al. Music perception in adult cochlear implant recipients. Acta Otolaryngol. 2003;123:826-35.

90. Gfeller K, Knutson JF, Woodworth G, et al. Timbral recognition and appraisal by adult cochlear implant users and normal-hearing adults. J Am Acad Audiol. 1998;9:1-19.

91. Gfeller K, Witt S, Woodworth G, et al. Effects of frequency, instrumental family, and cochlear implant type on timbre recognition and appraisal. Ann Otol Rhinol Laryngol. 2002;111:349-56.

92. Looi V, She JHK. Music perception of cochlear implant users: a questionnaire, and its implications for a music training program. Int J Audiol. 2010;49:116-28.

93. Looi V, McDermott H, McKay C, et al. Comparisons of quality ratings for music by cochlear implant and hearing aid users. Ear Hear. 2007;28:59S-61S.

94. Gfeller K, Christ A, Knutson J, et al. The effects of familiarity and complexity on appraisal of complex songs by cochlear implant recipients and normal hearing adults. J Music Ther. 2003;40:78-112.

95. Certo MV, Kohlberg GD, Chari DA, et al. Reverberation time influences musical enjoyment with cochlear implants. Otol Neurotol. 2015;36:e46-50.

96. Looi V, She JHK. Music perception of cochlear implant users: a questionnaire, and its implications for a music training program. Int J Audiol. 2010;49:116-28.

97. Drennan WR, Oleson JJ, Gfeller K, et al. Clinical evaluation of music perception, appraisal and experience in cochlear implant users. Int J Audiol. 2015;54:114-23.

98. Looi V, Gfeller K, Driscoll V. Music appreciation and training for cochlear implant recipients: a review. Semin Hear. 2012;33:307-34.

99. Gfeller K, Christ A, Knutson JF, et al. Musical backgrounds, listening habits, and aesthetic enjoyment of adult cochlear implant recipients. J Am Acad Audiol. 2000;11:390-406.

100. Looi V, She JHK. Music perception of cochlear implant users: a questionnaire, and its implications for a music training program. Int J Audiol. 2010;49:116-28.

101. Lassaletta L, Castro A, Bastarrica M, et al. Musical perception and enjoyment in post-lingual patients with cochlear implants. Acta Otorrinolaringol Esp. 2008;59:228-34.

102. Gfeller K, Witt S, Stordahl J, et al. The effects of training on melody recognition and appraisal by adult cochlear implant recipients. J Acad Rehabil Audiol. 2000;33:115-38.

103. Gfeller K, Witt S, Adamek M, et al. Effects of training on timbre recognition and appraisal by postlingually deafened cochlear implant recipients. J Am Acad Audiol. 2002;13:132-45.

104. Driscoll V, Oleson J, Jiang D, et al. The effects of training on recognition of musical instruments presented through cochlear implant simulations. J Am Acad Audiol. 2009;20:71-82.

105. Gfeller K, Driscoll V, Kenworthy M, et al. Music therapy for preschool cochlear implant recipients. Music Ther Perspect. 2011;29:39-49.

106. Hsiao F, Gfeller K. Music perception of cochlear implant recipients with implications for music instruction: a review of literature. Update Univ S C Dep Music. 2012;30:5-10.

107. Hsiao F, Gfeller K. How we do it: adaptation of music instruction for pediatric cochlear implant recipients. Cochlear Implants Int. 2011;12:205-08.

108. Trehub SE, Vongpaisal T, Nakata T. Music in the lives of deaf children with cochlear implants. Ann NY Acad Sci. 2009;1169:534-42.

109. Yucel E, Sennaroglu G, Belgin E. The family oriented musical training for children with cochlear implants: speech and musical perception results of two year follow-up. Int J Pediatr Otorhinolaryngol. 2009;73:1043-52.

110. Looi V, She JHK. Music perception of cochlear implant users: a questionnaire, and its implications for a music training program. Int J Audiol. 2010;49:116-28.

111. Kohlberg GD, Mancuso DM, Chari DA, et al. Music engineering as a novel strategy for enhancing music enjoyment in the cochlear implant recipient. Behav Neurol. 2015.

112. Looi V, She JHK. Music perception of cochlear implant users: a questionnaire, and its implications for a music training program. Int J Audiol. 2010;49:116-28.

113. Drennan WR, Oleson JJ, Gfeller K, et al. Clinical evaluation of music perception, appraisal and experience in cochlear implant users. Int J Audiol. 2015;54: 114-23.

Chapter 11

Contemporary Vestibular Testing

Steven D Rauch

OVERVIEW

This chapter presents a review of current means of testing the vestibular system and current patterns of vestibular test usage. Then, the chapter covers promising vestibular function tests that are just emerging in clinical use. Finally, the chapter considers new tests that are currently undergoing preclinical evaluation.

VESTIBULAR SYSTEM AND CURRENT VESTIBULAR DIAGNOSTIC TESTING

Sense of balance is different from all the other senses. Each of the other senses has only a single input: you hear with your ears, you see with your eyes, and you smell with your nose. Balance is different. Balance receives diverse inputs (Flowchart 11.1). The vestibular system receives input from the five inner ear balance organs, three semicircular canals to detect rotation, and two otolith organs to detect linear movements. The vestibular system also receives vision input that provides cues to spatial position, and it receives somatosensory inputs from joint and muscle proprioception. There are also autonomic inputs from lower extremity and gut vasculature that may play a significant role in certain settings. All these major inputs, inner ear, vision, and proprioception, converge in the vestibular brain stem. In the vestibular brain stem these signals are compared to see if they agree and they are integrated to create a sense of spatial orientation that we call balance. This comparison and sensory integration task was learned early in life, during infancy and toddlerhood, when young children are sitting, crawling, and walking. After sensory integration, the brain passes the signals for other processing and then to efferent pathways. Some of these go to the eyes to create the vestibulo-ocular reflexes (VOR) that allow us to maintain gaze fixation when the head is moving. Other signals go down the spine as vestibular spinal reflexes that help

Flowchart 11.1: Block diagram of the vestibular system

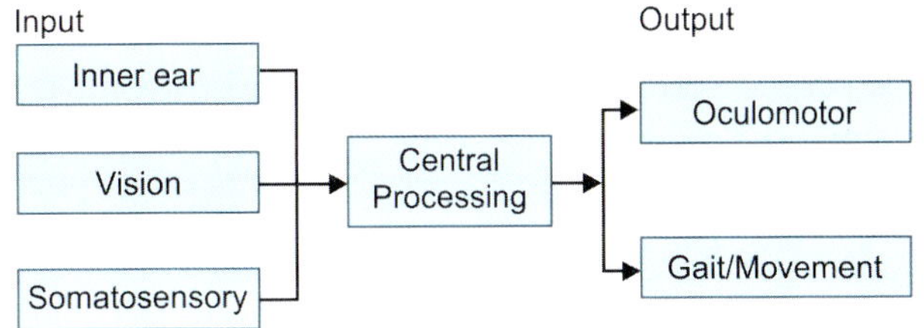

The vestibular system receives inputs on three "channels": inner ear, vision, and somatosensory (i.e. tactile and proprioception).

The inputs go to brainstem vestibular nuclei and to cerebellum for processing. At the central level, the inputs are compared and should corroborate each other. Disagreement (a.k.a. "sensory conflict") results in vertigo, dysequilibrium, and motion sickness.

Output to eye muscles enables gaze stabilization during motion. Output via vestibulospinal tracts enables control of locomotion.

maintain posture and gait stability. A disturbance anywhere in the sensory inputs, central processing, or the motor outputs may cause a sense of imbalance, vertigo, or dizziness.

One of the consequences of having diverse vestibular inputs and complex central integration of these inputs is that damage or loss of any one input can be managed by central adaptation or compensation to "recalibrate" and glean enough vestibular information to maintain acceptable balance. This is quite different from hearing, for example. When loss of an ear leaves a patient with a persistent hearing deficit, it is easily measurable with a behavioral audiogram. Measurements of vestibular function are indirect and poorly correlated with specific physical symptoms of dizziness or dysequilibrium. In the majority of standard vestibular function tests, a movement or motion input is provided and a postural or oculomotor output is measured. The normal input–output relationship of the vestibular system is well known. However, in a patient with vestibular pathology, an input can be provided and an output measured, but the output is highly ambiguous. Adaptation and central processing can compensate for damage to the input so that output measures are only a dim reflection of input damage. Standard vestibular function testing includes electro- and/or videonystagmography, sinusoidal vertical axis rotation testing, and computerized dynamic posturography. The objective of each of these tests is to determine the integrity of the sensory pathways of the inner ear vestibular organs and vestibular nerves. However, all the standard tests are measuring efferent reflexes, an indirect measure of input and central processing problems.

Clinicians face the challenge of determining who to test, when to test, and which of these tests is most applicable. There are four circumstances in which vestibular function testing is clinically useful. The first is for confirmation or hypothesis testing. In this instance, the clinician may have a general idea of the problem and would like to seek objective confirmation. An example would be a patient who has a report of episodic vertigo and some hearing loss on one side and appears to fit diagnostic criteria for Meniere's disease. The Vestibular test battery is expected to show peripheral vestibular hypofunction in the ear that is both symptomatically and audiometrically affected. A second indication for vestibular function test is to provide a more complete picture where a bedside examination may only provide a sketch. An auditory analogy would be the circumstance where a bedside ear examination with whispered speech and tuning forks makes it clear that a patient has a mild or moderate hearing loss that suggests presbycusis. Even though the clinical scenario seems clear-cut, it is standard practice to send the patient for a comprehensive audiogram, including air- and bone-conducted pure tone thresholds and word recognition scores. This more complete data set provides a richer picture of the objective aspects of the patient's auditory dysfunction, which the experienced clinician can correlate well with the patient's report of symptoms. A third indication for vestibular function testing is documentation. Patients who have suffered injuries coming up for medicolegal review or patients who are about to undergo invasive or irreversible ablative surgical procedures benefit from documentation to provide objective measures of the current status quo vis-à-vis vestibular function. For example, a patient who is going to receive intratympanic gentamicin for Meniere's disease is advised to have vestibular function testing, both to assess the degree of dysfunction in the affected ear and also to assess whether or not there is any occult dysfunction on the asymptomatic ear. This information helps the clinician to counsel the patient about the expected post-treatment recovery. Finally, vestibular function testing is indicated as a means of hunting for hints or clues when thorough medical history and physical examination fail to provide a clear-cut diagnosis. This may be the most common indication for vestibular function in use by inexperienced clinician, but is done with reluctance by experienced "dizzy doctors". There is high likelihood of the test battery identifying minor abnormalities that are not well correlated with clinical presentation and can lead one down a long path of uninformative diagnostic studies and consultations.

Despite the limitations of currently available vestibular function tests, vestibular diagnostic testing can still be extremely informative. The positive and negative predictive value of vestibular function tests is intimately related to the specificity of the diagnostic question that is posed. Imagine this radiologic analogy: If a patient is sent to the Radiology Department with a requisition stating, "Sick patient, please scan", the radiologist will be unable to offer very helpful diagnostic service. In contrast, if the requisition states "Febrile patient with left-sided pleuritic chest pain and productive cough, rule out pneumonia" the radiologist can offer a very precise series of X-rays or scans to isolate the problem and confirm the diagnosis. Likewise, if a dizzy patient is sent to the vestibular laboratory with a requisition stating "Dizzy patient", the vestibular diagnostic laboratory provides only very limited feedback. A requisition stating, "Unilateral right side sensorineural hearing loss, episodic vertigo, rule out right side vestibular hypofunction", provides the laboratory all the information it needs to provide a very specific evaluation and assessment. Regrettably this style of very specific diagnostic questions submitted to the vestibular diagnostic laboratory is the exception rather than the rule. This is a matter of educating the physicians who are ordering the tests.

Ultimately, the standard vestibular test battery of videonystagmography (VNG), rotary chair testing, and dynamic posturography provides responses to a hierarchy of questions. The first question: Is there any vestibular pathology? In patients who have complaints of dizziness and imbalance, approximately two thirds of vestibular test batteries will identify some objective abnormality of central or peripheral vestibular function.[1] The second question: Is the pathology central, peripheral, or mixed? If the pathologic findings indicate a peripheral site, the third question: Is the abnormality right or left sided?

As stated above, the standard vestibular test battery comprises an electronystagmography (ENG)/VNG, sinusoidal vertical axis rotation with visual-vestibular interaction, and computerized dynamic posturography. The ENG/VNG testing has a component of voluntary and visually evoked eye movements to confirm normal ocular motility, a series of reflexive eye movements that are also oculomotor in nature (optokinetic nystagmus, saccadic pursuit, and sinusoidal gaze tracking), and finally, a series of evoked eye movements related to vestibular function, including positioning and positional testing (Dix-Hallpike test) and aphysiologic vestibular-evoked testing, the caloric test. Each of these components of the test gives important information about ocular motility, central vestibular function, and peripheral vestibular function. The caloric test, the best-known vestibular function test among otolaryngologists, is quite sensitive to actual peripheral vestibular pathology but prone to many false positives and negatives due to anatomic variations and technical issues in the administration of the test.[2] The bithermal water caloric is the reliability standard of this test, though many clinicians use warm and cool air stimuli. Air stimulation, however, may not transmit enough thermal stimulus through soft tissue and bone, especially if the temporal bone is well pneumatized. In cases of eardrum perforation or mucosalized areas in the ear canal or mastoid cavity, blowing warm air into a moist ear can produce evaporation and a paradoxical cool caloric. This creates eye movements in the "wrong" direction and confounds interpretation of the test. Even with the water caloric, there are inconsistencies due to anatomy or to difficulty properly positioning the irrigation catheter in the ear canal. Water calorics cannot be performed if there is an ear drum perforation. Neither air nor water calorics can be interpreted accurately if there has been tympanomastoid surgery.

Sinusoidal vertical axis rotation is a highly reliable test for detecting peripheral and central vestibular dysfunction.[3] It is far more specific than caloric testing but less sensitive. It also suffers from the problem that the stimulus is administered to both ears simultaneously. If the phase and gain outputs of eye movement during the sinusoidal testing are abnormal, it is often impossible to determine which is the pathologic ear. Ideally, the results of the vertical axis rotation test are interpreted in light of the caloric findings. If the caloric suggests pathology on one side and the vertical axis rotation test suggests peripheral hypofunction, these two facts are combined to confirm a unilateral peripheral abnormality. If there is no significant caloric asymmetry, but the rotation testing is abnormal, it is ambiguous if there is a unilateral loss or a partial bilateral loss. Visual-vestibular interaction testing is a supplement to the standard sinusoidal vertical axis rotation test. It provides visual stimuli while the patient is rotating in the chair. Normal performance on the test requires central integration of visual and vestibular inputs in both synergistic and antagonistic modes. Failure of these tests is an indication of central vestibular dysfunction. Computerized dynamic posturography is the one common test that measures vestibulo-spinal reflexes rather than VOR. It is a measure of static postural stability under a series of different challenges as the patient is deprived of other sensory signals or as those other sensory inputs are distorted. Unfortunately, the posturography test has been shown to have rather limited clinical application.[4] It is most effective as a means of detecting malingers. Poor performance on the test when deprived of visual and proprioceptive input, the so-called vestibular pattern, correlates somewhat with patient complaints of poor balance, but is of no help in determining the site of lesion or a specific diagnosis.

EMERGING CLINICAL VESTIBULAR DIAGNOSTIC TESTS

As noted above, the vestibular system receives input from five inner ear vestibular organs, the three semicircular canals and the two otolith organs. The standard vestibular diagnostic tests primarily test function of the horizontal semicircular canal. This is the case both for caloric and for rotary chair testing. There are two newer vestibular diagnostic tests that extend our ability to measure function in the other inner ear vestibular organs. These are the video head impulse test (vHIT) and the vestibular-evoked myogenic potential (VEMP).

Video Head Impulse Test

The vHIT is a means of measuring VOR in response to a very high velocity input. When the head is moved quickly in the plane of one of the semicircular canals, the eyes make a compensatory movement in the opposite direction in order to stabilize gaze. This is the so-called head impulse test developed by Halmagyi and Curthoys.[5] If the head thrust is made in the horizontal plane, the horizontal semicircular canal drives the reflexive eye movement. If the head is rotated slightly and pitched forward or back, it will stimulate either the superior semicircular canal or the contralateral posterior semicircular canal. In this way, each of the six semicircular canals can be tested independently.[6-10] If one of these canals is weak, head thrust in the appropriate plane and direction will evoke a weak eye response. A pair of head-mounted goggles with an accelerometer to read the head movement stimulus and with infrared camera to read the oculomotor response has been developed and is available from several manufacturers. The head movement and eye movement responses are sent from the goggles to a computer, which can display these movements as a video trace of the head movement versus the eye movement. The ratio of eye movement to head movement is referred to as gain. In a normal ear the gain approaches one. As the eye movement is reduced by inner pathology, this gain value gets smaller and smaller.

The equipment to administer the vHIT test is relatively inexpensive compared to many other types of vestibular function diagnostic equipment. The equipment is lightweight and portable. The training to properly administer and interpret the test is also relatively simple and straightforward. This is the first diagnostic test approach that has enabled isolation of each of the six semicircular canals. All these features combine to make vHIT a highly appealing test that has seen rapid adoption in the last few years throughout the developed world. It is important to note that the vHIT is measuring performance of the vestibular end organs at high velocity. It is a velocity that may be seen in real world situations, but it is measuring something quite different from the caloric test, which measures horizontal canal function at exceedingly low velocity created by inner ear fluid convection current. Thus, the caloric test and the vHIT are measuring different velocity extremes of end organ sensitivity and are thus complimentary. One does not replace the other. The sensitivity of the caloric test may be greater than the sensitivity fo the vHIT but the caloric test only measures the horizontal canal while the vHIT tests all six canals.

Vestibular-Evoked Myogenic Potentials

Vestibular-evoked myogenic potentials are electrical muscle potentials that can be recorded in the head and neck region in response to acoustic stimulation of the otolith organs. The first VEMP test to be brought to clinical application is the cervical VEMP, or cVEMP test.[11,12] In this study a train of high intensity tone pips is played into the ear and recordings are made at the ipsilateral sternocleidomastoid muscle (Fig. 11.1). Acoustic stimulation of the saccule evokes a signal that ascends in the inferior vestibular nerve to the vestibular brainstem. From there it exerts an inhibitory influence on descending motor signals to the ipsilateral sternocleidomastoid muscle. Electromyography recordings of the sternocleidomastoid can be signal averaged to identify these inhibitory influences.[13,14] The strengths of the cVEMP test derive from

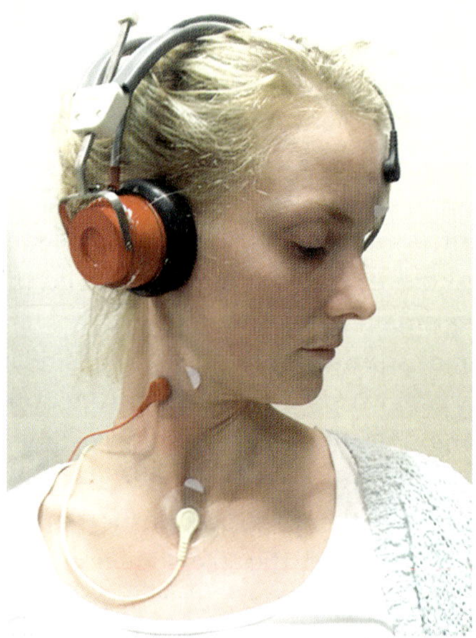

Fig. 11.1: cVEMP testing setup.

the fact that it arises exclusively from stimulation of the saccule and it is transmitted centrally exclusively by the inferior vestibular nerve. Weakness of the cVEMP test includes the fact that any degree of conductive hearing loss is likely to inhibit the response and, because the cVEMP is an inhibitory reflex, it can only be recorded when there is intense voluntary muscle retraction of the ipsilateral sternocleido-mastoid muscle. Patients with neck weakness or stiffness do not generate a reliable cVEMP response.

Response of the saccule to acoustic stimuli is frequency dependent. Although it is common in many centers to perform the cVEMP test with a 500 Hz tone burst and a recording of the cVEMP amplitude, it is much more clinically informative to perform the cVEMP with a range of tone burst frequencies (500 Hz, 750 Hz, and 1,000 Hz) and to record cVEMP threshold as the output. This is more time-consuming but provides a much more informative data set for detection or evaluation of peripheral dysfunction of the saccule and inferior vestibular nerve.[15]

In recent years, attention has also turned to ocular VEMP or oVEMP. The oVEMP is also generated by stimulation of otolith organs.[14] It is usually evoked with a bone conducted stimulus and the response arises predominately (but not exclusively) from the utricle. The signal is carried predominately (but not exclusively) by the superior vestibular nerve and crosses in the brainstem to evoke an excitatory response in the contralateral inferior oblique and inferior rectus muscles of the eye. During the test, the patient is instructed to look upward from neutral gaze in order to bring the inferior eye muscles in proximity to electrodes placed on or near the lower eyelid. A bone conduction stimulus is applied to the forehead and signal averaging is performed on the output at the eye muscle. Advocates of the oVEMP test note that its great advantage is that it enables measurement of otolith organ function even in the presence of conductive hearing loss because of the use of a bone conduction stimulus. However, the test is generally inferior to cVEMP because it does not arise exclusively from a single vestibular end organ and it does not ascend exclusively in a single vestibular nerve. It is a combination of utricular and saccular stimulation and both inferior and superior vestibular nerve transmission. Furthermore, there is some indication that the detectability of oVEMP falls off more rapidly with age than does the cVEMP.

Both oVEMP and cVEMP tests are seeing increased clinical use in recent years. However, the precise physiology being measured, the methodology for performing these measurements and the interpretation of the outputs are still evolving topics (Table 11.1). Implementation

Table 11.1: VEMP highlights.

	cVEMP	oVEMP
Sensory organ	Saccule	Utricle (mostly)
Best stimulus	Air-conducted tone burst	Bone-conducted tone burst
Neural pathway	Uncrossed/Inhibitory	Crossed/Excitatory
Recording site	Ipsilateral SCM muscle	Contralateral inferior oblique and rectus muscle

Flowchart 11.2: Vestibular psychophysics measures perception rather than reflex outputs.

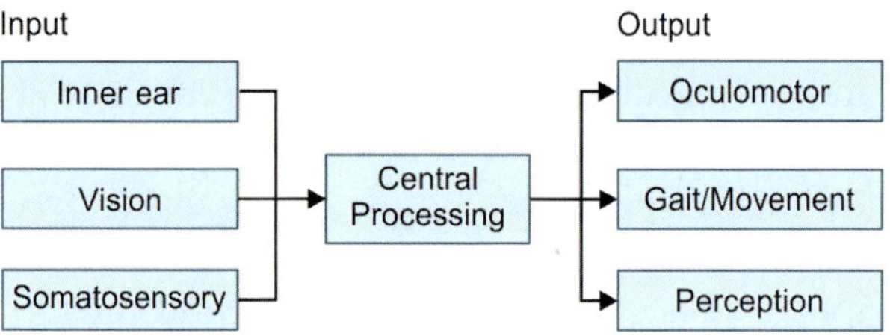

Perception is also an "output" of the vestibular system but it is an output to other higher brain centers rather than efferent neuromuscular pathways.

of their use in the clinical setting requires a significant commitment of time, resources, and personnel to develop the necessary expertise and good clinical practices to make the test most informative. There are no currently available commercial systems in the United States for performance of oVEMP and cVEMP testing. It is up to each clinical site to develop their own instrumentation and methodology.

FUTURE VESTIBULAR FUNCTION TESTING

The most promising new approach to assessment of vestibular function is vestibular psychophysical testing, a measure of perception rather than reflex output (Flowchart 11.2).[16] Psychophysical approaches have been used in hearing testing for decades. The behavioral audiogram is a psychophysical test where we measure perceptual thresholds for hearing. Detection of vestibular perceptual thresholds is challenging. It requires equipment that can deliver very subtle and very precise motion stimuli. The patient then raises a hand or presses a button to confirm that they are aware of the motion. The equipment must be able to deliver these stimuli in different planes of motion to test different parts of the vestibular system. Currently, this is only being done on a research basis. Preliminary results are quite promising. For example, Lewis and colleagues have demonstrated that this approach can differentiate patients with migraine-associated vertigo from normal subjects and from migraineurs without vertigo.[17] This is preliminary work and shows great promise but it remains to be seen if the findings can be validated in larger and more diverse patient populations. As noted above, the equipment for performing this testing is large and expensive. It is unclear if practical and cost-effective implementation of the approach will find its way into clinical practice.

As noted early in this chapter, current methods of vestibular function testing measure input–output characteristics of the vestibular system, but are poorly correlated with patient symptoms. One of the great strengths of psychophysical approach is that it is measuring features of vestibular function likely to be highly correlated with symptoms.

CONCLUSION

Standard vestibular function tests, including VNG, vertical axis rotation testing, and posturography are valuable adjuncts to evaluation of the dizzy patient. The more focused the clinical question that is posed to the vestibular laboratory, the more informative the interpretation of the vestibular function test results. Emerging approaches using vHIT and VEMP testing offer more precise localization of site of lesion in the vestibular end organs. The vHIT test measures each of the six semicircular canals independently. The cVEMP measures saccular function and the oVEMP measures predominately utricular function. While end organ site of lesion mapping is potentially informative and of substantial clinical value, all these tests still correlate poorly with patient's actual symptoms. Psychophysical measures of vestibular perceptual thresholds may soon enable us to make measurements that are more tightly correlated with patient symptoms and performance in daily life.

REFERENCES

1. Gordon CR, Shupak A, Spitzer O, et al. Nonspecific vertigo with normal otoneurological examination. The role of vestibular laboratory tests. J Laryngol Otol. 1996;110:1133-7.
2. Baloh R, Honrubia V. Clinical Neurophysiology of the Vestibular System, 3rd edition. Oxford University Press; 2001. pp. 171-208.
3. Priesol AJ, Cao M, Brodly CE, et al. Clinical vestibular testing assessed with machine-learning algorithms. JAMA Otolaryngol Head Neck Surg. 2015;141: 364-72.
4. Visser JE, Carpenter MG, van der Kooij H, et al. The clinical utility of posturography. Clin Neurophys. 2008;119:2424-36.
5. Halmagyi GM, Curthoys IS. A clinical sign of canal paresis. Arch Neurol. 1988;45: 737-9.

6. Weber KP, MacDougall HG, Halmagyi GM, et al. Impulsive testing of semi-circular-canal function using video-oculography. Ann N Y Acad Sci. 2009;1164: 486-91.

7. MacDougall HG, Weber KP, McGarvie LA, et al. The video head impulse test: diagnostic accuracy in peripheral vestibulopathy. Neurol. 2009;73:1134-41.

8. Macdougall HG, McGarvie LA, Halmagyi GM, et al. The video head impulse test (vHIT) detects vertical semicircular canal dysfunction. PLoS One. 2013;8: e61488.

9. MacDougall HG, McGarvie LA, Halmagyi GM, et al. Application of the video head impulse test to detect vertical semicircular canal dysfunction. Otol Neurotol. 2013;34(6):974-9.

10. McGarvie LA, MacDougall HG, Halmagyi GM, et al. The video head impulse test (vHIT) of semicircular canal function—age dependent normative values of VOR gain in healthy subjects. Front Neurol. 2015;6:154.

11. Colebatch JG, Halmagyi GM. Vestibular evoked potentials in human neck muscles before and after unilateral vestibular deafferentation. Neurology. 1992; 42:1635-6.

12. Ferber-Viart C, Dubreuil C, Duclaux R. Vestibular evoked myogenic potentials in humans: a review. Acta Otolaryngol (Stockh). 1999;119:6-15.

13. Curthoys IS, Manzari L. Otolithic disease: clinical features and the role of vestibular evoked myogenic potentials. Semin Neurol. 2013;33:231-7.

14. Curthoys IS, Vulovic V, Burgess AM, et al. Neural basis of new clinical vestibular tests: otolithic neural responses to sound and vibration. Clin Exp Pharmacol Physiol. 2014;41:371-80.

15. Rauch SD, Zhou G, Kujawa SG, et al. Vestibular evoked myogenic potentials (VEMPs) show altered tuning in patients with Meniere's disease. Otol Neurotol. 2004;25:333-8.

16. Merfeld DM, Priesol A, Lee D, et al. Potential solutions to several vestibular challenges facing clinicians. J Vestib Res. 2010;20:71-7.

17. Lewis RF, Priesol AJ, Nicoucar K, et al. Dynamic tilt thresholds are reduced in vestibular migraine. J Vestib Res. 2011;21:323-30.

Chapter 12

Recent Advances in Understanding the Pathogenesis of Acquired Cholesteatoma

Chin-Lung Kuo

OVERVIEW OF CHOLESTEATOMA

Cholesteatoma has been known for more than three centuries.[1] The disorder is commonly characterized as "skin in the wrong place",[2-4] given that it consists of a well-demarcated cystic lesion derived from an abnormal growth of "keratinizing squamous epithelium trapped within temporal bone".[5-7] Cholesteatoma is locally invasive and capable of causing the destruction of structures in the middle ear cleft. Associated intracranial complications can render cholesteatoma a cause of morbidity and death for individuals who lack access to suitable medical care.[8,9]

History and Etymology

The French anatomist Joseph-Guichard Du Verney first reported a cholesteatoma-like case in 1683.[10] In 1829, Cruveilhier first described the pathologic features of what he referred to as a pearly tumor (tumeur perlée), in reference to its pearl-white appearance.[11] However, it was the German anatomopathologist Johannes Mueller who first coined the term cholesteatoma (chole = cholesterol; stea = fat; oma = tumor) in 1838, based on the belief that cholesteatoma is a tumor, which is "greasy in nature".[7,12,13] Although further designations have also been proposed, such as "margaritoma" by Graigie in 1891[14] and "keratoma" by Schuknecht in 1974,[3] "cholesteatoma" has remained the most common term in clinical usage.[7,15,16] However, this is a misnomer because the lesion is neither composed of cholesterol crystals or fat nor is it of neoplastic nature.[7,15,17] These misunderstandings are the main reasons for the ambiguity associated with the term "cholesteatoma" in the medical community as well as in the population at large.

Histopathology of Cholesteatoma

Macroscopically, cholesteatoma presents as a whitish ovoid or round friable mass with a thin wall containing pultaceous or macerated

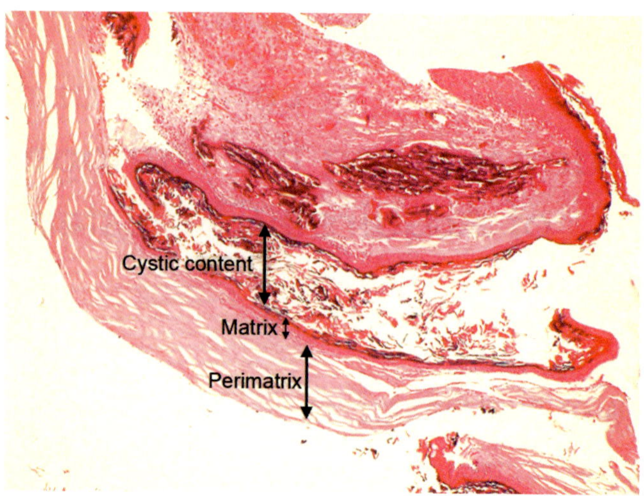

Fig. 12.1: Schematic illustration showing the structure of cholesteatoma. A mass of keratin material surrounded by a thin layer of stratified squamous epithelium and fibrous tissue with focal calcification (H&E, ×40).

material. Microscopically, the lesion can be divided into three layers: cystic content, matrix, and perimatrix (Fig. 12.1).[18]

The matrix of cholesteatoma possesses a morphology similar to that of the epidermis of regular skin, which is a keratinized stratified squamous epithelium composed of proliferating basal and differentiated suprabasal keratinocytes. The epidermis of regular skin typically comprises four or five layers, depending on the region of skin being considered (Fig. 12.2). The matrix of cholesteatoma is a stratified squamous epithelium, composed of a basal or germinal layer (stratum basale or germinativum), a spinous layer (stratum spinosum), a granular layer (stratum granulosum), a lucid layer (stratum lucidum, usually not detectable), and a cornified or horny layer (stratum corneum). The cornified layer of the matrix is hyperkeratotic and desquamating, and the lamellae of the keratin form the cystic content.[18] The cystic content is the central component of cholesteatoma and is composed of fully differentiated anucleate keratin squames mixed with sebaceous material and purulent and/or necrotic matter. The outermost layer is the perimatrix (lamina propria), which comprises inflamed subepithelial connective tissue (granulation tissue) containing collagen fibers, fibrocytes and inflammatory cells, such as lymphocytes, histiocytes, plasma cells, and neutrophilic leukocytes.[18-20]

Two Forms of Cholesteatoma: Congenital versus Acquired

Cholesteatoma is broadly divided into two types: (1) congenital, which is specific to childhood and (2) acquired, which affects children as

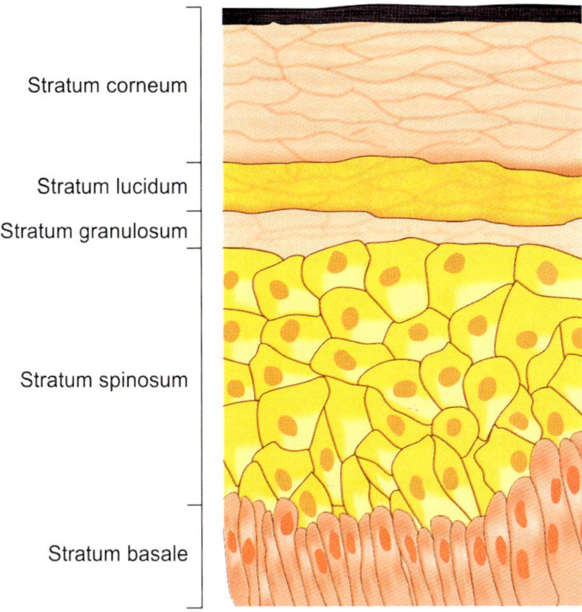

Fig. 12.2: Schematic representation showing the five layers in the epidermis of regular skin.

well as adults.[14] Congenital cholesteatoma arises as a nidus of trapped squamous epithelium behind an intact eardrum during embryogenesis and develops in children without a history of otitis media or previous otologic surgery. Congenital cholesteatoma is typically located in the anterior mesotympanum or the perieustachian tube area. Unlike congenital cholesteatomas, the acquired form typically develops as a result of chronic middle ear infection and may be associated with eardrum perforation.[21-23] To date, the mechanisms underlying the etiopathogenesis of acquired cholesteatoma remain a subject of competing hypotheses and debate. In this chapter, the author reviews previous research on acquired cholesteatoma and summarizes the evidence pertaining to its potential etiopathogenesis.

Epidemiology of Acquired Cholesteatoma

The annual incidence of acquired cholesteatoma ranges from approximately 9 to 12.6 cases per 100,000 adults and from 3 to 15 cases per 100,000 children.[14,24-27] The incidence of cholesteatoma is higher in males, with a male predominance (1.4:1).[16,28] The prevalence of cholesteatoma is highest among Caucasians, followed by Africans, and is seldom observed in non-Indian Asians.[20,29] Several families with multiple generations of affected individuals have recently been identified, which suggests that there may be an underlying genetic propensity for cholesteatoma.[30,31]

Clinical Presentations and Complications of Acquired Cholesteatoma

Patients with cholesteatomas often describe frequently recurring foul otorrhea, which is characterized by scant but purulent draining discharge. Hearing loss is usually progressive and can be conductive or sensorineural. Conductive hearing loss occurs when ossicles are impaired, and further damage to the cochlea may cause sensorineural hearing loss, occasionally complicated by tinnitus.[32] Destruction of the bone overlying the semicircular canals (particularly the horizontal canal) can lead to vertigo and balance dysfunction.[33] Violation of the facial nerve canal can lead to temporary or permanent facial paralysis.[34]

In the preantibiotic era, cholesteatomas were susceptible to secondary infections[35]; however, the recent widespread use of antibiotics has drastically reduced the incidence of these problems. Nonetheless, clinicians should be aware of the danger of infectious complications due to the fact that cholesteatomas seldom present signs of acute or chronic infection. Indeed, a failure to implement sufficient infection controls can lead to fatal complications, such as meningitis, brain abscess, epidural abscess, septic cavernous sinus thrombosis, and acute mastoiditis with subperiosteal abscess.[35-37]

In summary, cholesteatomas may exist in a nonaggressive state and remain undetected for years before the manifestation of potentially dangerous presentations.[38] Undiscovered or untreated cholesteatomas may grow dangerously large and/or invade intratemporal structures, leading to intra- and extracranial complications.[8,35-37,39-42] It is important to note that despite the fact that otalgia, headache, vomiting, and fever are not typical presentations of cholesteatoma, these occurrences are an indication of possible impending intratemporal or intracranial complications and thus require immediate assessment and treatment to minimize the likelihood of fatal consequences. Furthermore, recurrent or persistent otorrhea (for periods exceeding 2 weeks) and suspicious hearing impairments in previously operated ears should be treated as signs of potential cholesteatoma.[5]

PROMINENT THEORIES REGARDING THE ETIOPATHOGENESIS OF ACQUIRED CHOLESTEATOMA

Despite the fact that cholesteatoma has been known for more than three centuries, the nature of the disorder remains an issue of contention. Traditionally, four prominent theories have dominated the debate on the etiopathogenesis of acquired cholesteatoma: (1) squamous metaplasia theory, (2) epithelial invasion or migration theory (immigration theory), (3) basal cell hyperplasia theory (papillary ingrowth theory), and (4) invagination theory (retraction pocket theory).

Squamous Metaplasia Theory (Fig. 12.3)

The "squamous metaplasia theory" was most widely accepted among otologists of the 19th century. This theory was first proposed by Wendt in 1873, based on the assumption that metaplastic transformation of middle ear mucosa into keratinizing epithelium led to the formation of cholesteatoma.[43] The enlargement of cholesteatoma concurrent with infection and inflammation would lead to lysis and perforation of the tympanic membrane, resulting in the typical appearance of an attic cholesteatoma. Sadé provided evidence in support of this theory by demonstrating that chronic irritation can cause pluripotent mucosal epithelial cells to become keratinizing.[44,45] The "squamous metaplasia theory" has also been supported by animal studies.[46,47]

Epithelial Invasion or Migration Theory (Immigration Theory, Fig. 12.4)

"Epithelial invasion or migration theory" is another possible mechanism for the etiopathogenesis of primary acquired cholesteatoma. It was

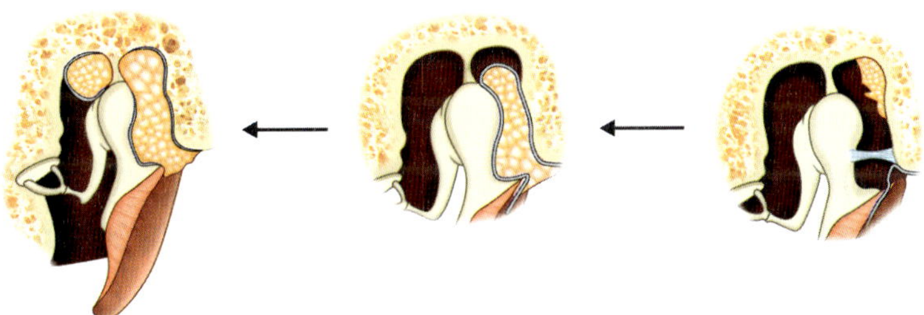

Fig. 12.3: Squamous metaplasia theory.

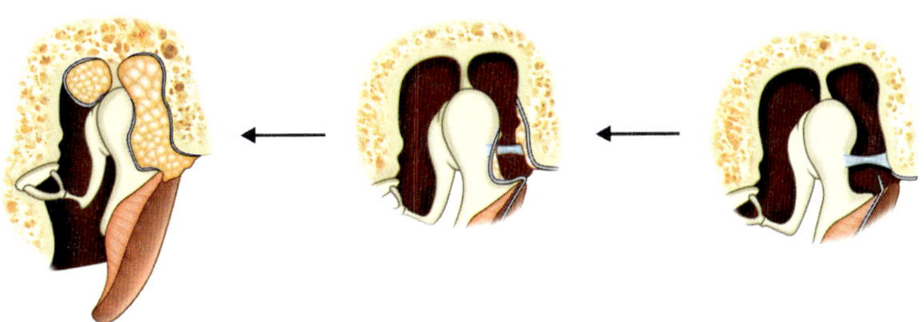

Fig. 12.4: Epithelial invasion or migration theory (immigration theory).

independently proposed by Habermann in 1888[48] and Bezold in 1890,[49] based on observations made during surgery. This theory is based on the assumption that the keratinizing squamous epithelium of the tympanic membrane invades or migrates into the middle ear through a defect in the tympanic membrane. The concept of the theory has been further strengthened by contemporary researchers. For example, following the examination of histologic sections of the temporal bones of 60 children, Karmody and Northrop found evidence that the squamous epithelium of the tympanic membrane actively migrates toward the middle ear in a medial direction.[50] Accordingly, a retraction pocket would not be regarded as the precursor of acquired cholesteatoma. This theory has also been corroborated in animal studies.[51,52]

Basal Cell Hyperplasia Theory (Papillary Ingrowth Theory, Fig. 12.5)

In 1925, Lange challenged the theory of squamous metaplasia with the "basal cell hyperplasia theory", which states that subepithelial tissue in Prussak's space is invaded by cholesteatoma microcysts within Shrapnell's membrane (pars flaccida).[53] Microcysts, buds, or pseudopods then form within the basal layer of the epithelium and fill with keratin.[54-57] This would preclude the need for perforations or a retraction pocket of the tympanic membrane to serve as prerequisites for the formation of an attic cholesteatoma. This theory would also help to account for the type of human cholesteatoma that occurs behind an intact tympanic membrane.[55,58,59] The hypothesis of squamous metaplasia has been substantiated in several clinical, experimental, and animal studies.[47,55,60,61]

Invagination Theory (Retraction Pocket Theory, Fig. 12.6)

Invagination theory (i.e. retraction pocket of tympanic membrane), first proposed by Wittmaack in 1933,[62] is currently the most widely

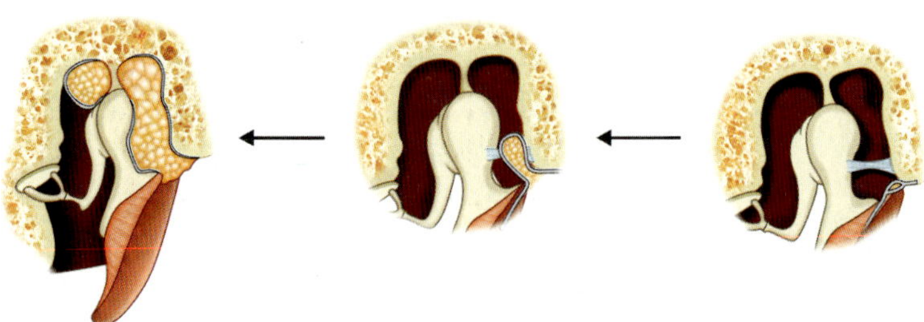

Fig. 12.5: Basal cell hyperplasia theory (papillary ingrowth theory).

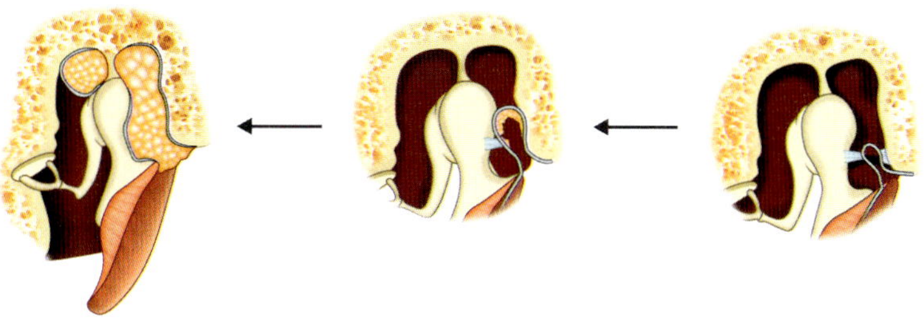

Fig. 12.6: Invagination theory (retraction pocket theory).

accepted explanation for acquired cholesteatoma. The theory states that a retraction pocket of the pars flaccida, which is less fibrous and less resistant to displacement than is pars tensa, is a precursor to cholesteatoma. The formation of the retraction pocket is due to negative pressure within the middle ear. This negative pressure may be induced by dysfunction of the Eustachian tube (hydrops ex vacuo), repeated inflammation, dysfunction in epitympanic recess ventilation, habitual sniffing, or a mastoid of small volume.[63-69] The retraction pocket deepens with the accumulation of desquamated keratin, whereupon the formation of a cholesteatoma obstructs the opening of the pocket, thereby inducing ingrowth expansion into the middle ear cleft.

Hybrid Theory

The retraction pocket theory is generally accepted as the most common pathogenic mechanism for cholesteatoma;[20] however, a number of otologists believe that the pathogenesis of this disorder is a complex hybrid process involving a combination of the abovementioned mechanisms and/or other mechanisms.[16,68,70] For example, in 2000, Sudhoff and Tos proposed a combination of the retraction pocket theory with the basal cell theory to explain the formation of retraction pocket cholesteatoma.[68]

In 2015, Jackler et al. proposed a new theory, referred to as the "mucosal traction theory" in which it was posited that mucosal membrane interactions are the driving force in cholesteatoma, wherein the sequential adhesion of opposing mucosal surfaces is induced by the retraction of bridging mucoid bands, as shown in Figure 12.7.[70] According to this theory, negative pressure within the middle ear causes deflation of the most pliant portions of the tympanic membrane; however, this would require that this retraction of the drum occurs in close proximity to the ossicles. The medial surface of the tympanic membrane and the lateral surface of the ossicles are then coapted, and the conjoined mucosal bilayer is reabsorbed, such that the coupling

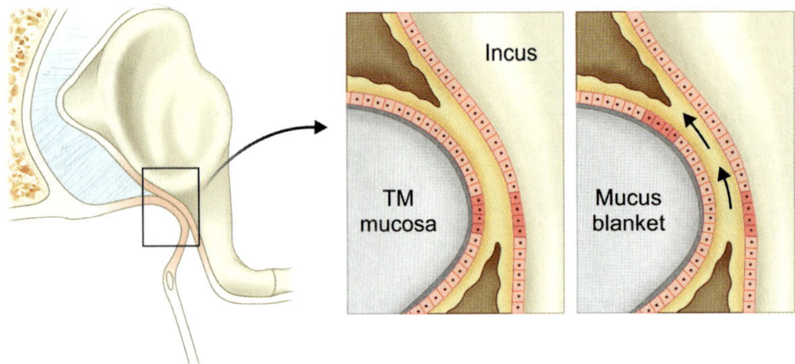

Fig. 12.7: Coupling of two opposing mucosal surfaces, resulting in the dragging of pliable tympanic membrane superiorly into the preformed mucosal cavities (middle ear and mastoid).

of the two opposing mucosal surfaces causes the pliable tympanic membrane to be dragged superiorly into the preformed mucosal cavities (the middle ear and mastoid). The trapping of mucosa and mucosal elements by this migration would lead to the production of proinflammatory cytokines, thereby promoting the proliferation and migration of keratinocytes.

The "mucosal traction theory" appears to explain the essential characteristics of most cases of acquired cholesteatoma and even provides a plausible explanation for the fact that some patients develop atelectasis while others develop a pouch. Nonetheless, a number of cases cannot be explained by this theory, such as those in which the tympanic membrane adheres to the medial wall of the middle ear with the ossicles warped within, which are referred to as adhesive otitis media. Regardless, only a small portion of adhesive otitis media (reportedly 25%) progress to cholesteatoma.[71] Conversely, cholesteatoma can develop even in cases where the tympanic membrane remains intact (i.e. without retraction).[55,58,59,72]

ADVANCES IN BIOMOLECULAR RESEARCH ON ETIOPATHOGENESIS

No single theory is able to explain the common clinical hallmarks of every type of cholesteatoma: uncoordinated hyperproliferation, invasion, migration, altered differentiation, aggressiveness, and recidivism.[16] However, a number of modern technologies, which examine biological properties at the molecular level, have been used to gain insight into the behavior of cholesteatoma. In the following section, the author summarizes recent important advances that have helped to elucidate the etiopathogenesis of acquired cholesteatoma.

Do Acquired Cholesteatomas Contain Cholesterol or Lipids?

For the past two decades, the term cholesteatoma (chole = cholesterol; stea = fat; oma = tumor) has been viewed as a misnomer due to the non-neoplastic nature of the disorder and the fact that cholesterol or lipids are no longer believed to be main constituents. However, a growing body of biochemical evidence implicates cholesterol as an essential component of cholesteatoma. Some studies have suggested that high concentrations of cholesterol may be synthesized from desmosterol and delta 7-cholestenol (lathosterol) in the matrix of cholesteatoma.[73,74] Recent biochemical analysis has also revealed that lipids in cholesteatoma are synthesized and stored in Odland bodies of the keratinocytes of the stratum granulosum, which comprises fatty acids, ceramides, and cholesterol.[16] Bloksgaard et al. recently applied multiphoton excitation fluorescence microscopy in their investigation into the morphology and intrinsic physical properties of acquired cholesteatoma.[75] Analysis of lipid composition in cholesteatoma has revealed the presence of all major classes of lipids in the stratum corneum of normal skin (ceramides, long-chain fatty acids, and cholesterol). Svane-Knudsen et al. also reported increased lipid metabolic activity in cholesteatoma.[76]

Nevertheless, the abovementioned observations may not be sufficient to draw a definitive conclusion as to the relationship between cholesterol and cholesteatoma. The fact that cholesterol has been found in the matrix of cholesteatomas does not necessarily mean that a cholesteatoma contains cholesterol. In fact, cholesterol crystals are commonly observed in the inflammatory magma of any long-standing middle ear inflammatory condition. Overall, this phenomenon may be viewed as a side-effect of local tissue breakdown, which provides a source of cholesterol in middle ear effusions and crystalline deposits.[77]

Genomic Instability in Acquired Cholesteatoma

Insufficient Evidence for Genomic Instability

The term cholesteatoma is also viewed as a misnomer because these growths are non-neoplastic and nonmetastatic in nature. There is insufficient evidence to suggest that cholesteatomas are premalignant or malignant lesions.[14,78,79] Cellular dysplasia, an early neoplastic process, does not appear to be a critical event in the genesis of cholesteatoma.[14,78-82] Several cytogenetic and histopathological studies have revealed that inherent genomic instability (in the form of abnormal or aneuploid quantities of DNA) is not always an essential feature of cholesteatoma.[78,79,83-85]

Connexin 26, also known as gap junction β-2 (GJB2), is one of the 21 structurally related transmembraneous proteins in humans that assemble to form intercellular channels, thereby allowing the rapid transport of selected ions and small molecules.[78,86] Connexin 26 is encoded by the *GJB2* gene, which is expressed in the cochlea and the skin. Mutations in the *GJB2* gene have been shown to cause congenital nonsyndromic sensorineural hearing loss and hyperkeratotic skin disorders.[87] Choung et al. identified the upregulation of connexin 26 in the epithelium of cholesteatoma in the human middle ear, compared with the levels observed in normal retroauricular skin and the skin of the ear canal.[86] Recent microarray analyses by Klenke et al. further revealed that the expression of *GJB2* is higher in cholesteatoma tissue than in the skin of the external auditory canal.[88] It would therefore be reasonable to assume that mutations in the *GJB2* gene could alter the development of cholesteatoma and/or influence the aggressiveness nature of the lesion. However, a prospective observational study by James et al. failed to identify any correlation between *GJB2* gene mutations and the severity of cholesteatoma (i.e. the extent of cholesteatoma growth and number of eroded ossicles).[87]

Potential Genomic Alterations in Cholesteatomas

Thus far, researchers have been unable to provide sufficient genomic evidence to support assertions related to premalignant or malignant processes in cholesteatoma. Nevertheless, a few cases of cholesteatoma-related carcinoma have been reported.[89-91] A growing number of researchers have been seeking to clarify the role of genomic instability in cholesteatoma.

First, alterations in the expression of proto-oncogenes (e.g. c-myc and c-jun) have been shown to contribute to the multifactorial pathogenesis of cholesteatoma.[14,92-96] Previous studies have revealed the down-regulation of several tumor suppressor genes (e.g. p53, p27, CDH18, 19 and ID4, PAX3, LAMC2, and TRAF2B) in cholesteatomas.[78,88,97,98] For instance, tumor protein p53, which is encoded by the *Tp53* gene, functions as a tumor suppressor. Tumor protein p53 protects the cell from genome mutation and/or the undesired propagation of DNA damage.[79,99,100] Mutations in the *p53* gene give rise to mutant p53 proteins, which are highly expressed in various types of cancer.[79,100] The expression of p53 in cholesteatoma appears to be higher than that in normal skin or the eardrum.[79]

Second, epidermal growth factor receptor (EGFR) is associated with keratinocyte proliferation to the basal layer in normal epidermis. The upregulation and activation of the EGFR, which has been observed in several tumor types, plays an important role in tumor initiation and progression.[101-104] A number of studies have identified alterations in the regulation of EGFR in cholesteatoma.[105,106] Furthermore, the over-expression of transforming growth factor α (TGF-α), a specific ligand involved in the activation of EGFR and a potent stimulator of cell growth, has also been found in cholesteatoma.[107]

In addition, cellular FLICE (FADD-like IL-1β-converting enzyme)–inhibitory protein (c-FLIP) is a master antiapoptotic regulator, which is highly expressed in human malignancies and benign hyperplastic epithelial disease.[108] An increase in the expression of c-FLIP has recently been observed in cholesteatoma, and the upregulation of c-FLIP appears to be positively correlated with that of Ki-67, a representative marker of hyperproliferation.[108]

E-cadherin and β-catenin are cell adhesion molecules essential to the maintenance of epithelial structure and function.[109] The increased invasiveness in squamous cell carcinoma is related to a reduction in the expression of E-cadherin and β-catenin,[110,111] which has also been observed in cholesteatoma. Notably, this reduction is more pronounced in acquired cholesteatoma than in the congenital form.[109] This difference in cell–cell adhesion between the acquired and congenital forms of cholesteatoma may explain the relatively aggressive nature of acquired cholesteatoma, compared with the congenital type.

The abovementioned research suggests the existence of a link between genomic alterations and the pathogenesis of cholesteatoma. However, it should be noted that existing evidence remains insufficient to make a definitive conclusion as to the actual underlying association between cholesteatoma and neoplasms.

Epigenetic Regulation in Cholesteatoma: The Role of MicroRNAs

Epigenetic regulation in cholesteatoma has been shown to play a critical role in the pathogenesis of cholesteatoma.[78] MicroRNAs are noncoding small RNA molecules (containing 22–24 nucleotides), which regulate the expression of post-transcriptional messenger RNA (mRNA).[78,112-116] Dysregulation of microRNA expression has been implicated in neoplastic and hyperproliferative diseases.[78,113,115]

For example, phosphatase and tensin homolog (PTEN) and pro-grammed cell death 4 (PDCD4) have been recognized as potent tumor suppressors, controlling various aspects of apoptosis, proliferation, invasion, and migration. Friedland et al. recently reported that the upregulation of microRNA-21 could lead to the suppression of PTEN and PDCD4, resulting in keratinocyte proliferation, migration, growth, and invasion in cholesteatoma.[115] Another study, performed by Chen and Qin, that examined the role of microRNAs in the pathogenesis of cholesteatomas, confirmed higher levels of microRNA-21 and a more pronounced reduction in PTEN and PDCD4 protein levels in cholesteatoma tissue, compared with that of normal skin, particularly among pediatric patients.[113]

Chen and Qin further compared cholesteatomas and normal skin tissue with regard to levels of microRNA-let-7a and its target protein, the high mobility group AT-hook 2 (HMGA2). HMGA2 has been identified as an oncogene, the overexpression of which is a common characteristic of neoplastic cells in both experimental and human models. They identified the upregulation of microRNA-let-7a concurrent with the downregulation of HMGA2 in cholesteatomas, compared with normal skin. This observation implies that microRNA-let-7a may inhibit the expression of HMGA2, leading to a reduction in the proliferation of cholesteatoma cells and increased keratinocyte apoptosis.

Over-Reaction of Host Immune Response to Inflammation

Researchers have been attempting to delineate the precise molecular and cellular dysfunctions involved in the pathogenesis of cholesteatomas. Recent advances in immunohistochemical analysis have revealed that interactions between matrix keratinocytes and perimatrix fibroblasts play an important role in the processes of homeostasis and tissue regeneration after inflammation.[117] Furthermore, the over-reaction of host immune response to inflammation via autocrine and paracrine signaling has recently been associated with the progression of cholesteatoma.[79,118-120] As shown in Figure 12.8, matrix keratinocytes secrete parathyroid-hormone-related proteins (PTHrPs) and proinflammatory cytokines, such as interleukin (IL)-1α, IL-1β, IL-6, and IL-8.[14,78,121] These keratinocyte-derived cytokines induce perimatrix fibroblasts to secrete several other cytokines, such as keratinocyte growth factor, granulocyte macrophage-colony stimulating factor, epidermal growth factor (EGF), tumor necrosis factor-α, platelet-derived growth factor, and TGF-α.[122-124] These fibroblast-derived cytokines in turn induce the differentiation, proliferation, and migration of matrix keratinocytes. In a form of autocrine signaling, TGF-α and TGF-β are constitutively expressed in hyperproliferative epithelium, regulating keratinocyte proliferation and differentiation.[14,78,125-127]

Recent studies have explored the role of the innate immune system in the etiopathogenesis and growth of cholesteatoma. In an

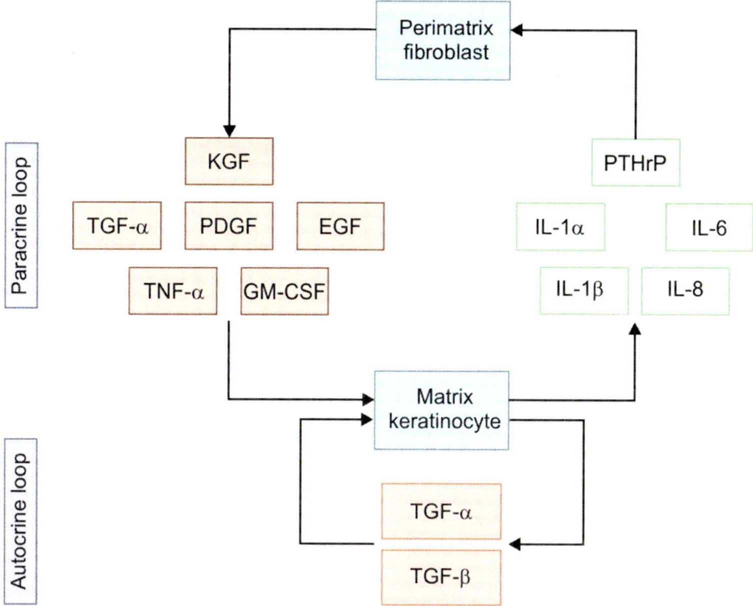

Fig. 12.8: Schematic representation showing paracrine and autocrine interactions between matrix keratinocytes and perimatrix fibroblasts.
(KGF: Keratinocyte growth factor; EGF: Epidermal growth factor; PDGF: Platelet-derived growth factor; TGF: Transforming growth factor; TNF: Tumor necrosis factor; GM-CSF: Granulocyte macrophage-colony stimulating factor; PTHrp: Parathyroid-hormone-related proteins; IL: interleukin).

inflammatory microenvironment, a variety of cells in the innate immune system (e.g. macrophages and neutrophils) express pattern recognition receptors (PRRs) for the identification of pathogens or pathogen-related molecular patterns. The Toll-like receptor (TLR) family is a major family of PRRs and is essential to the induction and activation of innate immunity during the course of an infection.[128,129] Szczepański et al. recently reported stronger expression of TLR-2, TLR-3, and TLR-4 in acquired cholesteatoma, compared with the weak expression of these receptors found in normal skin cells.[129] This evidence suggests that TLRs may play a role in the etiopathogenesis of cholesteatoma. Nucleotide-binding oligomerization domain (NOD) receptors and nod-like receptors (NLRs) are another major form of innate immune sensors, which are capable of responding immediately to pathogenic invasion.[130] Recent studies in gene association have revealed a relationship between enhanced NOD2 mRNA levels and the development of acquired cholesteatoma.[128,131] These findings indicate that the mediation of innate immune signaling by NLRs and TLRs may be involved in the etiopathogenesis and growth of cholesteatoma.

Bone Resorption in Acquired Cholesteatoma

Immunohistochemical analysis has recently revealed that the upregulation of cytokines in cholesteatoma may promote osteoclastogenesis via direct or indirect effects on osteoclasts, leading to inflammatory bone resorption. These cytokines include IL-1, IL-6, IL-17, interferon-β, and PTHrP.[16,78,132,133] Receptor activator of nuclear factor kappa-B ligand (RANKL), an osteoclast differentiation factor, has also been identified as an osteoimmune key regulator in bone physiology and pathology.[134] Osteoprotegerin (OPG), a soluble decoy receptor for RANKL, inhibits osteoclast formation by inhibiting interactions between RANKL and its membrane-bound receptor RANK. The RANKL/OPG/RANK axis has been shown to regulate bone remodeling, and more recently, this has been implicated in the bone remodeling of cholesteatoma.[135] A recent meta-analysis of five studies on the correlation of the RANKL/OPG/RANK system with middle ear cholesteatoma showed that a significantly positive correlation exists between increased RANKL expression and cholesteatoma, whereas OPG expression showed an inverse association with the disorder.[136]

Expansion of a cholesteatoma may lead to a rupturing of the cholesteatoma sac, resulting in the escape of keratinous substance and various proteolytic enzymes into the subepithelial layer (perimatrix).[18] The leaked content usually results in a marked granulomatous reaction to foreign bodies and bone destruction.[16,18,97] Matrix-metalloproteinases (MMPs) are important proteolytic enzymes in cholesteatoma, which have been shown to promote the aggressiveness of cholesteatoma with regard to the destruction of bony tissue.[16,97] Upregulated MMP expression (e.g. MMP1, MMP9, MMP10, and MMP12) and down-regulated expression of associated enzyme inhibitors (tissue inhibitor of metalloproteinases) constitute degradation of the extracellular matrix.[88] Pediatric cholesteatomas are generally more aggressive than their adult counterparts,[137] perhaps due to more severe inflammation and a greater number of metalloproteinases.[138]

Angiogenesis in Acquired Cholesteatoma

In addition to paracrine and autocrine regulatory mechanisms, angiogenesis in the perimatrix is also pivotal in the proliferation and aggressiveness of cholesteatoma. Angiogenesis is characteristic of middle ear inflammation, particularly in inflammatory granulation tissue and cholesteatoma.[139,140] Inflammatory cell populations (e.g. monocytes, macrophages, and infiltrating leukocytes) in the matrix and perimatrix release a variety of angiogenic growth factors, such as vascular endothelial growth factor (VEGF), IL-8, cyclooxygenase 2 (COX-2), EGF, platelet-derived growth factor, basic fibroblast growth factor, hepatocyte growth factor, and TGF-β.[14,78,140-142] These factors subsequently promote angiogenesis in the perimatrix, paving the way for the proliferation and increased aggressiveness of cholesteatoma through the provision of a new vascular network, similar to a scenario in tumor growth.[140] Among these angiogenic growth factors, VEGF, IL-8, and COX-2 are the most potent under inflammatory conditions found in the middle ear.[7,55,143,144] Recent studies have suggested that these three factors can be regulated by the transcription factor inhibitor of DNA binding (Id1),[140] which is active in the otitis media and the cholesteatomal perimatrix.[145,146] Therefore, Id1 may serve as a potential target for treatments addressing the progression of cholesteatoma in the middle ear cleft by downregulating the three aforementioned angiogenic growth factors and thereby inhibiting angiogenesis.

Role of Infection in Acquired Cholesteatoma

Recent breakthroughs suggest that middle ear infections may also influence the aggressiveness of cholesteatoma.[119] *Pseudomonas aeruginosa* is the bacteria most frequently identified with cholesteatoma.[147] The aerobic metabolism of *P. aeruginosa* induces the production of reactive oxygen species. Increases in oxidative stress and decreases in the level of antioxidants have recently been identified in cholesteatoma patients. An imbalance between oxidative processes and antioxidants increases biofilm production and appears to be involved in cholesteatoma pathogenesis.[148,149]

Furthermore, *P. aeruginosa* lipopolysaccharide (LPS) has been found to activate keratinocyte hyperproliferation in vitro,[119] which indicates that intracellular signal transduction cascades may be associated with cell proliferation in cholesteatoma. The presence of bacteria may prevent the cholesteatoma epithelium from activating the terminal differentiation program and returning to a state of quiescence. As a result, the on-going proliferative, migratory, and invasive behaviors tend to persist.[79]

Since the 1950s, researchers have been investigating the relevance of chemical lysis in bone destruction associated with cholesteatoma.[150] Kaneko et al. demonstrated that the acidic activity of escaped keratin debris from the cholesteatoma sac may play an important role in bone destruction.[151] These acids are derived from products of aerobic (e.g. *Staphylococcus aureus* and *Proteus* species) as well as anaerobic (e.g. *Peptococcus* and *Bacteroides* species) microorganisms.[152] In a recent laboratory study, Nguyen et al. indicated that the leakage of acid through the cholesteatoma epithelium may be caused by an increase in the permeability of the epithelium associated with a decrease in filaggrin expression.[153]

Other researchers have recently revealed that high concentrations of bacterial LPS associated with prolonged inflammation may evoke myeloperoxidase (MPO) activity in cholesteatoma.[154] The MPO is a hemeprotein and the key constituent of neutrophil azurophilic granules capable of producing hypohalous acids to carry out antimicrobial activity.[154,155] Researchers have shown that increased MPO expression is associated with the cholesteatoma-related destruction of bone.[154,156]

CONCLUSION

Recent advances in biomolecular research have deepened our understanding of the etiopathogenesis of acquired cholesteatoma. This chapter summarizes existing theories and presents the current state of research on etiopathogenesis. Unfortunately, existing evidence is insufficient to enable the formulation of any conclusions with regard to the true nature of cholesteatoma. It appears that the pathogenetic process of cholesteatoma is multifactorial, comprising several complex and dynamic pathophysiologic changes that involve extracellular as well as intracellular signal transduction cascades.

None of the numerous theories that have been posited are able to provide a comprehensive explanation of all aspects of the observed behavior of cholesteatoma. Indeed, the development of each proposed mechanism was based on individual empirical or experimental observations, i.e. descriptive accounts of how cholesteatomas behave under specific conditions. With further advances in the field of otology, our understanding of the etiopathogenesis and behavior of acquired cholesteatoma will no doubt continue to evolve. It is the opinion of the author that a single-minded quest to find a comprehensive theory capable of explaining the multifactorial pathogenesis of cholesteatoma should not be the aim of research efforts. Rather, the major challenge lies in identifying relationships among existing theories to produce a network of theories capable of furthering the development of improved treatment modalities.

REFERENCES

1. Kuo CL, Liao WH, Shiao AS. A review of current progress in acquired cholesteatoma management. Eur Arch Otorhinolaryngol. 2015;272(12):3601-9.
2. Moran WB Jr. Cholesteatoma. In: English GE (Ed). Otolaryngology. New York: Harper & Row; 1980.

3. Schuknecht HF. The Pathology of the Ear. Cambridge: Harvard University; 1974.
4. Robinson JM. Cholesteatoma: skin in the wrong place. J R Soc Med. 1997;90:93-6.
5. Isaacson G. Diagnosis of pediatric cholesteatoma. Pediatrics. 2007;120:603-8.
6. Semaan MT, Megerian CA. The pathophysiology of cholesteatoma. Otolaryngol Clin North Am. 2006;39:1143-59.
7. Dornelles C, Costa SS, Meurer L, et al. Some considerations about acquired adult and pediatric cholesteatomas. Braz J Otorhinolaryngol. 2005;71:536-45.
8. Prescott CA. Cholesteatoma in children—the experience at The Red Cross War Memorial Children's Hospital in South Africa 1988-1996. Int J Pediatr Otorhinolaryngol. 1999;49:15-9.
9. Diom ES, Cisse Z, Tall A, et al. Management of acquired cholesteatoma in children: a 15 year review in ENT service of CHNU de FANN Dakar. Int J Pediatr Otorhinolaryngol. 2013;77:1998-2003.
10. Du Verney JG. Traité de l'organe de l'ouie. Paris: E. Michaillet, 1683.
11. Cruveilhier J. Anatomie Pathologique du Corps Humain. Paris: Baillière, 1829.
12. Müller J. Über den feineren Bau und die Formen der krankhaften Geschwülste. Erste Lieferung. Berlin: G. Reimer, 1838.
13. Soldati D, Mudry A. Knowledge about cholesteatoma, from the first description to the modern histopathology. Otol Neurotol. 2001;22:723-30.
14. Kuo CL, Shiao AS, Yung M, et al. Updates and knowledge gaps in cholesteatoma research. Biomed Res Int. 2015;2015:854024.
15. Barath K, Huber AM, Stampfli P, et al. Neuroradiology of cholesteatomas. AJNR Am J Neuroradiol. 2011;32:221-9.
16. Olszewska E, Wagner M, Bernal-Sprekelsen M, et al. Etiopathogenesis of cholesteatoma. Eur Arch Otorhinolaryngol. 2004;261:6-24.
17. Sie KC. Cholesteatoma in children. Pediatr Clin North Am. 1996;43:1245-52.
18. Ferlito A. A review of the definition, terminology and pathology of aural cholesteatoma. J Laryngol Otol. 1993;107:483-8.
19. Lim DJ, Saunders WH. Acquired cholesteatoma: light and electron microscopic observations. Ann Otol Rhinol Laryngol. 1972;81:1-11.
20. Vital V. Pediatric cholesteatoma: personal experience and review of the literature. Otorhinolaryngol Head Neck Surg. 2011;45:5-14.
21. Spilsbury K, Miller I, Semmens JB, et al. Factors associated with developing cholesteatoma: a study of 45,980 children with middle ear disease. Laryngoscope. 2010;120:625-30.
22. Kuo CL, Lien CF, Shiao AS. Mastoid obliteration for pediatric suppurative cholesteatoma: long-term safety and sustained effectiveness after 30 years' experience with cartilage obliteration. Audiol Neurootol. 2014;19:358-69.
23. Kuo CL, Lien CF, Chu CH, et al. Otitis media with effusion in children with cleft lip and palate: a narrative review. Int J Pediatr Otorhinolaryngol. 2013;77:1403-9.
24. Aquino JE, Cruz Filho NA, de Aquino JN. Epidemiology of middle ear and mastoid cholesteatomas: study of 1146 cases. Braz J Otorhinolaryngol. 2011;77:341-7.
25. Louw L. Acquired cholesteatoma pathogenesis: stepwise explanations. J Laryngol Otol. 2010;124:587-93.
26. Kemppainen HO, Puhakka HJ, Laippala PJ, et al. Epidemiology and aetiology of middle ear cholesteatoma. Acta Otolaryngol. 1999;119:568-72.

27. Tos M. Incidence, etiology and pathogenesis of cholesteatoma in children. Adv Otorhinolaryngol. 1988;40:110-7.
28. Nelson M, Roger G, Koltai PJ, et al. Congenital cholesteatoma: classification, management, and outcome. Arch Otolaryngol Head Neck Surg. 2002;128:810-4.
29. Nevoux J, Lenoir M, Roger G, et al. Childhood cholesteatoma. Eur Ann Otorhinolaryngol Head Neck Dis. 2010;127:143-50.
30. Prinsley P. Familial cholesteatoma in East Anglia, UK. J Laryngol Otol. 2009;123: 294-7.
31. Homoe P, Rosborg J. Family cluster of cholesteatoma. J Laryngol Otol. 2007;121: 65-7.
32. Kuo CL, Shiao AS, Liao WH, et al. Can long-term hearing preservation be expected in children following cholesteatoma surgery? Results from a 14-year-long study of atticotomy-limited mastoidectomy with cartilage reconstruction. Audiol Neurootol. 2012;17:386-94.
33. Shohet JA, de Jong AL. The management of pediatric cholesteatoma. Otolaryngol Clin North Am. 2002;35:841-51.
34. Kuo CL, Liao WH, Li WY, et al. Deceptive facial nerve variant may cloud otologists' judgment: a dilemma in middle ear surgery. Int Adv Otol. 2014;10:291-3.
35. Migirov L, Yakirevitch A, Kronenberg J. Mastoid subperiosteal abscess: a review of 51 cases. Int J Pediatr Otorhinolaryngol. 2005;69:1529-33.
36. Prasad SC, Shin SH, Russo A, et al. Current trends in the management of the complications of chronic otitis media with cholesteatoma. Curr Opin Otolaryngol Head Neck Surg. 2013;21:446-54.
37. Maksimovic Z, Rukovanjski M. Intracranial complications of cholesteatoma. Acta Otorhinolaryngol Belg. 1993;47:33-6.
38. Shihada R, Brodsky A, Luntz M. Giant cholesteatoma of the temporal bone. Isr Med Assoc J. 2006;8:718-9.
39. Mustafa A, Heta A, Kastrati B, et al. Complications of chronic otitis media with cholesteatoma during a 10-year period in Kosovo. Eur Arch Otorhinolaryngol. 2008;265:1477-82.
40. Smith JA, Danner CJ. Complications of chronic otitis media and cholesteatoma. Otolaryngol Clin North Am. 2006;39:1237-55.
41. Matanda RN, Muyunga KC, Sabue MJ, et al. Chronic suppurative otitis media and related complications at the University Clinic of Kinshasa. B-ENT. 2005;1: 57-62.
42. Greenberg JS, Manolidis S. High incidence of complications encountered in chronic otitis media surgery in a U.S. metropolitan public hospital. Otolaryngol Head Neck Surg. 2001;125:623-7.
43. Wendt H. Desquamative entundung des mittelohrs (Cholesteatom des Felsenbeins). Arch Heilkunde. 1873;14:428.
44. Sade J, Babiacki A, Pinkus G. The metaplastic and congenital origin of cholesteatoma. Acta Otolaryngol. 1983;96:119-29.
45. Sade J. Retraction pockets and attic cholesteatomas. Acta Otorhinolaryngol Belg. 1980;34:62-84.
46. Kuijpers W, Vennix PP, Peters TA, et al. Squamous metaplasia of the middle ear epithelium. Acta Otolaryngol. 1996;116:293-8.
47. Yamamoto-Fukuda T, Takahashi H, Koji T. Animal models of middle ear cholesteatoma. J Biomed Biotechnol. 2011;2011:394241.

48. Habermann J. Zur Entstehung des Cholesteatoms des Mittelohres. Arch Ohrenheilkd. 1888;27:43-51.

49. Bezold F. Cholesteatom, Perforation derMembrana flaccida Shrapnelli und Tubenverschluss Zeitschrift fuer Ohrenheilkunde. 1890;20:5-29.

50. Karmody CS, Northrop C. The pathogenesis of acquired cholesteatoma of the human middle ear: support for the migration hypothesis. Otol Neurotol. 2012; 33:42-7.

51. Jackson DG, Lim DJ. Fine morphology of the advancing front of cholesteatoma—experimental and human. Acta Otolaryngol. 1978;86:71-88.

52. Masaki M, Wright CG, Lee DH, et al. Experimental cholesteatoma. Epidermal ingrowth through tympanic membrane following middle ear application of propylene glycol. Acta Otolaryngol. 1989;108:113-21.

53. Lange W. über die Entstehung der Mittelohrcholesteatoma. Z Hals Nasen Ohrenheilkd. 1925;11:250–271.

54. Eavey RD, Camacho A, Northrop CC. Chronic ear pathology in a model of neonatal amniotic fluid ear inoculation. Arch Otolaryngol Head Neck Surg. 1992;118: 1198-203.

55. Chole RA, Tinling SP. Basal lamina breaks in the histogenesis of cholesteatoma. Laryngoscope. 1985;95:270-5.

56. Ruedi L. Pathogenesis and treatment of cholesteatoma in chronic suppuration of the temporal bone. Ann Otol Rhinol Laryngol. 1957;66:283-305.

57. Steinbach E, Gruninger G. Experimental production of cholesteatoma in rabbits by using non-irritants (skin tolerants). J Laryngol Otol. 1980;94:269-79.

58. Mills RP, Padgham ND. Management of childhood cholesteatoma. J Laryngol Otol. 1991;105:343-5.

59. Mills R. Cholesteatoma behind an intact tympanic membrane in adult life: congenital or acquired? J Laryngol Otol. 2009;123:488-91.

60. Ruedi L. Cholesteatosis of the attic. J Laryngol Otol. 1958;72:593-609.

61. Wright CG, Bird LL, Meyerhoff WL. Tympanic membrane microstructure in experimental cholesteatoma. Acta Otolaryngol. 1991;111:101-11.

62. Cawthorne T, Pickard B. The pathology and treatment of cholesteatoma auris. J Laryngol Otol. 1965;79:945-51.

63. Steinbach E, Pusalkar A, Heumann H. Cholesteatoma—pathology and treatment. Adv Otorhinolaryngol. 1988;39:94-106.

64. Magnuson B. Tubal closing failure in retraction type cholesteatoma and adhesive middle ear lesions. Acta Otolaryngol. 1978;86:408-17.

65. Falk B, Magnuson B. Evacuation of the middle ear by sniffing: a cause of high negative pressure and development of middle ear disease. Otolaryngol Head Neck Surg. 1984;92:312-8.

66. Lindeman P, Holmquist J. Mastoid volume and eustachian tube function in ears with cholesteatoma. Am J Otol. 1987;8:5-7.

67. Sade J. Cellular differentiation of the middle ear lining. Ann Otol Rhinol Laryngol. 1971;80:376-83.

68. Sudhoff H, Tos M. Pathogenesis of attic cholesteatoma: clinical and immuno-histochemical support for combination of retraction theory and proliferation theory. Am J Otol. 2000;21:786-92.

69. Marchioni D, Mattioli F, Alicandri-Ciufelli M, et al. Prevalence of ventilation blockages in patients affected by attic pathology: a case-control study. Laryngoscope. 2013;123:2845-53.

70. Jackler RK, Santa Maria PL, Varsak YK, et al. A new theory on the pathogenesis of acquired cholesteatoma: mucosal traction. Laryngoscope. 2015;125(Suppl 4): S1-14.

71. Mansour S, Magnan J, Haidar H, et al. Tympanic Membrane Retraction Pocket: Overview and Advances in Diagnosis and Management. Cham, Switzerland: Springer International Publishing; 2015.

72. Zechner G. Adhesive process and cholesteatoma in the sequel of tubal dysfunction (author's transl). Laryngol Rhinol Otol (Stuttg). 1980;59:179-84.

73. Nomura Y. Cholesterol metabolism in cholesteatoma and cholesterol granuloma. Ann Otol Rhinol Laryngol Suppl. 1984;112:129-32.

74. Hayashida T, Iwamori M, Kitsuwa T, et al. Biochemical study of cholesteatoma and cholesterol granuloma—occurrence of delta 7-cholestenol in the tissues of cholesteatoma. ORL J Otorhinolaryngol Relat Spec. 1984;46:242-7.

75. Bloksgaard M, Svane-Knudsen V, Sorensen JA, et al. Structural characterization and lipid composition of acquired cholesteatoma: a comparative study with normal skin. Otol Neurotol. 2012;33:177-83.

76. Svane-Knudsen V, Halkier-Sorensen L, Rasmussen G, et al. Altered permeability barrier structure in cholesteatoma matrix. Eur Arch Otorhinolaryngol. 2002;259:527-30.

77. Sade J, Teitz A. Cholesterol and cholesteatoma. Acta Otolaryngol. 1983;95: 547-53.

78. Kuo CL. Etiopathogenesis of acquired cholesteatoma: prominent theories and recent advances in biomolecular research. Laryngoscope. 2015;125:234-40.

79. Albino AP, Kimmelman CP, Parisier SC. Cholesteatoma: a molecular and cellular puzzle. Am J Otol. 1998;19:7-19.

80. Bassiouny M, Badour N, Omran A, et al. Histopathological and immunohistochemical characteristics of acquired cholesteatoma in children and adults. Egypt J Ear Nose Throat Allied Sci. 2012;13:7-12.

81. Welkoborsky HJ, Jacob RS, Hinni ML. Comparative analysis of the epithelium stroma interaction of acquired middle ear cholesteatoma in children and adults. Eur Arch Otorhinolaryngol. 2007;264:841-8.

82. Mallet Y, Nouwen J, Lecomte-Houcke M, et al. Aggressiveness and quantification of epithelial proliferation of middle ear cholesteatoma by MIB1. Laryngoscope. 2003;113:328-31.

83. Caglar O, Bulbul F, Sennaroglu L. Incidence of otitis media with effusion and long-term clinical findings in children with cleft lip and palate types. Kulak Burun Bogaz Ihtis Derg. 2013;23:268-74.

84. Uchida N, Ito S, Hirano M. Localization of proliferating cell nuclear antigen in aural cholesteatoma. Kurume Med J. 1993;40:225-8.

85. Bollmann R, Knopp U, Tolsdorff P. DNA cytometric studies of cholesteatoma of the middle ear. HNO. 1991;39:313-4.

86. Choung YH, Park K, Kang SO, et al. Expression of the gap junction proteins connexin 26 and connexin 43 in human middle ear cholesteatoma. Acta Otolaryngol. 2006;126:138-43.

87. James AL, Chadha NK, Papsin BC, et al. Pediatric cholesteatoma and variants in the gene encoding connexin 26. Laryngoscope. 2010;120:183-7.

88. Klenke C, Janowski S, Borck D, et al. Identification of novel cholesteatoma-related gene expression signatures using full-genome microarrays. PLoS One. 2012;7:e52718.

89. Rothschild S, Ciernik IF, Hartmann M, et al. Cholesteatoma triggering squamous cell carcinoma: case report and literature review of a rare tumor. Am J Otolaryngol. 2009;30:256-60.

90. Takahashi K, Yamamoto Y, Sato K, et al. Middle ear carcinoma originating from a primary acquired cholesteatoma: a case report. Otol Neurotol. 2005;26:105-8.

91. Westerman ST, Sylvia LC, Tepper E. Carcinoma arising out of a primary acquired cholesteatoma. J Med Soc N J. 1981;78:600-2.

92. Palko E, Poliska S, Csakanyi Z, et al. The c-MYC protooncogene expression in cholesteatoma. Biomed Res Int. 2014;2014:639896.

93. Ecsedi S, Rakosy Z, Vizkeleti L, et al. Chromosomal imbalances are associated with increased proliferation and might contribute to bone destruction in cholesteatoma. Otolaryngol Head Neck Surg. 2008;139:635-40.

94. Ozturk K, Yildirim MS, Acar H, et al. Evaluation of c-MYC status in primary acquired cholesteatoma by using fluorescence in situ hybridization technique. Otol Neurotol. 2006;27:588-91.

95. Shinoda H, Huang CC. Expressions of c-jun and p53 proteins in human middle ear cholesteatoma: relationship to keratinocyte proliferation, differentiation, and programmed cell death. Laryngoscope. 1995;105:1232-7.

96. Holly A, Sittinger M, Bujia J. Immunohistochemical demonstration of c-myc oncogene product in middle ear cholesteatoma. Eur Arch Otorhinolaryngol. 1995;252:366-9.

97. Maniu A, Harabagiu O, Perde Schrepler M, et al. Molecular biology of cholesteatoma. Rom J Morphol Embryol. 2014;55:7-13.

98. Bayazit YA, Karakok M, Ucak R, et al. Cycline-dependent kinase inhibitor, p27 (KIP1), is associated with cholesteatoma. Laryngoscope. 2001;111:1037-41.

99. Hartwell LH, Kastan MB. Cell cycle control and cancer. Science. 1994;266:1821-8.

100. Muller PA, Vousden KH, Norman JC. p53 and its mutants in tumor cell migration and invasion. J Cell Biol. 2011;192:209-18.

101. Rusch V, Klimstra D, Linkov I, et al. Aberrant expression of p53 or the epidermal growth factor receptor is frequent in early bronchial neoplasia and coexpression precedes squamous cell carcinoma development. Cancer Res. 1995;55:1365-72.

102. Stanton P, Richards S, Reeves J, et al. Epidermal growth factor receptor expression by human squamous cell carcinomas of the head and neck, cell lines and xenografts. Br J Cancer. 1994;70:427-33.

103. Reinartz JJ, George E, Lindgren BR, et al. Expression of p53, transforming growth factor alpha, epidermal growth factor receptor, and c-erbB-2 in endometrial carcinoma and correlation with survival and known predictors of survival. Hum Pathol. 1994;25:1075-83.

104. Khazaie K, Schirrmacher V, Lichtner RB. EGF receptor in neoplasia and metastasis. Cancer Metastasis Rev. 1993;12:255-74.

105. King LE, Jr, Gates RE, Stoscheck CM, et al. The EGF/TGF alpha receptor in skin. J Invest Dermatol. 1990;94:164S-70S.

106. Vassar R, Fuchs E. Transgenic mice provide new insights into the role of TGF-alpha during epidermal development and differentiation. Genes Dev. 1991; 5:714-27.

107. Ergun S, Zheng X, Carlsoo B. Expression of transforming growth factor-alpha and epidermal growth factor receptor in middle ear cholesteatoma. Am J Otol. 1996;17:393-6.

108. Chung JH, Lee SH, Park CW, et al. Expression of Apoptotic vs Antiapoptotic Proteins in Middle Ear Cholesteatoma. Otolaryngol Head Neck Surg. 2015 Jun 29. doi: 10.1177/0194599815591810 [Epub ahead of print].

109. Lee DW, Chung JH, Lee SH, et al. Comparative analysis of the expression of E-cadherin, β-catenin, and β1 integrin in congenital and acquired cholesteatoma. Eur Arch Otorhinolaryngol. 2015 Apr 12. doi: 10.1007/s00405-015-3621-x [Epub ahead of print].

110. Schonborn I, Zschiesche W, Behrens J, et al.. Expression of E-cadherin/catenin complexes in breast cancer. Int J Oncol. 1997;11:1327-34.

111. Andrews NA, Jones AS, Helliwell TR, et al. Expression of the E-cadherin-catenin cell adhesion complex in primary squamous cell carcinomas of the head and neck and their nodal metastases. Br J Cancer. 1997;75:1474-80.

112. Rudnicki A, Avraham KB. microRNAs: the art of silencing in the ear. EMBO Mol Med. 2012;4:849-59.

113. Chen X, Qin Z. Post-transcriptional regulation by microrna-21 and let-7a microRNA in paediatric cholesteatoma. J Int Med Res. 2011;39:2110-8.

114. Hui AB, Lenarduzzi M, Krushel T, et al. Comprehensive MicroRNA profiling for head and neck squamous cell carcinomas. Clin Cancer Res. 2010;16:1129-39.

115. Friedland DR, Eernisse R, Erbe C, et al. Cholesteatoma growth and proliferation: posttranscriptional regulation by microRNA-21. Otol Neurotol. 2009;30: 998-1005.

116. Bartel DP. MicroRNAs: genomics, biogenesis, mechanism, and function. Cell. 2004;116:281-97.

117. Yoshikawa M, Kojima H, Yaguchi Y, et al. Cholesteatoma fibroblasts promote epithelial cell proliferation through overexpression of epiregulin. PLoS One. 2013;8:e66725.

118. Ferlito A, Devaney KO, Rinaldo A, et al. Clinicopathological consultation. Ear cholesteatoma versus cholesterol granuloma. Ann Otol Rhinol Laryngol. 1997; 106:79-85.

119. Preciado DA. Biology of cholesteatoma: special considerations in pediatric patients. Int J Pediatr Otorhinolaryngol. 2012;76:319-21.

120. Kojima H, Tanaka Y, Tanaka T, et al. Cell proliferation and apoptosis in human middle ear cholesteatoma. Arch Otolaryngol Head Neck Surg. 1998;124:261-4.

121. Cheshire IM, Blight A, Ratcliffe WA, et al. Production of parathyroid-hormone-related protein by cholesteatoma cells in culture. Lancet. 1991;338:1041-3.

122. Yetiser S, Satar B, Aydin N. Expression of epidermal growth factor, tumor necrosis factor-alpha, and interleukin-1alpha in chronic otitis media with or without cholesteatoma. Otol Neurotol. 2002;23:647-52.

123. Chung JW, Yoon TH. Different production of interleukin-1alpha, interleukin-1beta and interleukin-8 from cholesteatomatous and normal epithelium. Acta Otolaryngol. 1998;118:386-91.

124. Schilling V, Negri B, Bujia J, et al. Possible role of interleukin 1 alpha and interleukin 1 beta in the pathogenesis of cholesteatoma of the middle ear. Am J Otol. 1992;13:350-5.

125. Raynov AM, Choung YH, Park HY, et al. Establishment and characterization of an in vitro model for cholesteatoma. Clin Exp Otorhinolaryngol. 2008;1:86-91.

126. Lang S, Schilling V, Wollenberg B, et al. Localization of transforming growth factor-beta-expressing cells and comparison with major extracellular components in aural cholesteatoma. Ann Otol Rhinol Laryngol. 1997;106:669-73.

127. Schulz P, Bujia J, Holly A, et al. Possible autocrine growth stimulation of cholesteatoma epithelium by transforming growth factor alpha. Am J Otolaryngol. 1993;14:82-7.

128. Leichtle A, Klenke C, Ebmeyer J, et al. NOD-like receptor signaling in cholesteatoma. Biomed Res Int. 2015;2015:408169.

129. Szczepanski M, Szyfter W, Jenek R, et al. Toll-like receptors 2, 3 and 4 (TLR-2, TLR-3 and TLR-4) are expressed in the microenvironment of human acquired cholesteatoma. Eur Arch Otorhinolaryngol. 2006;263:603-7.

130. Fukata M, Vamadevan AS, Abreu MT. Toll-like receptors (TLRs) and Nod-like receptors (NLRs) in inflammatory disorders. Semin Immunol. 2009;21:242-53.

131. Lee HY, Park MS, Byun JY, et al. Expression of pattern recognition receptors in cholesteatoma. Eur Arch Otorhinolaryngol. 2014;271:245-53.

132. Haruyama T, Furukawa M, Kusunoki T, et al. Expression of IL-17 and its role in bone destruction in human middle ear cholesteatoma. ORL J Otorhinolaryngol Relat Spec. 2010;72:325-31.

133. Ahn JM, Huang CC, Abramson M. Third place—Resident Basic Science Award 1990. Interleukin 1 causing bone destruction in middle ear cholesteatoma. Otolaryngol Head Neck Surg. 1990;103:527-36.

134. Kawai T, Matsuyama T, Hosokawa Y, et al. B and T lymphocytes are the primary sources of RANKL in the bone resorptive lesion of periodontal disease. Am J Pathol. 2006;169:987-98.

135. Jeong JH, Park CW, Tae K, et al. Expression of RANKL and OPG in middle ear cholesteatoma tissue. Laryngoscope. 2006;116:1180-4.

136. Chen AP, Wang B, Zhong F, et al. Expression levels of receptor activator of nuclear factor-kappaB ligand and osteoprotegerin are associated with middle ear cholesteatoma risk. Acta Otolaryngol. 2015;135:655-66.

137. Kuo CL, Shiao AS, Liao WH, et al. How long is long enough to follow up children after cholesteatoma surgery? A 29-year study. Laryngoscope. 2012;122:2568-73.

138. Dornelles Cde C, da Costa SS, Meurer L, et al. Comparison of acquired cholesteatoma between pediatric and adult patients. Eur Arch Otorhinolaryngol. 2009; 266:1553-61.

139. Olszewska E, Chodynicki S, Chyczewski L. Role of angiogenesis in the pathogenesis of cholesteatoma in adults. Otolaryngol Pol. 2004;58:559-63.

140. Fukudome S, Wang C, Hamajima Y, et al. Regulation of the angiogenesis of acquired middle ear cholesteatomas by inhibitor of DNA binding transcription factor. JAMA Otolaryngol Head Neck Surg. 2013;139:273-8.

141. Sudhoff H, Dazert S, Gonzales AM, et al. Angiogenesis and angiogenic growth factors in middle ear cholesteatoma. Am J Otol. 2000;21:793-8.

142. Ferrara N, Davis-Smyth T. The biology of vascular endothelial growth factor. Endocr Rev. 1997;18:4-25.

143. Lee YW, Chung Y, Juhn SK, et al. Activation of the transforming growth factor beta pathway in bacterial otitis media. Ann Otol Rhinol Laryngol. 2011;120: 204-13.

144. Juhn SK, Jung MK, Hoffman MD, et al. The role of inflammatory mediators in the pathogenesis of otitis media and sequelae. Clin Exp Otorhinolaryngol. 2008; 1:117-38.

145. Zhang QA, Hamajima Y, Zhang Q, et al. Identification of Id1 in acquired middle ear cholesteatoma. Arch Otolaryngol Head Neck Surg. 2008;134:306-10.

146. Hamajima Y, Komori M, Preciado DA, et al. The role of inhibitor of DNA-binding (Id1) in hyperproliferation of keratinocytes: the pathological basis for middle ear cholesteatoma from chronic otitis media. Cell Prolif. 2010;43:457-63.

147. Ricciardiello F, Cavaliere M, Mesolella M, et al. Notes on the microbiology of cholesteatoma: clinical findings and treatment. Acta Otorhinolaryngol Ital. 2009;29:197-202.

148. Garca MF, Aslan M, Tuna B, et al. Serum myeloperoxidase activity, total antioxidant capacity and nitric oxide levels in patients with chronic otitis media. J Membr Biol. 2013;246:519-24.

149. Baysal E, Aksoy N, Kara F, et al. Oxidative stress in chronic otitis media. Eur Arch Otorhinolaryngol. 2013;270:1203-8.

150. Walsh TE, Covell WP, Ogura JH. The effect of cholesteatosis on bone. Ann Otol Rhinol Laryngol. 1951;60:1100-13.

151. Kaneko Y, Yuasa R, Ise I, et al. Bone destruction due to the rupture of a cholesteatoma sac: a pathogenesis of bone destruction in aural-cholesteatoma. Laryngoscope. 1980;90:1865-71.

152. Iino Y, Hoshino E, Tomioka S, et al. Organic acids and anaerobic microorganisms in the contents of the cholesteatoma sac. Ann Otol Rhinol Laryngol. 1983;92:91-6.

153. Nguyen KH, Suzuki H, Ohbuchi T, et al. Possible participation of acidic pH in bone resorption in middle ear cholesteatoma. Laryngoscope. 2014;124: 245-50.

154. Celebi O, Paksoy M, Aydin S, et al. Myeloperoxydase activity in the pathogenesis of cholesteatoma. Ind J Otolaryngol Head Neck Surg. 2010;62:32-5.

155. Klebanoff SJ. Myeloperoxidase: friend and foe. J Leukoc Biol. 2005;77:598-625.

156. Ozlem CE, Sanli A. Is there a relationship between myeloperoxidase activity and conductive hearing loss in chronic otitis media complicated by cholesteatoma? Ear Nose Throat J. 2015;94:166-92.

Chapter 13

Degenerative Disorders of the Cervical Spine: Special Consideration of ENT Aspects

Ermioni Touli, Oliver N Hausmann

INTRODUCTION

Cervical degenerative disorders are part of the normal aging of the cervical spine and represent a variety of distinct pathologies, including intervertebral disk herniation, cervical spondylosis, and cervical arthrosis. Clinical manifestations of neck pain, radiculopathy, and myelopathy can occur as a result of foraminal or central stenosis with compromise of the nerve roots or the spinal cord. Some atypical symptoms of these conditions like dysphagia or vertigo can lead the patient to refer to an ENT specialist. The clinical practitioner must keep in mind these conditions and readdress the patient accordingly. There is a variety of nonoperative and operative treatment options available according to the underlying pathology.

The cervical spine of the human extends between the base of the skull and the thoracic vertebrae and consists of seven individual vertebrae, the smallest of the spinal column, and the intervertebral disks between them. The C1 vertebra is named atlas and the C2 vertebra axis, as it provides the axis upon which the skull and atlas rotate. Above each vertebra exits a pair of spinal nerves with the same number as the vertebra below, with the exception of C8, which emerges below the vertebra C7. The posture of a normal human cervical spine is convex forward in the sagittal plane and follows a parallel line in the coronal plane, in contrast with the four-legged mammals in which the spine is parallel to the axial plane. The main functions of the cervical spine are to provide controlled three-dimensional mobility, to transfer loads from the head, and to protect the spinal cord. Seven spinal ligaments around each pair of adjacent vertebrae restrict the range of movement.

NECK PAIN

In a considerable number of patients, muscular and ligamentous factors may be the cause of neck pain. Therefore, axial neck pain may be attributed to posture, poor ergonomics, stress, and chronic muscle fatigue. Neck pain as a result of degenerative changes in the cervical disks or facet joints is controversial; however, in recent studies it appears that cervical disks and facet joints can be pain generators.[1]

According to available studies, the 1-year incidence of neck pain is estimated between 10.4% and 21.3% with a higher incidence among office and computer workers. At 1 year, between 33% and 65% of people have recovered from an episode of neck pain; however, recurrences are common since neck pain is frequently characterized from an episodic course over an individual's lifetime.[2] The natural history of neck pain has been evaluated by Gore et al. in a 10-year follow-up study. The results showed that 79% of the patients had a regression of pain and 43% a complete relief of symptoms; however, 32% reported persistent moderate or severe pain.[3]

RADICULOPATHY

Cervical radiculopathy is the result of irritation of the cervical spinal nerve root due to compression and local inflammation, associated with a cytokine response including an increased release of the tumor necrosis factor-alpha factor.[4] Cervical radiculopathy affects patients mainly in the fourth and fifth decade of life and has a reported prevalence of 3.3 cases per 1,000 people.[5] The two most frequent sites of radiculopathy are the C6 and C7 nerve roots.[6] Cervical radiculopathy can be due to disk herniation, cervical stenosis, or segmental instability.

The most frequent symptom is neck pain associated with predominant sharp radiating arm pain following a dermatomal, myotomal, or/and sclerotomal distribution. There are a number of tests that contribute to the diagnosis by provoking (axial compression test, Spurling's test) or relieving (shoulder abduction test) the pain as they change the available space of the neuroforamen. Aggravation of the pain may occur with neck extension or rotation toward the symptomatic side (Spurling's sign) or by maneuvers that increase the intradural pressure, such as coughing, sneezing, and valsalva.

Sensory disturbances, such as paresthesias, dysesthesias, and numbness, consistent with a dermatomic pattern and segmental motor deficits may be present according to the affected level. Reflex deficits are also usual, whereas motor symptoms are more often associated with a soft herniated disk and sensory symptoms with a hard herniated disk.[7] Vegetative disturbances, including vertigo, tinnitus, and cervical migraine, are also reported.[8] Cervical radiculopathy can result to cervical angina by mimicking coronary ischemic disease, whereas less frequently persistent breast pain may present as a primary symptom.[1,9]

Table 13.1: Cervical radicular syndrome.			
Nerve root	*Pain and sensory deficit*	*Motor deficit*	*Reflex*
C5	Shoulder	Muscle deltoid	–
C6	Arm, radial forearm, Dig I	Muscle biceps, wrist extensors	Biceps reflex (BSR)
C7	Dig II and III, scapular pain	Muscle triceps, finger extensors, wrist flexors	Triceps reflex (TSR)
C8	Dig IV and V	Finger flexors	–
T1	Ulnar forearm	Finger abductors	–

Involvement of the C3, C4, and C5 nerve roots may lead to unilateral or bilateral diaphragmatic weakness with dyspnea or orthopnea (Table 13.1).[10]

Cervical Disk Herniation

Disk herniations can be characterized as "soft" or "hard" disk herniations. Generally, a soft herniation is more acute, where age-related alterations of the intervertebral disk like disk dehydration tear and cleft formation lead to loss of the viscoelastic properties, decrease of the disk height, and prolapse of the inner core of the disk (nucleus pulposus) through the outer protective fibers (annulus) into the spinal canal, resulting to progressive motion segment degeneration. In contrast, spondylosis is a more chronic condition associated with the appearance of secondary degenerative changes and is referred to as a hard disk herniation. Moreover, similar signs and symptoms like radiculopathy, cervicocephalgia, or myelopathy can be caused by soft or hard disk herniations, through the local mechanical or chemical irritation of neural structures.

Central, lateral, or combined neurocompression may occur within the spinal canal, involving only the spinal cord, only the nerve roots, or both. Spontaneous resorption is possible and depends on the phase and position of the extrusion (Figs. 13.1A to C).[11]

Cervical Spondylosis

As the normal aging of the spine occurs, the segment degeneration continues. In parallel to loss of the disk height, reactive bone may present along the posterior vertebral bodies, so called spondylosis. Osteophytes of the endplates, facet, and uncovertebral joints develop, followed by hypertrophy and buckling of the posterior longitudinal ligament and the ligamentum flavum into the spinal canal. These hard disk herniations often lead to radicular entrapments and decrease the diameter of the spinal canal.

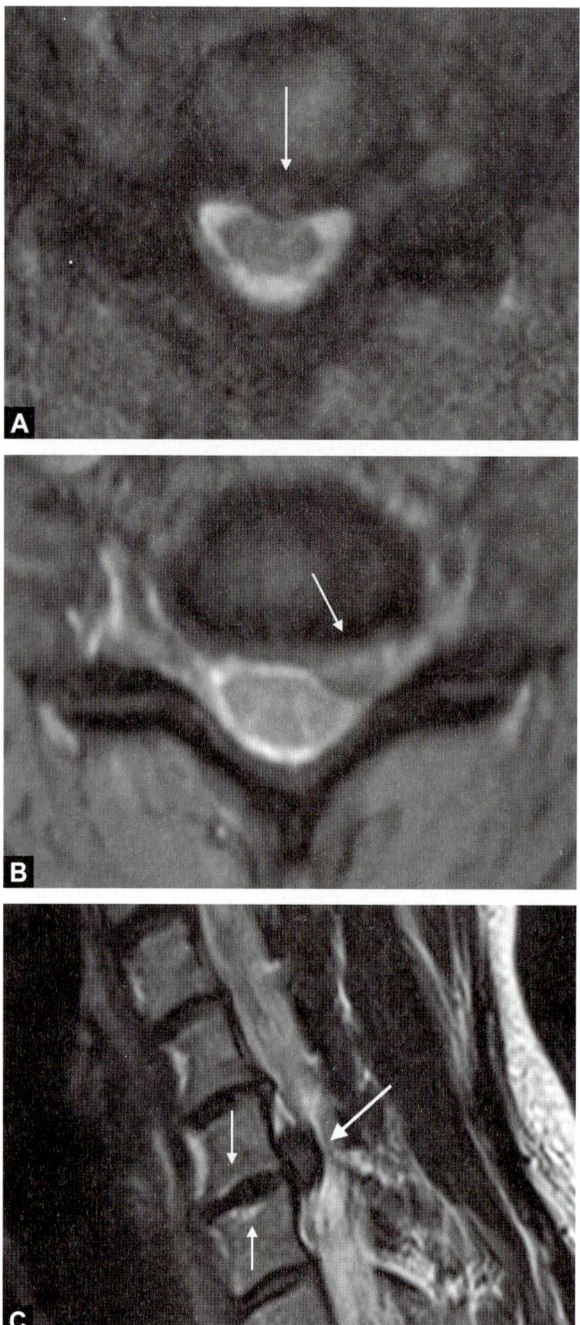

Figs. 13.1A to C: (A) Axial magnetic resonance imaging (MRI) image of a central cervical herniation (arrow) with rupture of the posterior ligament. Neurocompression of the spinal cord but not of the nerve roots. (B) Axial MRI image of a well hydrated, left posterolateral cervical herniation (arrow) at the C5/C6 level with compression of the left C6 root. (C) Sagittal MRI image of the same patient as in image (B). Cervical herniation at the C5/C6 level (large arrow). Osteochondrosis (small arrows) of the 5th and 6th cervical vertebrae.

The spondylotic neck pain is attributed to disk degeneration, facet joint osteoarthritis, and segmental instability. It is often associated with nonradicular arm and shoulder pain and is aggravated through movement and specific positions. Stiffness of the neck and limitation of cervical motion are also common. Other concomitant symptoms of spondylosis are headaches, vertigo, dizziness, and other nonspecific sympathetic symptoms, which may include tinnitus, nausea, heart throb, hypomnesia, and gastroenterologic discomfort.[12]

Dysphagia, dyspnea, or dysphonia may present as a result of pressure on the esophagus, larynx, or trachea by osteophytes along the anterior vertebral bodies.[1,13] Cervical osteophytes may also be the cause of transient vertebrobasilar insufficiency resulting to vertigo, loss of balance, and syncope associated with rotation of the head to the affected side.[14,15] Pressure on the upper and middle parts of the cervical spinal cord may lead to secondary craniofacial pain or paresthesias associated with cervical pain due to involvement of the spinal nucleus of the trigeminal nerve (Figs. 13.2A to C).[1,16]

Cervical Spinal Instability

Cervical spinal instability is clinically considered to be the inability of the cervical spine, under physiological loads, to maintain relations between vertebrae in such a way that neither the spinal cord nor nerve roots are damaged or irritated without any consecutive deformity or pain.[17] However, the definition of instability has been a subject of considerable debate and has not been clearly established. Prevention of excessive movement and stability of the segment is provided through ligaments, facet joints, and the intervertebral disk, consecutively damage to one of these elements influences the other two.

The risk factors leading to cervical spinal instability include history of trauma, congenital collagenous diseases (e.g. Down syndrome),[18] and inflammatory arthritides (e.g. rheumatoid arthritis).[19] Grisel's syndrome, a rather rare disease, involves the nontraumatic subluxation of the atlantoaxial joint due to inflammatory ligamentous laxity and is associated with several common otolaryngeal conditions like upper respiratory tract infections (e.g. pharyngitis, adenotonsillitis, cervical abscess, tonsillar abscess, and otitis media) and head/neck surgery (e.g. tonsillectomy, adenoidectomy, pharyngoplasty, otoplasty, and mastoidectomy).[20,21]

Although rare in comparison with the instability of the lumbar spine, instability of the cervical spine usually occurs as a spondylolisthesis (forward displacement of the cephalad vertebra on the caudal one). Unstable degenerative spondylolisthesis of the cervical spine

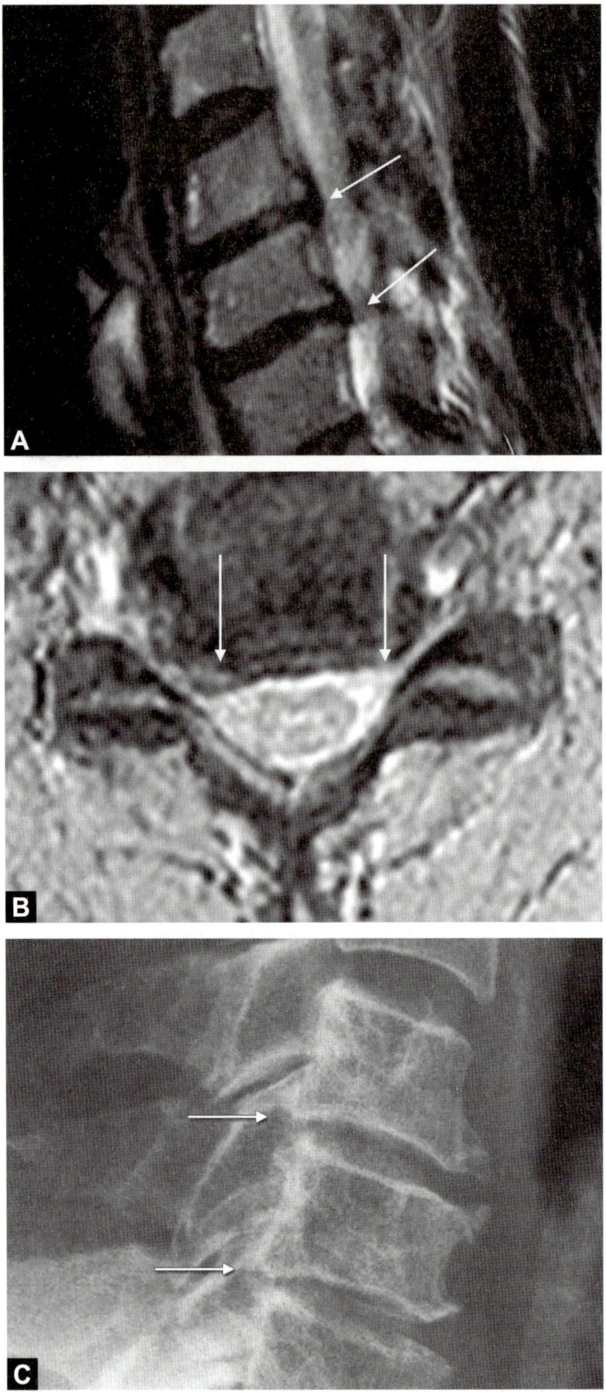

Figs. 13.2A to C: (A) Sagittal magnetic resonance imaging (MRI) image showing a hard disk herniation/spondylosis (arrows) C5/C6 and C6/C7. (B) Axial MRI image C6/C7 of the same patient. Note preforaminal entrapment of both C7 nerv roots (arrows). (C) Lateral radiography of the same patient showing the bony spurs (arrows).

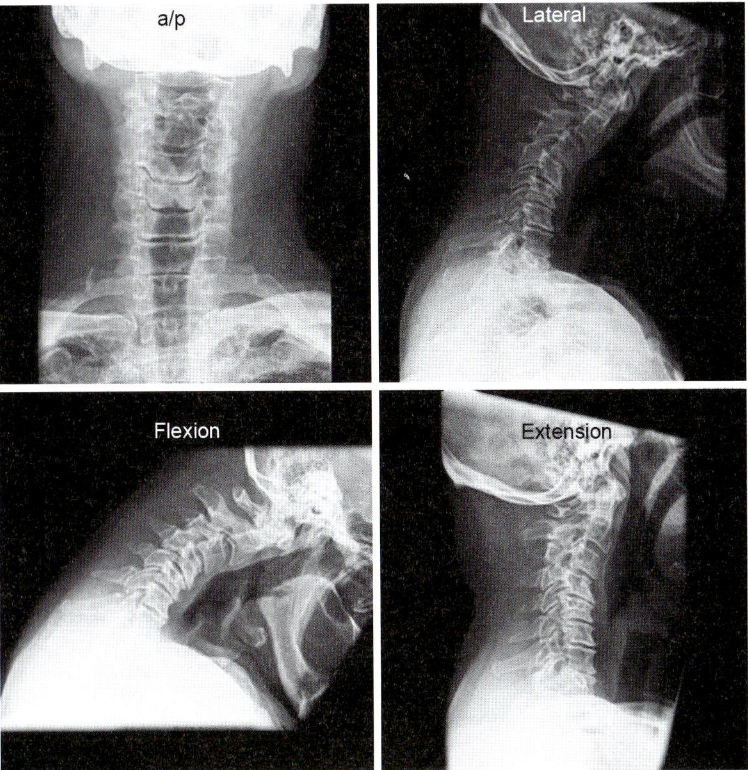

Fig. 13.3: Cervical spine instability of the C3/C4 level shown in neutral (anteroposterior, lateral) and flexion/extension radiographies.

usually occurs at the C3/C4 or C4/C5 levels (Fig. 13.3). Other sites of instability within the cervical spine are the atlantoaxial and the subaxial plane. The disease may manifest with a spectrum of symptoms including neurological deficits (radiculopathy, myelopathy) or only with axial neck pain.[22,23]

CERVICAL MYELOPATHY

Cervical myelopathy is the result of direct compression of the spinal cord resulting to chronic spinal cord injury. Although exact numbers of prevalence and incidence worldwide are not known, the prevalence of surgically treated cervical spondylotic myelopathy is estimated as 1.6 per 100,000 inhabitants.[24] In a national cohort study of eastern Asia, the incidence of cervical spondylotic myelopathy-caused hospitalization was 4.04 per 100,000 person-years, with higher incidences observed in older and male patients.[25] The natural history of the disease is variable and unpredictable. It may manifest with episodic

Table 13.2: Pathophysiological factors of cervical myelopathy.

Static factors	Dynamic factors	Biomechanical factors
Spondylosis	Changes in neck flexion/extension, which narrows cervical spinal canal dynamically ($\rightarrow$ repetitive injury, repetitive ischemia)	Ischemic injury due to chronic compression of the spinal cord vasculature
Disk degeneration		Glutamate-mediated excitotoxicity
Ossification of the posterior longitudinal ligament		Oligodendrocyte and neuronal apoptosis
Ossification of the ligamentum flavum		Disruption of the neurovascular unit
Congenital stenosis		

progression with periods of quiescence or as slow steady progression. Sometimes, there is a rapid onset of symptoms followed by a longer period of stability.[1]

The pathobiology of cervical myelopathy is similar to that occurring after traumatic spinal cord injury. It includes static factors that narrow the diameter of the spinal canal and dynamic compression factors leading to repetitive injury to the spinal cord. As a result, direct injury to neurons and glia occurs, as well as disruption of the neurovascular unit due to a secondary cascade of events including ischemia, excitotoxicity, and apoptosis (Table 13.2).[26]

Usual causes include disk herniation, cervical spondylosis, trauma, and ossification of the posterior longitudinal ligament (OPLL) or of the ligamentum flavum (OLF); both disorders are characterized by progressive ectopic bone formation within the posterior longitudinal ligament or the ligamentum flavum, respectively (Figs. 13.4A and B). Both are multifactorial diseases where environmental and genetic factors interact, making the pathophysiology not yet fully understood. The OLF occurs mainly in the lower thoracic region and rarely in the cervical region, whereas OPLL may extend from C2 to sacrum.[27,28]

The symptoms of myelopathy are variable and may present after impairment of the long tracts, which may be accompanied with impairment of the segmental nerves since central and foraminal stenosis are often combined. Difficulty in walking, with changes in balance and gait disturbances, occurs often combined with stiffness and power loss of the lower extremities. The characteristic gait includes decreased

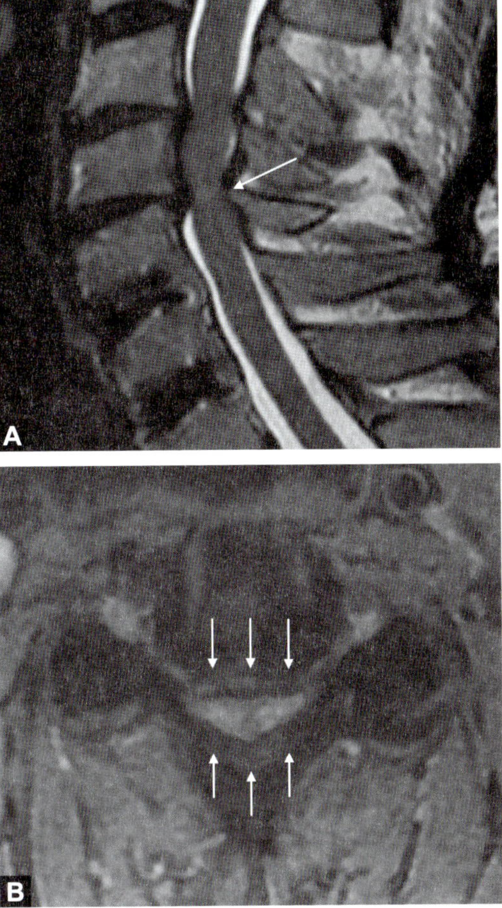

Figs. 13.4A and B: Adjacent segment stenosis C3/C4 and C4/C5 with consecutive myelopathy, after pre-existing fusion of the lower cervical spine, C5/C6 and C6/C7. (A) Sagittal image with high-signal change of spinal cord (arrow). (B) Axial image C4/C5 with severe compression of the spinal cord itself (arrows).

velocity and stride length as well as increased double support time, changes that may be attributable to impaired proprioception and stability in the lower extremities.[29] These gait characteristics are associated with a greater risk of fall in older patients, even in those without other concomitant health issues.[30]

Numb, clumsy hands with disturbance of the fine motor skills (i.e. writing, eating with chopsticks) are initially observed. In patients with cervical spondylosis, wasting and weakness of the extrinsic and intrinsic hand muscles, not associated with either sensory loss or spastic tetraparesis, may be seen.[31] The degree of neck pain and of sensory disturbances like loss of pain, positional sense, vibration, and temperature varies widely. Spasticity, clonus, and hyper-reflexia may be present in upper and lower extremities, whereas hyporeflexia

Table 13.3: Magnetic resonance imaging findings in cervical myelopathy.

Loss of cerebrospinal fluid space

Critical anteroposterior distance <9 mm

Suspected when <11 mm dynamic canal space in extreme flexion and extension

Banana shape of spinal cord

Increased signal of the spinal cord in T2-weighted image

may present at the level of the compression. At later stages, symptoms of tetraparesis or bowel and bladder dysfunction may present. Long tract signs like Babinski, Oppenheimer, and Gordon, indicating an upper motor neuron lesion, as well as Hoffmann's and Lhermitte sign may be positive.

Diagnosis of Degenerative Disk Diseases

The diagnosis of the degenerative disk diseases depends mainly on the history and the clinical examination. However, neuroradiologic imaging is crucial to the physician for the evaluation of the symptomatic patient.

The initial imaging study includes the conventional radiographies. The anteroposterior and lateral views are used for the evaluation of the sagittal profile and spinal canal diameter. Subluxations and malalignments as well as osteophyte formations and disk space narrowing must be evaluated according to the clinical findings. Developmental abnormalities and osteoarthritis may also be demonstrated. The oblique views are helpful for the evaluation of the facet joints and the neuroforamina. Flexion and extension radiographs may be of use for the evaluation of the mobility and stability of the spine in the upright position.

Computed tomography (CT) is a frequent method in current practice, mainly because it provides detailed information about osseous compressive alterations as well as in cases of magnetic resonance imaging (MRI) contraindications. Nonetheless after spinal surgery with instrumentation, the CT is the appropriate method for the accurate assessment of the hardware positioning and the evaluation of the degree of osseous fusion.

However, the method of choice for the visualization of the spine is the MRI, as it is characterized from very high sensitivity and provides direct information regarding the nerve roots and the spinal cord. The morphology of the cord as well as intramedullary changes is visible (Table 13.3 and Fig. 13.5). The MRI enables to evaluate the degree of degeneration of the disk (chondrosis, rupture of annulus or the

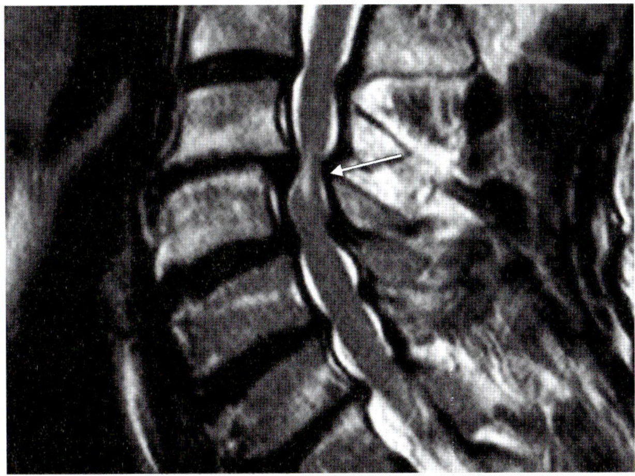

Fig. 13.5: Characteristic magnetic resonance imaging alterations with loss of cerebrospinal fluid space and increased signal in T2-weighted image in a patient suffering from cervical myelopathy.

posterior ligament) and/or of the vertebral body (osteochondrosis). The most important limitation of the MRI is the lack of accurate depiction of osseous structures.

In cases with atypical findings, neurophysiological investigations (electromyography/nerve conduction studies/somatosensory-evoked potential/motor-evoked potential) may be useful, as well as in cases difficult to differentiate between root and peripheral nerve damage. Injection studies such as discography contribute limited to the diagnosis.

TREATMENT OF DEGENERATIVE DISORDERS OF THE CERVICAL SPINE

The spectrum of treatments for cervical degenerative disorders varies according to the severity of symptoms and the underlying pathology. The main objectives of any treatment are to relieve the pain, to prevent or to improve any neurological deficits, and to restore the mobility of the patient. Usually, there is a multidisciplinary discussion for the decision of the best treatment strategy. Physiotherapists, chiropractors, general practitioners, pain specialists, and neuro- and orthopedic spine surgeons may be involved. Surgical options are usually considered after an adequate trial of conservative treatment.

Conservative Treatment

Chronic neck pain is a frequent symptom in the general population and can be of multifactorial etiology. As a result, the best initial

Table 13.4: Methods of conservative treatment.	
Medication	*Spinal manipulation*
Physical therapy	Transcutaneous electrical nerve stimulation (TENS)
Taping	Traction
Chiropractic	Radiofrequency denervation
Epidural injection or facet block	Infrared laser therapy
Bracing	Posture training

management is through nonoperative treatments. Especially, therapies involving manual therapy and exercise are considered more effective than alternative treatments.[32] Conservative management is the most appropriate initial treatment in almost all cases of cervical radiculopathy (Table 13.4). Patients with mild myelopathy are occasionally initially treated conservatively (e.g. collar immobilization), which may prove beneficial. However, careful monitoring of these patients is necessary as deterioration may occur despite the conservative treatment. In contrast, the role of conservative care in cases of moderate or severe cervical myelopathy is limited.[33]

Operative Treatment

Conservative measures must be exhausted for an adequate trial period in patients with neck pain before surgery is considered. Coexistence of a radiographic abnormality at the symptomatic level is also essential.[34]

In specific patients, surgery is effective for symptoms of cervical radiculopathy. Especially for cervical radiculopathy without evidence of myelopathy, surgery is recommended when all of the following criteria are present: (1) visualization of cervical root compression on MRI or CT, (2) symptoms and signs of cervical root-related dysfunction and/or pain, (3) progressive motor deficit, and (4) persistence of pain despite conservative treatment for at least 6–12 weeks.[35]

Surgical interventions are usually recommended to patients with moderate/severe or progressive myelopathy associated with radiographic findings. Surgery is considered to arrest the progression of myelopathy and may lead to functional improvement; especially early surgery is believed to improve the prognosis. Furthermore, patients with myelopathy are at an increased risk of spinal cord injury after mild traumatisms.[36] Cervical degenerative disorders can be treated with a variety of surgical techniques using a ventral, a posterior, or a combined approach.

Surgical Approach

There is debate whether the anterior or the posterior approach is more appropriate. Each of these techniques has advantages and disadvantages, and it is up to the surgeon to make the right choice according to the target pathology. However, the anterior cervical approach is currently more frequently used than the posterior as it poses certain advantages over the last one.

A ventral approach allows for decompression in kyphotic, neutral, or lordotic spines and simultaneously restores the normal cervical lordosis, in contradiction with the posterior approach, which is limited to patients with neutral or lordotic alignment.[37] Furthermore, it avoids the pain associated with a posterior paraspinal musculature stripping, as neck and shoulder pain is a usual complaint after posterior cervical spine surgery.[38]

In contrast to anterior approaches, posterior approaches avoid exposure and injury to critical neck structures including the esophagus, recurrent laryngeal nerve, and carotid artery. Through a posterior approach, there is less risk of tear of the dura and cerebrospinal fluid (CSF) leak in patients with OPLL where the ventral dura may be adnated with the posterior ligament. Posterior approach may also be used where the anterior approach can pose certain difficulties like in obese patients or in patients with short thick necks.[37] In addition, procedures involving a posterior approach limit adjacent segment disease and avoid the costs and potential complications of instrumentation.[39]

Nevertheless, the location of the stenosis must also be considered. For patients with cervical spine stenosis that primarily results from dorsal compression or where direct visualization and decompression of nerve roots is necessary, a posterior approach is preferred. Patients with ventral pathological entities, however, benefit more from a ventral procedure.[40,41] The number of involved levels poses also a limitation for the anterior approach alone, as an increase in the number of levels increases also the risk of graft failure and other surgical complications. More specific, the anterior cervical decompression with corpectomy can only be advised if the involved levels are one or two and the anterior cervical decompression with fusion until three levels.[39,42]

Anterior Approach

For the anterior approach, the patient is in a supine position and the arms and shoulders may be pulled caudally. Gardner-Wells tongs may be used for spinal traction. The procedure can be performed from the left or the right side. Although a left-sided approach is associated with fewer recurrent nerve complications, the thoracic duct may be exposed. The skin incision may be either transverse or longitudinal, with the transverse approach being more frequently preferred because of its better cosmetic results. After the incision of the platysma, the deep cervical fascia is divided while the sternocleidomastoid muscles with the carotid are placed laterally and the prelaryngeal muscles with the esophagus and the trachea medially. Extra caution must be given to avoid damage of the possibly exposed structures like the inferior or superior thyroid arteries and the inferior or superior laryngeal as well as the hypoglossal nerve.

Anterior Cervical Discectomy with Fusion

After adequate exposure of the cervical vertebral column, with preservation of the longus colli muscle, the anterior disk annulus is incised and the intervertebral disk is carefully removed to the posterior longitudinal ligament posteriorly. In cases of disk extrusion or myelopathy, the removal of the last is also necessary. The disk space is then distracted, and direct neural decompression can be achieved. The endplates of the adjacent vertebras are drilled to provide a flat surface for the intervertebral graft (Fig. 13.6).

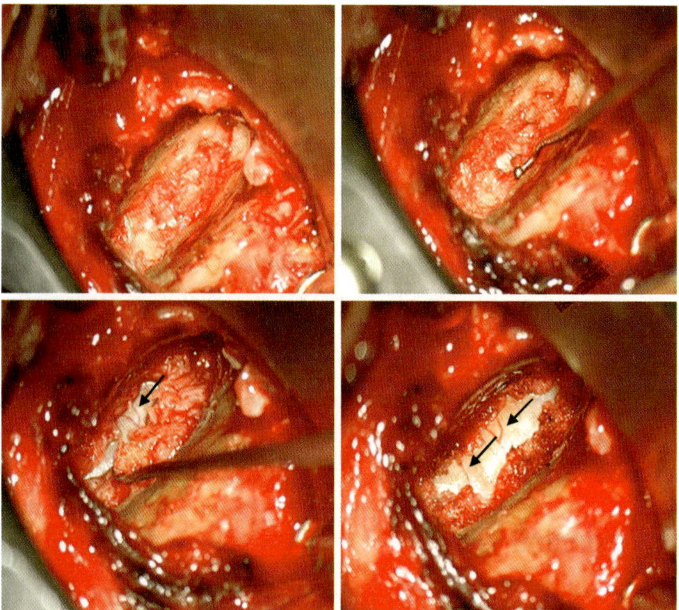

Fig. 13.6: Anterior discectomy with exposure of the dura: distraction of the disk space with pins and distractors and gradual removal of the intervertebral disk. Lastly, removal of the posterior longitudinal ligament (elevated by hooklet). The cervical dura and the dural vessels are visible (arrows).

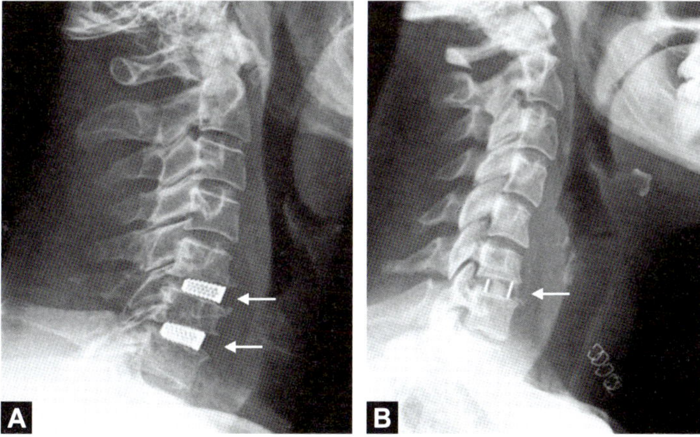

Figs. 13.7A and B: Anterior discectomy with fusion using (A) Titan cage, (B) polyetheretherketone cage.

Several techniques of anterior cervical discectomy with fusion (ACDF) have been described according to the various grafts that may be used. The most classic method involves the use of tricortical bone autograft harvested from the iliac crest. Autogenous bone graft has the advantage of being accessible during the procedure and can function as an osteoinductive signal or as an osteoconductive bridge. However, harvesting autogenous bone lengthens the procedure. Furthermore, it is associated with chronic donor site pain and long-term functional impairment as well as a significant number of complications unrelated to the principal procedure.[43,44] To avoid these complications, allograft may be used although the fusion rates are reported to be lower than those after the use of autograft.[45] Anterior cervical plating may be used after one or two-level ACDF with allograft to improve the fusion.[46]

In the last years, the use of cages for the fusion and stabilization of the cervical spine has become the most popular method. The cages can consist of various materials (titanium, hydroxyapatite coated, carbon, polyetheretherketone) and may be used empty or filled with bone or bone graft substitutes (Figs. 13.7A and B). The clinical outcome is considered to be equivalent with that after ACDF with autograft.[47] Except of the elimination of complications associated with the donor site, the cages can restore the disk height and the cervical lordosis; however, a higher pseudarthrosis rate may be observed.[48]

Anterior Discectomy without Fusion

Anterior discectomy is possible with partial preservation of the intervertebral disk. This technique can be used in soft disk herniation or sequestration without signs of spondylosis or segmental instability.

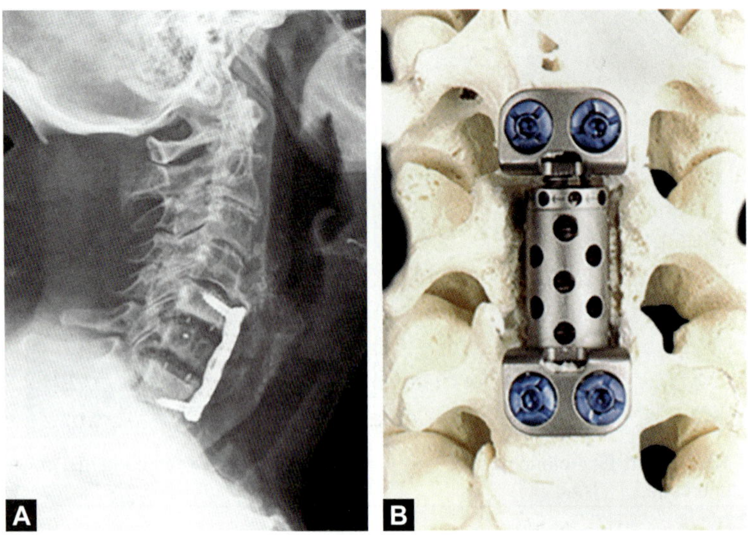

Figs. 13.8A and B: (A) Corpectomy C6 and anterior plating C5–C7. (B) Titan cage for corpectomy reconstruction in a bone model.

The procedure is considered to be safe with success rates comparable with those of ACDF especially when used in young individuals and for monosegmental disease,[49,50] however, usually an ACDF is performed.

Several techniques have been developed for the removal of the disk herniation without removing the intervertebral disk including lateral and combined lateral/anterior approaches.[51] Minimally invasive and percutaneous endoscopic techniques have also been developed including microsurgical anterior foraminotomy and the use of a transdiscal route for the removal of the herniation.[52]

Anterior Corpectomy with Fusion (ACCF)

In cases of narrow spinal canal or where access to the posterior side of the vertebra is required, an anterior discectomy may not be sufficient and a partial or complete corpectomy may be necessary (Figs. 13.8A and B).

After anterior discectomy of the cervical disk above and below the vertebra, the vertebral body is excised. The underlying pathology defines the degree of preservation of the involved anatomical structures, whereas for maximum decompression the posterior longitudinal ligament must also be removed.

Except of a more radical decompression, the evidence suggests that anterior corpectomy provides also higher fusion rates in comparison with multilevel ACDF as the fused surfaces are fewer in total.[53] However, surgical managements of three or four levels for cervical spondylotic myelopathy by ACDF or ACCF are considered equal in terms of clinical outcome, whereas ACDF presents less blood loss, better restoration of cervical lordosis, and fewer graft complications.[54] Anterior plating is recommended to increase fusion rate regardless of the number of levels fused. Autografts have been used for one-level corpectomies and allografts for longer reconstructions. The past years cages have gained in popularity as they prevent the site donor complications.

Anterolateral partial oblique corpectomy does not require the use of graft as more than half of the vertebral body is preserved. The aim of this procedure is the decompression of the spinal cord without fusion and the prevention of the patient from graft-, instrument-, and fusion-related complications.[55]

Total Disk Arthroplasty

The main disadvantage of spinal fusion is the postoperative segmental rigidity, possibly leading to adjacent segment degeneration. To preserve the segmental mobility, the total disk arthroplasty (TDA) for one or two levels has been developed. After the anterior discectomy has been performed, prosthesis is inserted into the intervertebral space (Figs. 13.9A and B).

The aim of any prosthesis is to provide the viscoelastic behavior of a healthy intervertebral disk and re-establish the function of the spinal segment. Various designs (Figs. 13.10A to D), consisting of implants with metal on metal or metal on polymer articulations or of one piece implants with metal endplates, have been developed to achieve this goal (Fig. 13.11).

The clinical studies of the various prosthesis used in the treatment of cervical degenerative disorders have shown that the TDA is a safe and effective surgical treatment for monosegmental cervical degenerative disk disease, and clinical outcomes are considered equivalent or superior to those after fusion.[56,57] Furthermore, in the short- and mid-term, the segmental motion can be preserved, and the procedure is associated with fewer reoperations compared to ACDF.[57]

In cases of multilevel cervical degenerative disk disease, a hybrid operation may be performed, which includes the combination of ACDF with TDA (Fig. 13.12). The TDA is performed in the segment with the better preoperative mobility, whereas ACDF is performed in the more rigid segment. With this procedure segment motion is obtained at the arthroplasty level and immobilization at the fused level (Table 13.5). However, more trials are necessary for the final evaluation of this technique.[58]

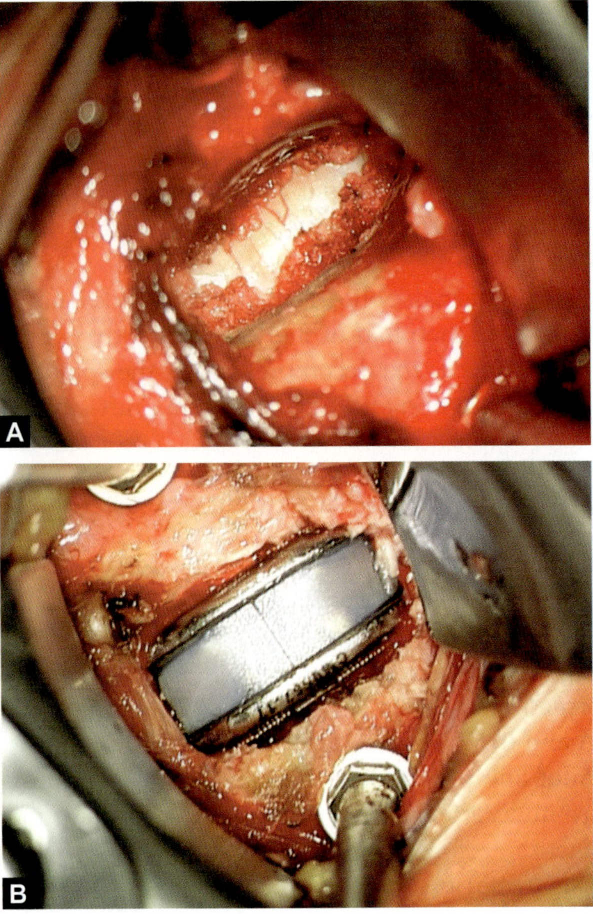

Figs. 13.9A and B: Total disk arthroplasty using the Freedom prosthesis. View of the cervical spine (A) before and (B) after the placement of the prosthesis.

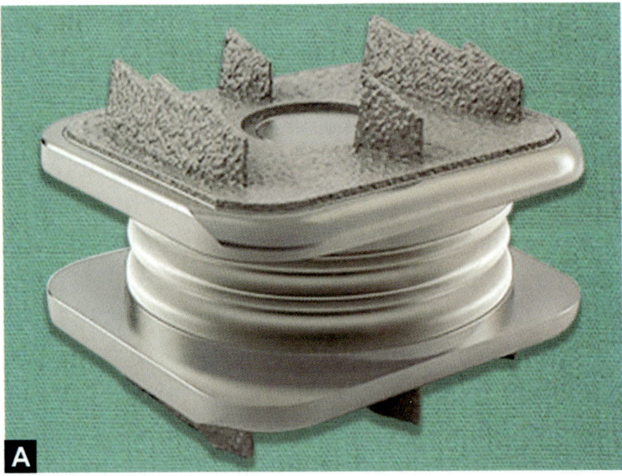

Fig. 13.10A

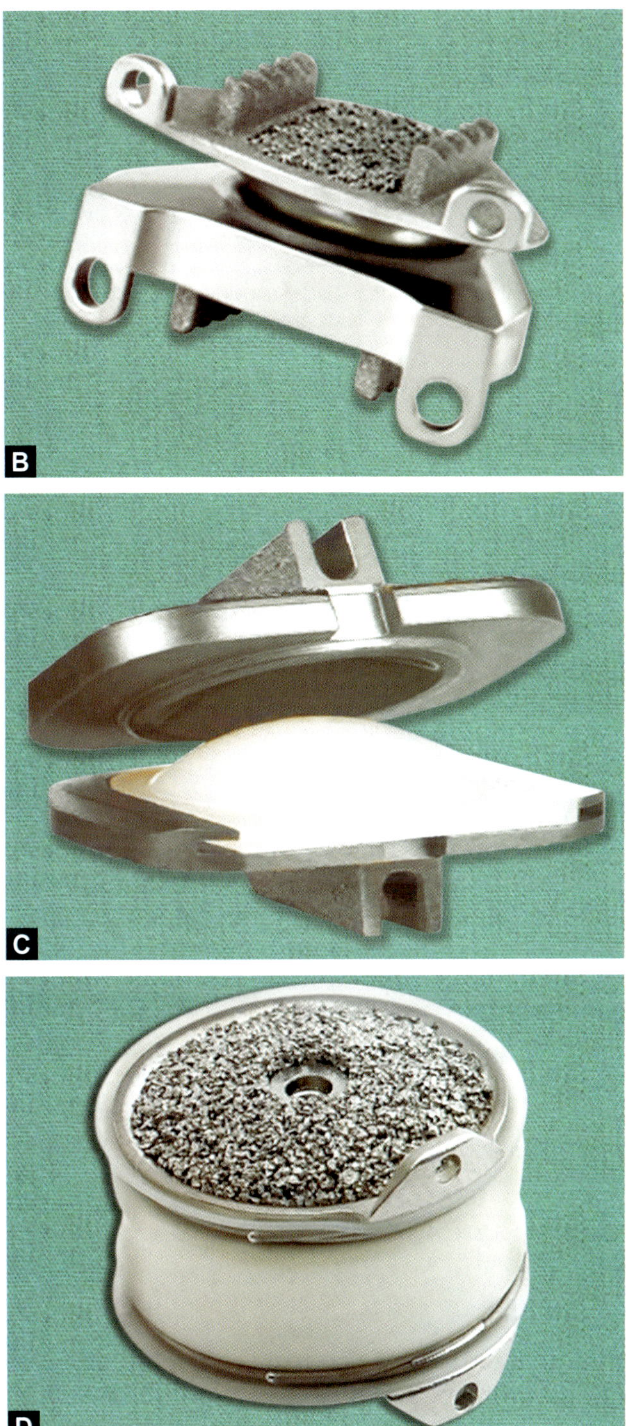

Figs. 13.10A to D: (A) M6 prosthesis. (B) Prestige prosthesis. (C) Prodisc C prosthesis. (D) Bryan prosthesis.

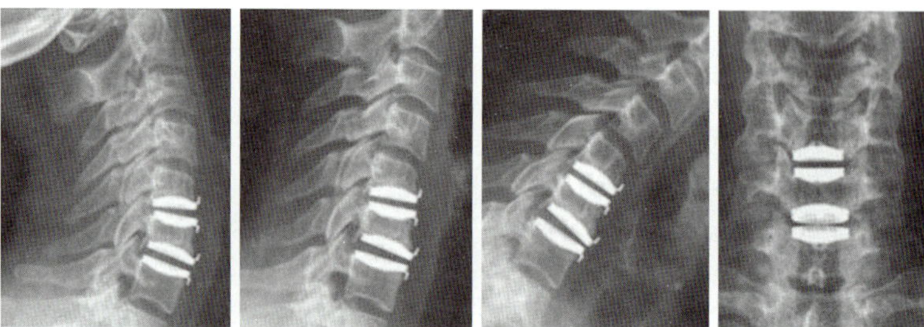

Fig. 13.11: Cervical spine mobility after C5/C6 and C6/C7 total disk arthroplasty in extension, lateral, flexion, and anteroposterior radiographs.

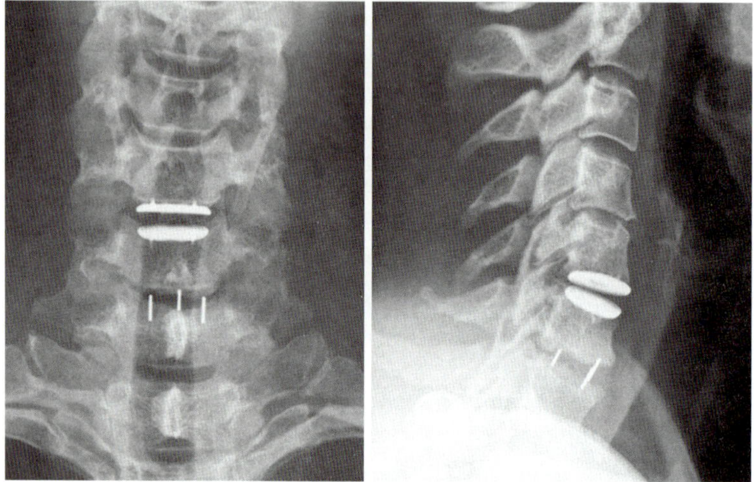

Fig. 13.12: Anteroposterior and lateral radiography after a hybrid operation using a Freedom prosthesis C5/C6 and a polyetheretherketone cage C6/C7.

Table 13.5: Indications of TDA versus ACDF.	
Prosthesis	*Cage*
Intraoperative mobility	Severe degeneration
Active patient	Osteodiscogenic spondylosis
Younger biological age	Age > 60 years
Soft disk	Myelopathy

(TDA: Total disk arthroplasty; ACDF: Anterior cervical discectomy with fusion).

Posterior Approach

For the posterior approach, the patient is in a prone position with the head stabilized by Mayfield skull tongs. A skin incision in the midline is performed, and the paraspinal muscles are separated from the cervical spine. The ligamentum nuchae is then in the midline incised, and the dissection continues along the spinal processes and lamina.

Laminectomy

The posterior laminectomy includes the removal of the lamina and the spinous process so that the spinal cord has more space posteriorly. It is used only when the cervical lordosis is preserved, mainly in cases of multilevel cervical myelopathy, especially in elderly patients or where the neural compression is located posteriorly. The procedure can be combined with a foraminotomy in cases of radiculopathy. The main disadvantage of this method is its limited application only in cases of lordosis as well as a possible postoperative deformity and instability. For this reason, posterior instrumentation can be added to the procedure for extra stability and correction of the kyphosis.[59]

Foraminotomy

Posterior cervical foraminotomy is used only in cases of unilateral radiculopathy without neck pain involvement. For this procedure, part of the superior and inferior lamina is removed as well as part of the facet. Sometimes, partial removal of the intervertebral disk is also necessary. To prevent postoperative neck pain, minimally invasive and endoscopic techniques have been developed for posterior foraminotomy and/or discectomy.

Laminoplasty

The purpose of laminoplasty is the relief of pressure on spinal cord by enlarging the spinal canal. It is mainly indicated in cases of multilevel stenosis of the cervical spinal canal. Its main advantage in comparison with laminectomy is the preservation of the posterior bony structures to preserve the postoperative stability. In addition, laminoplasty has showed lower surgery complication and reoperation rate compared to the cervical decompression with corpectomy when three or more levels are involved.[42]

Several methods of laminoplasty have been developed, but two are the fundamental techniques. The expansive door laminoplasty involves cutting the lamina partially on both sides, creating a trough on one side and an opening on the other side. Then the lamina is lifted up on this side, and a spacer may be inserted to prevent a recurrence of the stenosis. For the French open door laminoplasty, troughs are created on both sides of the lamina and an opening in the center of it, followed by elevation of both sides.

Combined Anterior and Posterior Approach

Despite associated with a higher complications rate, the combination of anterior and posterior approach can be the most beneficial technique

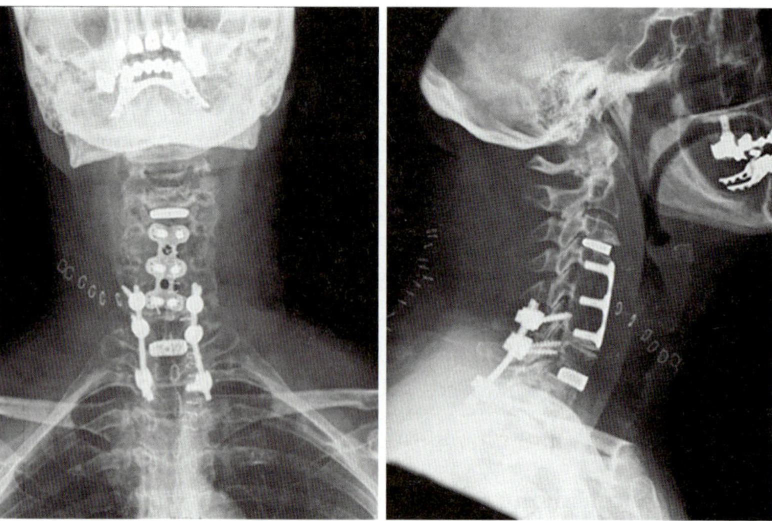

Fig. 13.13: Combined anterior and posterior approach in a patient with cervical spine instability.

for some patients with complex cervical spine disorders[60] (Fig. 13.13). This can be performed as one-stage procedure or with some time interval. Especially, patients who undergo multilevel surgery or patients with a higher risk for instability and pseudarthrosis with proof of poor bone quality or with metabolic disorders can be candidates for a combined procedure.[86]

COMPLICATIONS

Various complications have been reported after surgical treatment of cervical degenerative disk disorders. The occurrence of perioperative complications is associated with increased age, combined anterior–posterior procedures, increased operative time, and increased operative blood loss.[61] The most important complications include:

- Recurrent laryngeal nerve palsy and unilateral vocal fold paralysis with dysphonia is the most common otolaryngologic complication after anterior cervical spine surgery with an incidence that varies widely among the existing studies. In the majority of cases, it is temporary, but it can also be permanent, accompanied with or without hoarseness, and it is more frequently associated with anterior cervical reoperations. There is controversy weather techniques like monitoring of endotracheal cuff pressure released after retractor placement, and left-sided approach may reduce the incidence of this complication.[62,63] Preoperative ENT evaluation of the patients undergoing anterior cervical spine surgery would be extremely helpful in patients with pre-existing silent unilateral vocal cord paralysis, since the operation could place the functional vocal cord in danger and provoke respiratory insufficiency.[64]

- Arytenoid dislocation is a very rare complication of anterior cervical spine operations and occurs mainly due to the intubation. It is important that in cases of postoperative prolonged hoarseness, arytenoid dislocation is also considered in the differential diagnosis, so that it is not misdiagnosed as vocal fold paresis due to laryngeal nerve lesion.[65]

- Laryngeal dislocation is an extremely rare complication after anterior cervical spine surgery and may present as postoperative neck swelling. If more common causes have been excluded, it should be considered in the differential diagnosis, and imaging studies may be necessary before extubation to confirm the diagnosis.[66]

- Dysphagia is the most common early complication after anterior cervical spine surgery, but it is even more common with combined anterior–posterior procedures. It occurs possibly due to neurological or/and soft-tissue injuries. Its incidence decreases significantly with the time, and it appears to be influenced by the duration of pre-existing pain and by the number of vertebral levels involved in the surgical procedure.[61,67]

- Hypopharyngeal diverticulum is rare after anterior cervical spine surgery but must be considered in cases of persistent postoperative dysphagia. It may present as a delayed complication and thus long-term follow-up with imaging studies is necessary. Association has been found with revision surgeries and infections.[68]

- Retropharyngeal hematoma postcervical spine operation is rare but may be proven fatal. It is mainly formed in the early post-operative period. The most important risk factors are considered to be the presence of diffuse idiopathic skeletal hyperostosis or of OPLL, therapeutic heparin use, and longer operative time with involvement of greater number of surgical levels.[69]

- Esophageal perforations are rare after anterior cervical spine surgery and may result from minor complications to mediastinitis and death. There are case reports of esophageal penetrations after failure of lateral distraction devices or due to pressure from them. The most frequent symptoms are neck and throat pain, odynophagia, dysphagia, hoarseness, and aspiration.[70]

- Spinal infection and abscess formation is uncommon after cervical spine surgery and is mainly present after esophageal perforations. In cases of persistent dysphagia or deterioration of pre-existed dysphagia, the patient should be evaluated for esophageal perforation and consecutive spinal infection.[71]

- Sleep apnea after anterior cervical spine surgery is very rare. Central sleep apnea is reported in only two cases in the literature as a transient early or delayed complication after posterior laminectomy for the treatment of cervical myelopathy.[72]
- Horner's syndrome is associated with ptosis, ipsilateral miosis, and anhydrosis and is the result of damage of the sympathetic trunk during the anterior approach to the lower cervical spine. In the lower cervical spine, the sympathetic trunk is situated closer to the medial border of the longus colli muscle and thus more susceptible to injuries.[73]
- Hypoglossal nerve palsy with dysarthria and dysphagia is a very rare complication after anterior surgery of the upper cervical spine. Although the functional impairment may resolve spontaneously, the palsy is considered to be rather permanent.[74]
- Cerebrospinal fluid leak due to cervical dural tears has a reported prevalence of 0.5–3% and can be present after anterior or posterior procedures. The main risk factors for its development are the presence of an ossified posterior longitudinal ligament and an anterior revision surgery. Furthermore, cervical CSF leak is associated with the risk of meningitis, CSF fistel, or pseudomeningocele.[75]
- Intracranial epidural hemorrhage after spinal surgery is extremely uncommon but may develop secondary due to cerebrospinal fluid leak and intracranial hypotension. It should be considered in cases of cervical spine surgery with delayed restoration of consciousness and respiration after anesthesia, especially in adolescents.[76]
- Spinal epidural hematoma may occur in patients undergoing posterior or anterior cervical spine surgery. It presents with postoperative neurologic deterioration and often occurs the first 24 hours after surgery. It may extend to adjacent nonoperated levels. Avoidance of postoperative nonsteroidal anti-inflammatory drugs may decrease the risk in contrast with higher level of comorbidities, which appears to be a risk factor.[77,78]
- Segmental root palsy is one of the commonest complications of anterior or posterior cervical decompression surgery. Especially, common is the postoperative C5 palsy leading to a variety of symptoms. The pathology of this condition is not fully understood, although many hypotheses have been proposed.
- Vertebral artery injury is a rare complication, which occurs mainly after anterior cervical decompression or posterior atlantoaxial transarticular screw fixation. Potential risk exists also in cases of cervical pedicle screw or C1 lateral mass screw fixation.[79] Rare cases of vertebral arteriovenous fistula are also reported after anterior surgery.[80]

- Respiratory insufficiency is a rare but potentially lethal complication after anterior cervical spine surgery. It is mostly attributed to edema of the pharyngeal wall or of the arytenoids and more frequent in patients with prolonged procedures, with greater blood loss, where more than three vertebral levels are involved.[81]
- Tetraparesis or tetraplegia is one of the most feared complications after cervical spine operations, and it occurs mainly due to epidural hematoma.[82] Other possible causes are iatrogenic traumatisms, abscess formation, or a vascular insult such as the ischemia and reperfusion injury.
- Death due to cervical spine surgery is considered rather rare. The overall incidence is believed to be 0.42%.[83]
- Surgical site infection is a common complication after cervical spine surgery with an incidence that varies widely among the various studies. Higher rates have been reported after posterior procedures compared with anterior procedures and when a neck collar is used.[84]
- Adjacent segment disease is not really a complication as it is more of a natural consequence of some cervical spine operations. It involves many pathologies including instability, listhesis, herniation, stenosis, arthritis, scoliosis, and vertebral compression fracture. After fusion extra stress is added to the adjacent segments, especially to the more mobile regions, leading to degeneration.[85]
- Instrumentation failure, graft dislocation, or collapse and nonfusion are all complications dependent on the procedure that has been followed.

REFERENCES

1. Rao R. Neck pain cervical radiculopathy and cervical myelopathy. Pathophysiology natural history and clinical evaluation. J Bone Joint Surg Am. 2002; 84(10):1872-81.
2. Hoy DG, Protani M, De R, Buchbinder R. The epidemiology of neck pain. Best Pract Res Clin Rheumatol. 2010;24(6):783-92.
3. Gore DR, Sepic SB, Gardner GM, et al. Neck pain: a long-term follow-up of 205 patients. Spine. 1987;12(1):1-5
4. Rothman SM, Huang Z, Lee KE, et al. Cytokine mRNA expression in painful radiculopathy. Pain J. 2009;10(1):90-9.
5. Wainner RS, Gill H. Diagnosis and nonoperative management of cervical radiculopathy. J Orthop Sports Phys Ther. 2000;30(12):728-40.
6. Radhakrishnan K, Litchy WJ, O'Fallon WM, et al. Epidemiology of cervical radiculopathy. A population-based study from Rochester, Minnesota, 1976 through 1990. Brain. 1994;117(Pt 2):325-35.
7. Connell MD, Wiesel SW. Natural history and pathogenesis of cervical disk disease. Orthop Clin North Am. 1992;23:369-80.

8. Yonenobu K. Cervical radiculopathy and myelopathy: when and what can surgery contribute to treatment? Eur Spine J. 2000;9(1):1-7.

9. LaBan MM, Meerschaert JR, Taylor RS. Breast pain: a symptom of cervical radiculopathy. Arc Phys Med Rahebil. 1979;60(7):315-7.

10. Abbed, KM, Coumans, JV. Cervical radiculopathy pathophysiology, presentation and clinical evaluation. Neurosurgery. 2007; 60(1):28-34.

11. Mochida K, Komori H, Okawa A, et al. Regression of cervical disc herniation observed on magnetic resonance images. Spine (Phila Pa 1976). 1998;23(9): 990-5: discussion 996-7.

12. Hong L, Kawaguchi Y. Anterior cervical discectomy and fusion to treat cervical spondylosis with sympathetic symptoms. J Spinal Disord Tech. 2011;24:11-4.

13. Bauer F. Dysphagia due to cervical spondylosis. J Laryngol Otol. 1953;67(10): 615-30.

14. Smith DR, Vanderark GD, Kempe LG. Cervical spondylosis causing vertebrobasilar insufficiency: a surgical treatment. Neurol Neurosurg Psychiatry. 1971;34(4):388-92.

15. Bulsara KR, Velez DA, Villavizenzio A. Rotational vertebral artery insufficiency resulting from cervical spondylosis: case report and review of the literature. Surg Neurol. 2006;65(6):625-7.

16. Browne P, Clark G, Kuboki T, et al. Concurrent cervical and craniofacial pain. Oral Surg Oral Med Oral Pathol Oral Radiol. 1990;88(6):633-40.

17. White AA, Johnson RM, Panjabi MM, et al. Biomechanical analysis of cervical stability in the cervical spine. Clin Orthop Relat Res. 1975;109:85-96.

18. Pueschel SM, Scola FH. Atlantoaxial instability in individuals with Down syndrome: epidemiologic, radiographic, and clinical studies. Pediatrics. 1987; 80(4):555-60.

19. Dreyer SJ, Boden SD. Natural history of rheumatoid arthritis of the cervical spine. Clin Orthop Relat Res. 1999;366:98-106.

20. Karkos PD, Benton J, Leong SC, et al. Grisel's syndrome in otolaryngology: a systematic review. Int J Pediatr Otorhinolaryngol. 2007;71(12):1823-7.

21. Bocciolini C, Dall'Olio D, Cunsolo E, et al. Grisel's syndrome: a rare complication following adenoidectomy. Acta Otorhinoraringol Ital. 2005; 25(4):245-9.

22. Zahrai A, Rhee J. Cervical and thoracic degenerative spinal instability. Semin Spine Surg. 2013;25(2):83-91.

23. Deburge A, Mazda K, Guigui P. Unstable degenerative spondylolisthesis of the cervical spine. J Bone Joint Surg. 1995;77B(1):122-5.

24. Boogaarts HD, Bartels RH. Prevalence of cervical spondylotic myelopathy. Eur Spine J. 2015;24(Suppl 2):139-41.

25. Wu JC, Ko CC, Yen YS, et al. Epidemiology of cervical spondylotic myelopathy and its risk of causing spinal cord injury: a national cohort study. Neurosurg Focus. 2013;35(1):E10.

26. Baptiste DC, Fehlings MG. Pathophysiology of cervical myelopathy. Spine J. 2006;6(6):190-7.

27. Inamasu J, Guiot BH, Sachs DC. Ossification of the posterior longitudinal ligament: an update on its biology, epidemiology and natural history. Neurosurgery. 2006;58(6):1027-39.

28. Inoue H, Seichi A, Kimura A, et al. Multiple-level ossification of the ligamentum flavum in the cervical spine combined with calcification of the cervical ligamentum flavum and posterior atlanto-axial membrane. Eur Spine J. 2013;22 (3):416-20.

29. Lee JH, Lee SH, Seo IS. The characteristics of gait disturbance and its relationship with posterior tibial somatosensory evoked potentials in patients with cervical myelopathy. Spine. 2011;36(8):524-30.

30. Mignadort JB, Deschamps T, Barrey E, et al. Gait disturbances as specific predictive markers of the first fall onset in elderly people: a two-year prospective observational study. Front Aging Neurosci. 2014;6:22.

31. Ebara S, Yonenobu K, Fujiwara K, et al. Myelopathy hand characterised by muscle wasting. A different type of myelopathy hand in patients with cervical spondylosis. Spine (Phila Pa 1976). 1998;13(7):785-91.

32. Hurwit E, Carragee E, Van der Velde G, et al. Treatment of neck pain: noninvasive interventions: results of the bone and joint decade 2000-2010 Task Force of Neck Pain and Its Associated Disorders. J Manipulative Physiol Ther. 2009; 32(2):141-75.

33. Boyce RH, Wang JC. Evaluation of neck pain, radiculopathy and myelopathy: imaging, conservative treatment, and surgical indications. Instr Course Lect. 2003;52:489-95.

34. Bambakidis NC, Feiz-Erfan I, Klopfenstein JD, et al. Indications for surgical fusion of the cervical and lumbar motion segment. Spine. 2005;30(16):S2-6.

35. Carette S, Fehlings MG. Clinical practice cervical radiculopathy. N Engl J Med. 2005;353(4):392-9.

36. Edwards CC 2nd, Riew KD, Anderson PA, et al. Cervical myelopathy: current diagnosis and treatment strategies. Spine J. 2003;3:68-81.

37. Epstein N. Posterior approaches in the management of cervical spondylosis and ossification of the posterior longitudinal ligament. Surg Neurol. 2002;58 (3-4):194-207; discussion 207-8.

38. Hosono N, Yonenobu K, Ono K. Neck and shoulder pain after laminoplasty: a noticeable complication. Spine J. 1996;21(17):1969-73.

39. Hsu W, Dorsi MJ, Witham TF. Surgical management of cervical spondylotic myelopathy. Neurosurg Q. 2009;19(4):302-7.

40. Alvin M, Lubelski D, Benzel E, et al. Ventral fusion versus dorsal fusion. Neurosurg Focus. 2013;35(1):e5.

41. Komotar R, Mocco J, Kaiser M. Surgical management of cervical myelopathy; indications and techniques for laminectomy and fusion. Spine J. 2006;6(6): 252S-67S.

42. Liu X, Min S, Zhang H, Zhou Z, et al. Anterior corpectomy versus posterior laminoplasty for multilevel cervical myelopathy: a systematic review and meta-analysis. Eur Spine J. 2014;23:362-7.

43. Georgia Hand and Microsurgery Clinic, Atlanta, GA. Iliac crest autogenous bone grafting: donor site complications. J South Orthop Assoc. 2000;9(2):91-7.

44. Silber JS, Anderson DG, Daffner SD, et al. Donor site morbidity after anterior iliac crest bone harvest for single-level anterior cervical discectomy and fusion. Spine. 2003;28(2):134-9.

45. Malloy K, Hilibrand A. Autograft versus allograft in degenerative cervical disease. Curr Orthop Pract. 2002;394:27-38.

46. Kaiser M, Haid R, Subach B, et al. Anterior cervical plating enhances arthrodesis after discectomy and fusion with cortical allograft. J Neuroserg. 2002;50(2): 229-38.

47. Hacker RJ, Cauthen JC, Gilbert TJ, et al. A prospective randomised multicenter clinical evaluation of an anterior cervical fusion cage. Spine. 2000;25(20): 2646-55.

48. Vavruch L, Hedlund R, Javid D, et al. A prospective randomised comparison between the Cloward procedure and a carbon fiber cage in the cervical spine: a clinical and radiologic study. Spine. 2002;27(16):1694-701.

49. Savolainen S, Rinne J, Hernesniemi J. A prospective randomized study of anterior single-level cervical disc operations with long-term follow up: surgical fusion is unnecessary. Neurosurgery. 1998;43(1):51-5.

50. Bertalanffy H, Eggert HR. Clinical long-term results of anterior discectomy without fusion for treatment of cervical radiculopathy and myelopathy. Acta Neurochir. 1998 (Wien);90:127-35.

51. Hakuba A. Trans-unco-discal approach: a combined anterior and lateral approach to cervical discs. J Neurosurg. 1976;45(3):284-91.

52. Jho HD. Microsurgical anterior cervical foraminotomy for radiculopathy: a new approach to cervical disc herniation. J Neurosurg. 1996;84(2):155-60.

53. Fraser JF, Härtl R. Anterior approaches to fusion of the cervical spine: a meta-analysis of fusion rates. J Neurosurg Spine. 2007;6(4):298-303.

54. Lin Q, Zhou X, Wang X, et al. A comparison of anterior cervical discectomy and corpectomy in patients with multilevel cervical spondylotic myelopathy. Eur Spine J. 2012;21(3):474-81.

55. Kiris T, Kilinçer C. Cervical spondylotic myelopathy treated by oblique corpectomy: a prospective study. Neurosurg J. 2008;62(3):674-82.

56. Murrey D, Janssen M, Delamarter R, et al. Results of the prospective, randomized, controlled multicenter Food and Drug Administration investigational device exemption study of the ProDisc-C total disc replacement versus anterior discectomy and fusion for the treatment of 1-level symptomatic cervical disc disease. Spine J. 2009;9(4):275-86.

57. Mummaneni PV, Burkus JK, Haid RW, et al. Clinical and radiographic analysis of cervical disc arthroplasty compared with allograft fusion: a randomized controlled clinical trial. Neurosurg J. 2007;6(3):198-209.

58. Jia Z, Mo Z, Ding F, et al. Hybrid surgery for multilevel cervical degenerative disc diseases: a systematic review of biomechanical and clinical evidence. Eur Spine J. 2014;23(8):1619-32.

59. Abumi K, Kaneda K, Shono Y, et al. One-stage posterior decompression and reconstruction of the cervical spine by using pedicle screw fixation systems. Neurosurg J. 1999;90(1):19-26.

60. Schultz KD, McLaughlin MR, Haid RW, et al. Single-stage anterior—posterior decompression and stabilization for complex cervical spine disorders. J Neurosurg.. 2000;93(2 Suppl):214-21.

61. Fehlings MG, Smith JS, Kopjar B, et al. Perioperative and delayed complications associated with the surgical treatment of cervical spondylotic myelopathy based on 302 patients from the AO Spine North America Cervical Spondylotic Myelopathy Study. Neurosurg J. 2012;16(5):425-32.

62. Apfelbaum RI, Kriskovich MD, Haller JR. On the incidence, cause, and prevention of recurrent laryngeal nerve palsies during anterior cervical spine surgery. Spine J. 2000;25(22):2906-12

63. Beutler WJ, Sweeney CA, Connolly PJ. Recurrent laryngeal nerve injury with anterior cervical spine surgery: risk with laterality of surgical approach. Spine J. 2001;26(12):1337-42.

64. Manski TJ, Wood MD, Dunsker SB. Bilateral vocal cord paralysis following anterior cervical discectomy and fusion: Case report. Neurosurg J. 1998;89(5):839-43.

65. Goz V, Qureshi S, Hecht AC. Arytenoid dislocation as a cause of prolonged hoarseness after cervical discectomy and fusion. Global Spine J. 2013;3(1):47-50.

66. Krauel J, Winkler D, Münscher A, et al. Laryngeal dislocation after ventral fusion of the cervical spine. Indian J Anaesth. 2013;57(3):285-8.

67. Riley LH III, Skolasky RL, Albert TJ, et al. Dysphagia after anterior cervical decompression and fusion: prevalence and risk factors from a longitudinal Cohort study. Spine J. 2005;30(22):2564-9.

68. Allis TJ, Grant NN, Davidson BJ. Hypopharyngeal diverticulum formation following anterior discectomy and fusion: case series. Ear Nose Throat J. 2010;89(11):E4-9.

69. O'Neill KR, Neuman B, Peters C, et al. Risk factors for postoperative retropharyngeal hematoma after anterior cervical spine surgery. Spine (Phila Pa 1976). 2014;39(4):246-52.

70. Gaudinez RF, English GM, Gebhard JS, et al. Esophageal perforations after anterior cervical surgery. Spinal Disord J. 2000;13(1):77-84.

71. Korovessis P, Repantis T, Vitsas V, et al. Cervical spondylodiscitis associated with oesophageal perforation: a rare complication after anterior cervical fusion. Eur J Orthop Surg Traumatol. 2013;23(Suppl 2):S159-63.

72. Massimiliano V, Della Pepa GM, Giuseppe B, et al. Reversible and delayed isolated central sleep apnea after cervical laminectomy: report of the first case. Acta Neurochir. 2014;156(2):267-8.

73. Ebraheim NA, Lu J, Yang H, et al. Vulnerability of the sympathetic trunk during the anterior approach to the lower cervical spine. Spine J. 2000;25(13):1603-6.

74. Sengupta DK, Grevitt MP, Mehdian SMH. Hypoglossal nerve injury as a complication of anterior surgery to the upper cervical spine. Eur Spine J. 1999;8(1):78-80.

75. Hannallah D, Lee J, Khan M, et al. Cerebrospinal fluid leaks following cervical spine surgery. J Bone Joint Surg Am. 2008;90(5):1101-5.

76. Li ZJ, Sun P, Dou YH, et al. Bilateral supratentorial epidural hematomas: a rare complication in adolescent spine surgery. Neurol Med Chir (Tokyo). 2012;52(9):646-8.

77. Goldstein CL, Bains I, Hurlbert RJ. Symptomatic spinal epidural hematoma after posterior cervical surgery: incidence and risk factors. Spine J. 2015 Jun;15(6):1179-87.

78. Song XH, Xu RM, Sun SH, et al. Analysis of epidural hematoma formative reason and its preventive measure after anterior cervical operation. Zhongguo Gu Shang. 2013;26(3):197-200.

79. Neo M, Fujibayashi S, Miyata M, et al. Vertebral artery injury during cervical spine surgery: a survey than more 5600 operations. Spine J. 2008;33(7):779-85.

80. Cosgrove GR, Théron J. Vertebral arteriovenosous fistula following anterior cervical spine surgery: report of two cases. Neurosurg J. 1987;66(2):297-9.

81. Sagi HC, Beutler W, Carroll E, et al. Airway complications associated with surgery on the anterior cervical spine. Spine J. 2002;27(9):949-53.

82. Jang JW, Lee JK, Seo BR, et al. Spontaneous resolution of tetraparesis because of postoperative cervical epidural hematoma. Spine J. 2010;10(12):e1-5.

83. Skolasky RL, Thorpe RJ Jr, Wegener ST, et al. Complications and mortality in cervical spine surgery: racial differences. Spine (Phila Pa 1976). 2014;39 (18):1506-12.

84. Barnes M, Liew S. The incidence of infection after posterior cervical spine surgery: a 10 year review. Global Spine J. 2012;2(1):3-6.

85. Virk SS, Niedermeier S, Yu E, et al. Adjacent segment disease. Orthopedics. 2014; 37(8):547-55.

86. König SA, Spetzger U. Surgical management of cervical spondylotic myelopathy—indications for anterior, posterior or combined procedures for decompression and stabilization. Acta Neurochir. 2014;156(2):253-8.

Chapter 14

An Update on Hearing Aid Technology

Mark Williams, Rekesh Patel

INTRODUCTION

In 2011, the World Health Organization estimated that 360 million people worldwide (15 years of age or over) were living with some disabling degree of hearing loss.[1] At the time of writing, this estimate would have equated to 5.3% of the world population who would benefit from medical/surgical intervention, implantable technology, or hearing aid use. The leading causes of bothersome hearing loss, which affect the international adult population, have been reported as being presbycusis and noise-induced hearing loss;[2] which result in a sensorineural hearing deficit that cannot, currently, be managed by medical means.

It is well documented that hearing loss can severely impair an individual's communication ability and, consequently, reduce their quality of life.[3] In older adults (>53 years old), it has been reported that hearing loss can amplify the general decline/frailty that, typically, occurs with the advancement of years leading to an increase in difficultly when engaging in daily living activities.[4] Large scale patient surveys have also revealed that these combined challenges can increase the risk of individuals experiencing isolationism and negative emotional states such as depression.[5] However, it is important to note that the negative impact of hearing loss can be ameliorated by the regular use of prescribed hearing aids. Multiple studies have demonstrated that hearing aid use can significantly reduce hearing loss-induced depression in addition to improving communication, cognitive function, and social interaction ability.[6,7] It is probable that the above factors have served to inspire the research and development effort that hearing aid manufacturers have invested in over the last 20 years.

Since the commercialization of the first fully digital hearing aid system from Widex A/S in the mid-1990s (Fig. 14.1), technology has dramatically evolved in order to meet the needs of individuals with

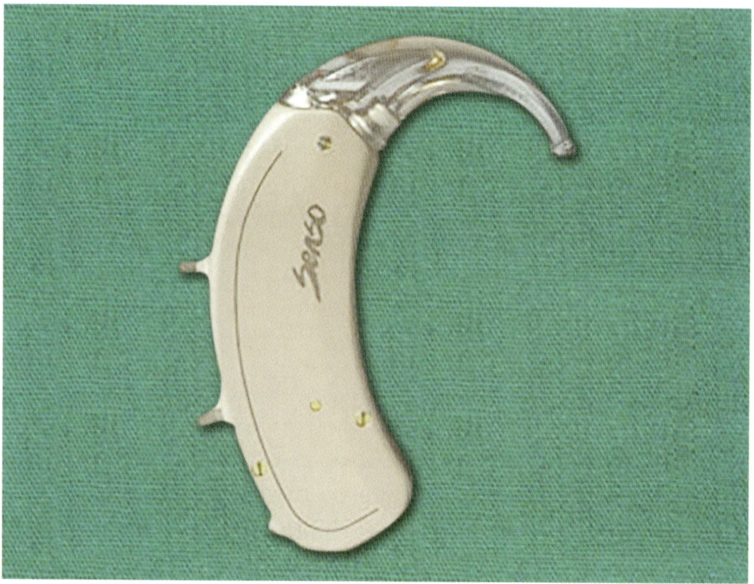

Fig. 14.1: Widex Senso behind-the-ear hearing aid. The first fully digital hearing aid by Widex A/S in the mid-1990s.
Courtesy: Widex A/S Lynge, Denmark.

hearing impairment and, more recently, bothersome tinnitus. As of 2015, the transition of use from analog to digital hearing aid technology appears to be almost complete with the vast majority of instrument manufactures no longer providing analog technology options for aiding. This is due to the fact that digital hearing aids have many clear advantages over analog instruments. The prime advantage of digital signal processing being that it can provide an incredibly high degree of sound signal manipulation that can translate into real audibility, comfort, and signal in noise detection improvements for the user. This enhancement in functionality is also achieved without excessive battery current requirements while also enabling the physical size of digital hearing instruments to actually be reduced. Manufactures have taken advantage of this increased flexibility to enable the development of specific algorithms that serve to manipulate a number of instrument processing parameters, simultaneously, in order to improve the listening experience and speech discrimination ability of the end user. The ability of user instruments to wirelessly interface directly with one another and other devices like smartphones, televisions, and audio equipment has also been made possible as a result of the inception of digital hearing aid technologies.

Presently, all hearing aid manufacturers offer instruments that really have evolved into intelligent, self-adapting systems that utilize a variety of algorithms that strive to address a user's listening requirements in specific environmental situations. Over the past two decades, manufacturer algorithms have proliferated in number and advanced in complexity as rival companies strive to improve their products. The number of instrument styles and shells has also increased dramatically. This chapter will serve to review current hearing aid technology features and examine how they can be applied clinically for the benefit of patients.

HOW HEARING AIDS WORK

Before reviewing contemporary hearing aid technology in detail, it is important to review some general points regarding amplification. Irrespective of the great variety of styles available, all digital hearing aids have the same core components: a microphone, a digital signal processor, an amplifier, a receiver (or speaker), and a battery cell. The microphone picks up sound signals and converts (or transduces) them into electrical signals. The amplifier then magnifies the electrical signal, to an appropriate degree, pursuant to the user's hearing requirements. The receiver then finally transduces the amplified electrical signals back into sound signals that are conveyed to the eardrum. The battery cell simply provides the power for the circuit process (Fig. 14.2).

It is useful to understand some basic terminologies that relate to the above process:

- *Input*: This refers to the sound pressure level (SPL) at the microphone port of a hearing aid and is expressed in dBSPL.
- *Output*: This refers to the SPL that is delivered to the ear from the receiver and is expressed in dBSPL.
- *Gain*: This refers to the level of amplification that is applied to the input signal by the hearing aid amplifier. It is the difference between the output SPL and the input SPL and is expressed in dB.

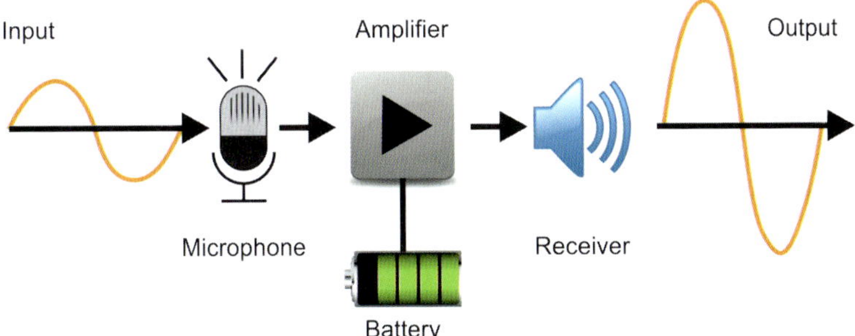

Fig. 14.2: Basic components of a hearing aid: microphone, amplifier, receiver, and battery. *Courtesy*: Starkey Hearing Technologies Minnesota, USA.

- *Compression*: Sensorineural hearing loss is, typically, associated with recruitment that results in individuals having difficulty in hearing low-intensity sounds while experiencing loud sounds as being just as unpleasant to a person with normal hearing function. This range of hearing between a subject's threshold audibility and threshold discomfort is referred to as their dynamic range. Therefore, if an instrument provides the same gain to all input SPLs of a certain frequency range, irrespective of them being soft or loud, high-intensity noises are going to be perceived as painful and may be damaging to the user. Equally very soft noises may be inaudible if the gain is lowered to protect the user from loud sounds. To overcome this, hearing aids utilize compression systems that lower (or compress) the gain applied to input signals in accordance with the input signal SPL. The degree of gain decreases as the input signal intensity increases. This enables all processed sounds to "fit" proportionately with the dynamic range so that soft noises are audible (but still soft) while loud sounds are perceived as loud but never loud enough to cause pain or discomfort. The input SPL level that induces the aid to actively compress the gain is known as the threshold kneepoint (TK).
- *Gain channel*: All contemporary digital hearing aids are able to divide sound into different frequency bands, called channels. The level of gain and compression in each channel can be adjusted independently, in order to enable certain frequency ranges to be amplified more than others. This is essential to enable proportional amplification to be applied appropriately in-line with the user's audiometric configuration (i.e. for presbycusis high gain for high-frequency signals and low gain for lower-frequency signals). This concept is very similar to graphic equalizer settings on other digital audio equipment. More channels usually enable the instrument to compensate for the user's hearing loss with greater precision. Also, the instrument's scene analysis, of the acoustic environment, can be more accurate that has the potential to enhance the efficacy of other algorithms. However, the theoretical benefits of channel numbers are not always translated into an improved listening experience by users.

INSTRUMENT STYLES

Hearing aids come in various shapes, sizes, and colors. Users choose devices for a variety of reasons, but decisions are primarily based on cosmetic appeal and the usability advantages that specific devices provide. The platforms utilized to enable signal processing within hearing aids are either digital or analog. As mentioned previously, analog hearings aids are being phased out due to the superiority of the evolving digital platforms that provide clients with improved functionality and adaptive parameter options for the auditory environment that they are in. A description of the different hearing aid styles has been detailed below starting with the least conspicuous devices.

Behind-the-Ear Hearing Aids

These are hearing aids where the mechanical body of the device sits behind the ear (BTE) and is connected to a silicone or acrylic mold via a hollow plastic tube as portrayed in Figures 14.3A and B. The mold is manufactured from an impression of the client's ear, and is made to occupy the concha along with part of the outer auditory meatus. The mold is bespoke for the client and specific for each ear. These types of devices can be used to treat individuals with mild to profound hearing losses. The size and shape of both the hearing aid body and mold will vary depending on the degree of hearing loss that requires aiding. These devices ensure durability and reliability as they typically possess water and cerumen repellent protection systems. This ensures that the hearing aids can be worn in a variety of environments for long periods of time.

Behind-the-ear hearing aids can also be fitted with "open ear" insertion tips whereby the clinician utilizes a small, soft earpiece/dome at the tip of a thinner hollow plastic tubing that inserts into the ear. This replaces the need for an ear mold and makes the setting aesthetic. Unfortunately, it is only suitable for mild or moderate hearing losses due to the limitations of most feedback suppression circuits. Open fittings reduce the risk of users experiencing the sometimes unwelcome sensation of blocking, or occlusion, which can cause the client's voice to sound resonant; particularly when pronouncing low-frequency speech phonemes.

Pros:
- Suitable for aiding a variety of hearing losses
- Durable
- Batteries last longer
- Open ear fittings are, acoustically, more comfortable for clients at risk of experiencing occlusion effects.

Cons:
- Size of the mold and tubing makes the device more noticeable
- Requires regular maintenance due to hardening of the plastic tubing that can impact on acoustic quality
- Body of the device is generally larger
- Feedback suppression is less robust.

Receiver-in-Canal Hearing Aids

The devices look similar to BTE aids, with the main difference being that the receiver sits directly within the auditory meatus rather than in the mechanical body BTE as portrayed in Figures 14.3C and D. This enables the overall device to be smaller than a BTE device, while also enabling it to be suitable for a variety of hearing losses. Moving the receiver away from the microphone not only reduces its size but also reduces the chance of feedback. A receiver-in-canal (RIC) device, also known as receiver in-the-ear hearing aid, benefits the client by providing an aesthetic look and lighter feel as the receiver is connected to the body of the device with a very thin discreet wire. Also, as the main body of RIC instruments is very small, compared to BTEs, the devices are normally cosmetically appealing to most individuals.

Pros:

- Suitable for aiding a variety of hearing losses
- Durable
- Device is cosmetically appealing
- Better feedback suppression than BTE.

Cons:

- Batteries have a lower capacity compared to BTEs.

Molded Hearing Aids

These are devices where the body of the instrument is entirely contained within the ear mold shell. These hearing aids are entirely bespoke and are molded to fit the patient's auditory meatus and cavum concha. Unlike the BTE and RIC aids, there is no portion that sits BTE thus giving the system the opportunity to take advantage of the natural resonant properties of the pinna, to provide directionality, as the microphones are physically located within the ear canal/concha. Molded hearing aids are subject to a greater amount of wear and tear due to the electronics being exposed to potentially high levels of condensation and cerumen due to the instrument's location within the ear. Where possible, patients tend to prefer these devices as some models are generally more cosmetically appealing than BTE models. There are various types of molded hearing aids that vary in size and functionality.

In-the-Ear Hearing Aids

These devices were first developed in the mid-1950s and were the first molded hearing devices designed to fit entirely in the ear canal and cavum concha as portrayed in Figures 14.3E and F. The electronic components are wholly contained within the ear mold shell. They were initially designed to only aid mild hearing losses but with technological advances they have now evolved to be able to provide aiding for severe degrees of hearing loss. Due to their size, they have fewer functionality options, such as a volume control, and often have a limited ability to communicate with other wireless technologies.

Pros:

- Able to utilize resonant properties of the Pinna for improved natural directionality
- Cosmetically appealing compared to some BTE devices
- Ability to aid a variety of hearing losses.

Cons:

- Subject to wear and tear due to the mechanical components in closer contact to condensation and cerumen
- Not as cosmetically appealing as compared to completely-in-the-canal (CIC) and in-the-canal (ITC) devices.

ITC Hearing Aids

After in-the-ear (ITE) hearing aids were created, hearing aid technology and design improved further that enabled the miniaturization of the ITE device so that all components could fit into a shell that sits in the auditory meatus with only a slight protrusion into the cavum concha. The device is, consequently, less visible than the ITE as portrayed in Figures 14.3G and H. Due to the size, ITC devices are used to treat individuals with mild-to-severe hearing losses, but lose some features such as a volume control option and program interface. The ITC devices also have an improved ability to take advantage of the natural resonant properties of the pinna.

Pros:

- More aesthetic than both the ITE and BTE devices
- Able to utilize the natural acoustic properties of the pinna and the cavum concha
- Modern systems are able to treat individuals with a severe hearing loss.

Cons:

- Due to the size, battery life is often compromised
- Reduced ability for the client to alter the device amplification and program parameters
- Generally has no wireless capability

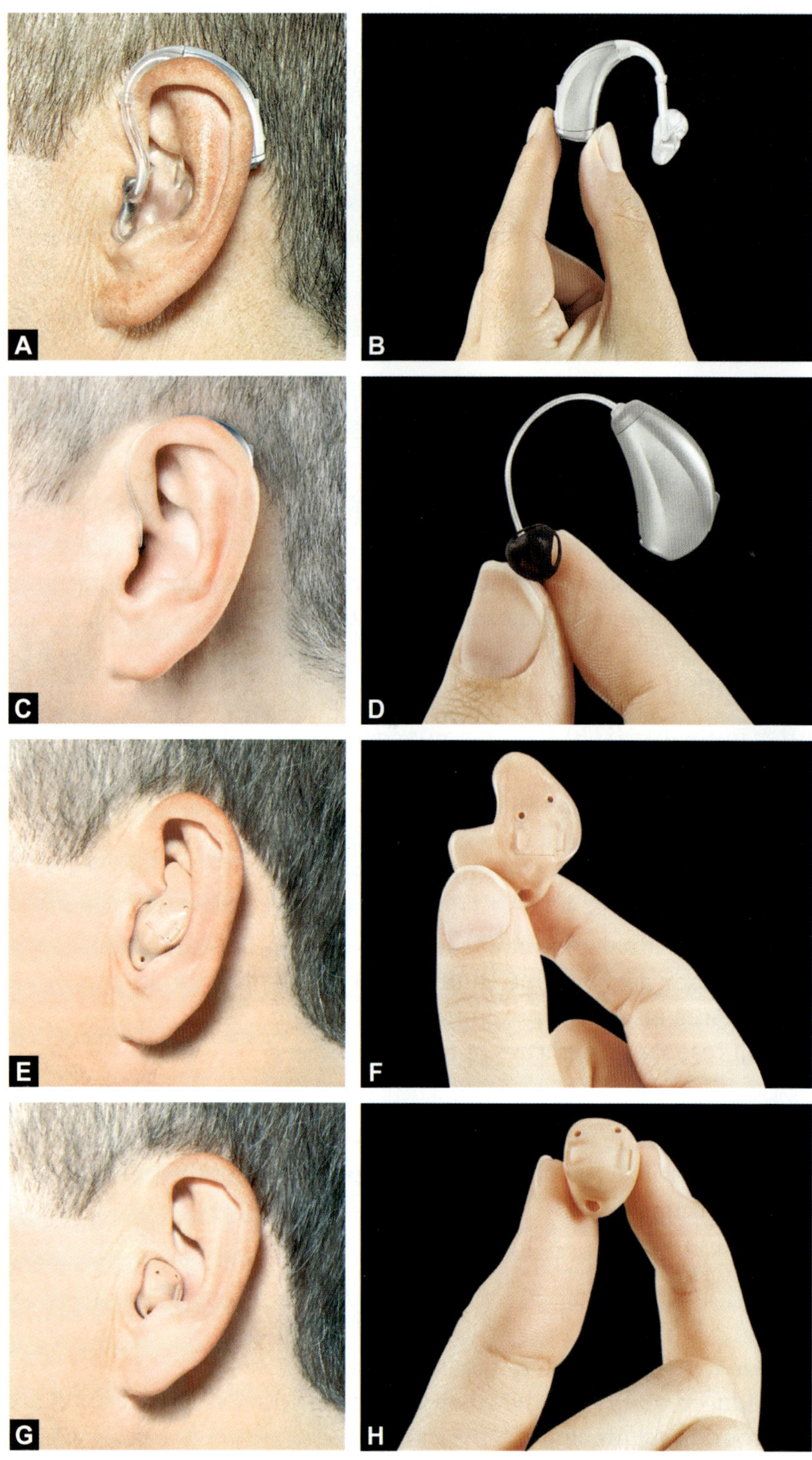

Figs. 14.3A to H

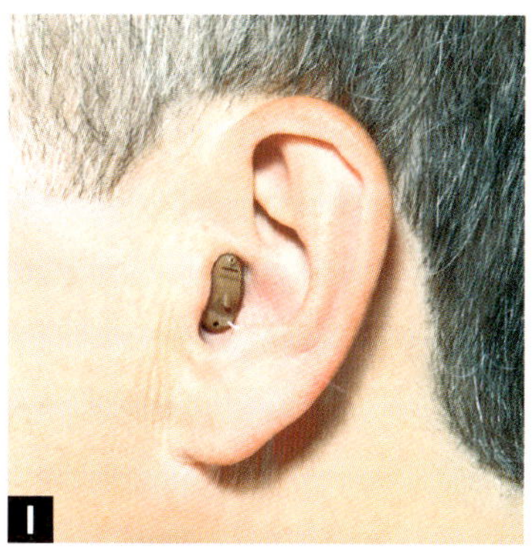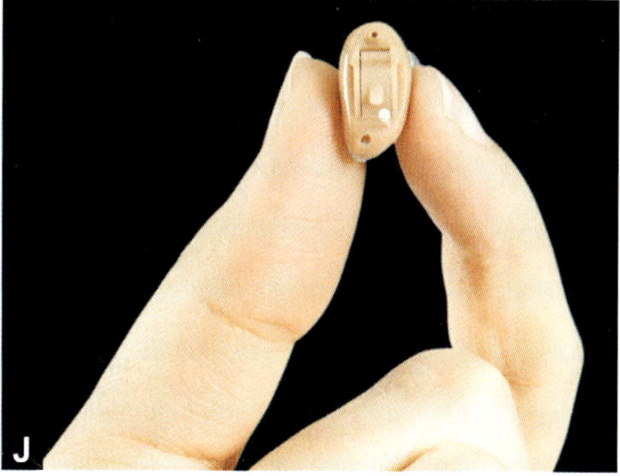

Figs. 14.3A to J: Different styles of hearing aid instruments displayed on and off the ear: (A and B) Behind-the-ear hearing aid. (C and D) Receiver-in-canal hearing aid. (E and F) In-the-ear hearing aid. (G and H) In-the-canal hearing aid. (I and J) Completely-in-the-canal hearing aid.
Courtesy: Starkey Hearing Technologies Minnesota, USA.

- An appropriate ear canal size is required, and hence it is not suitable for all individuals
- Subject to wear and tear.

CIC Hearing Aids

The CIC hearing aid is a smaller version of the ITE device, and is generally invisible if inserted deep enough into the auditory meatus as portrayed in Figures 14.3I and J. Apart from the obvious benefits of being cosmetically appealing, the CIC device is advantageous in many other areas. It maximizes the full effect of the natural resonance provided by the pinna and concha giving individuals a true sense of directionality. Due to its deeper setting, wind noise is less of a problem and it is easier to use with telephones and mobiles. Due to the small size of the device, patients may lose some functionality due to the limited shell.

Pros:

- More cosmetically appealing than the ITC
- Able to fully utilize the natural resonance from the pinna and cavum concha
- Provides an improved sense of natural directionality
- Wind noise is less problematic.

Cons:

- Changes in the auditory meatus will have long-term usability issues, particularly with respect to feedback suppression
- Loss of wireless capabilities

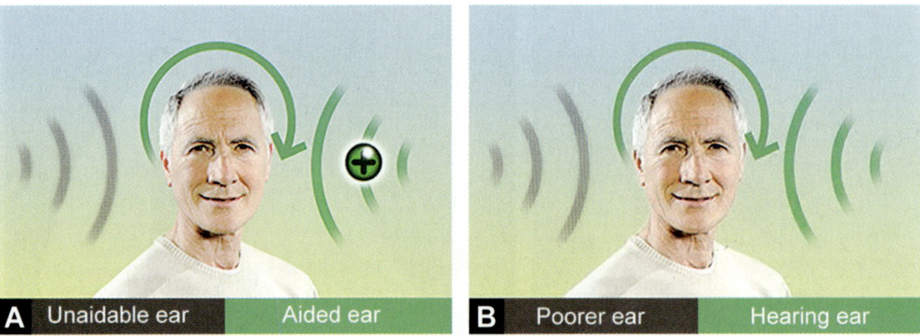

Figs. 14.4A and B: Contralateral routing of offside signal and bilateral contra routing of signal hearing aids instrument for the aiding for profound unilateral hearing losses. *Courtesy*: The Tinnitus Clinic Ltd. London, UK.

- Appropriate ear canal size is required, and hence is not suitable for all individuals
- Subject to greater wear and tear.

Contralateral Routing of Offside Signal and Bilateral Contra Routing of Signal Hearing Aids

Contralateral routing of offside signal (CROS) hearing aids were first created in the mid-1960s to try and cater for individuals who had profound single-sided hearing losses. Contralateral routing of offside signal aids are comprised of two components: the microphone, which is placed on the impaired ear and the receiver that is placed on the ear with normal hearing. The CROS device works by transmitting sound from the microphone to the receiver, which is placed on the good ear, thereby giving the user the ability to hear sounds originating from the nonfunctional side as illustrated in Figure 14.4A. The signals were generally routed via wired system, but due to technological advances these systems are now fully wireless.

As individuals with unilateral hearing losses often present with a degree of loss on their better ear, CROS aids were expanded to have the ability to provide acoustic information from the nonfunctional side of the head, while also aiding the better ear (Fig. 14.4B); these systems became known as bilateral contra routing of signal hearing aids. The system utilized often looked very similar to the CROS instruments.

Pros:

- Improves the client's ability to localize sound after training and nullifies the head shadow effect
- Discreet system if utilizing fully wireless technology
- Provides the user with better signal-to-noise ratio (SNR).

Cons:

- Battery life on the fully wireless system can be relatively short.

IMPROVING THE LISTENING IN NOISE EXPERIENCE

The most frequent complaint that audiologists are challenged with by patients, who have hearing impairment, is that of reduced clarity in noisy situations. The majority of people, with normal auditory function, are able to selectively focus their attention on specific acoustic signals while being able to filter out unwanted stimuli.[8] This ability has traditionally been referred to as the "cocktail party effect" and is highly dependent upon normative binaural auditory processing.[9] It has long been acknowledged that hearing loss does not only solely reduce an individual's audibility but also serves to impair normal auditory processing by inducing a variety of unwelcome psychoacoustic effects that can result in subjects experiencing a dramatic increase in difficulty when trying to hear selective sounds in noise.[10] This results in listeners requiring a much higher SNR in order to allow them to separate speech from noise.[11] The ability to attend to signals of interest, which emerge from a competing noise floor, is of great importance with respect to being able to socially function in any noisy situation. It is this very impairment that has been causatively linked to deafened individuals avoiding challenging situations that can result in pronounced isolation that may erode human quality of life.[12] It is, therefore, unsurprising that this has historically been a salient research issue for the hearing aid industry with new generation instruments that possessed adaptive directionality and automatic noise reduction capabilities becoming available for the first time in the early noughties (2000s).

To understand these systems, we first have to appreciate what directionality, or the reduction of sound processing at specific angles, actually is. One way of visually comprehending hearing aid directionality is to record the microphone polar plot (output of the hearing aid compared to input over a 0°–360° spatial map). The spatial areas that provide the highest reduction in sound pick up (or nulls) provide a representation of the instrument's directional capability. An omnidirectional setting provides an equal output at all angles surrounding the hearing aid (Fig. 14.5A), while a standard directional mode is most likely to resemble a hypercardioid (Fig. 14.5B) that induces a null at between 110° and 270°.[13] From the polar plot, a measure called the directivity index (DI) can be obtained. This quantifies how sensitive a microphone is to sounds arriving from the front (0° azimuth) relative to sounds arriving from other directions. For example, an omnidirectional

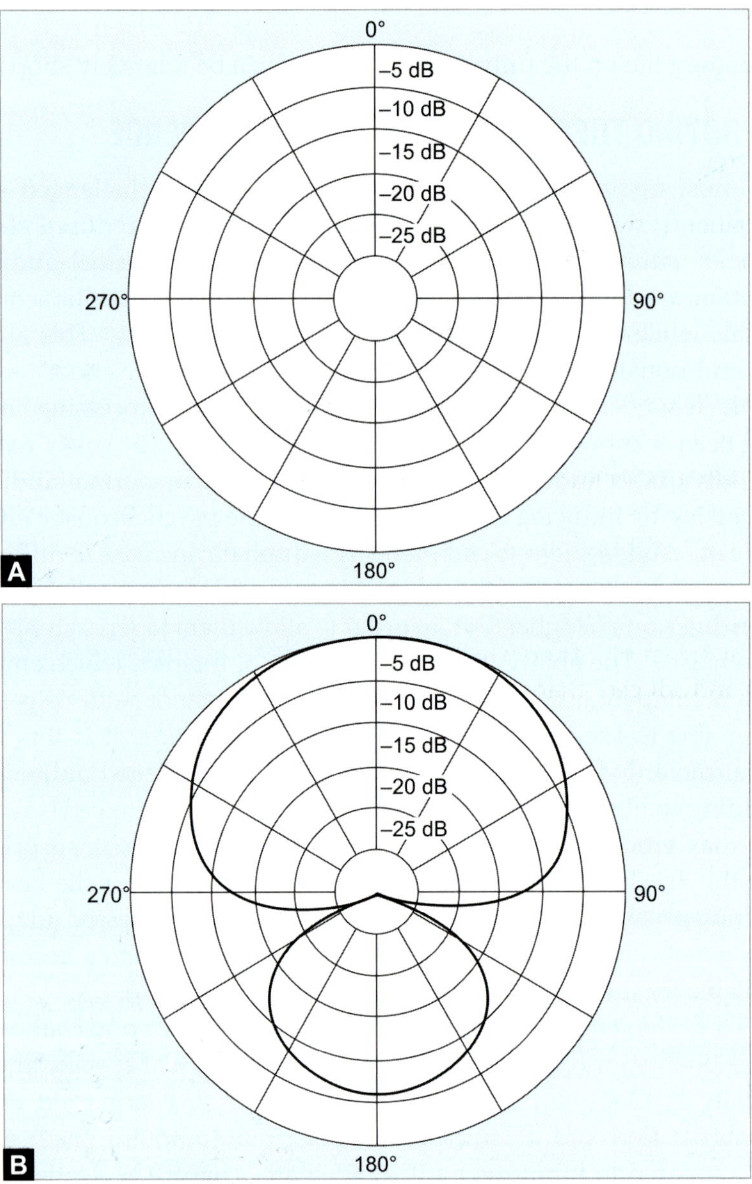

Figs. 14.5A and B: Microphone polar plots displaying omnidirectional (A) and directional (hyper cardioid) (B) sensitivity patterns.

microphone would have a DI of 0 dB when measured in a test chamber while an exceptional directional microphone may possess a value of up to 6 dB when measured under laboratory conditions.[14] All modern RIC and BTE instruments possess dual microphone systems that provide a number of directional functions that can be both directly controlled by the user or simply left to run automatically as a background feature. These dual mics work synergistically to alter their polar plots in response to challenging acoustic environments with the goal of enhancing the user's SNR.

AUTOMATIC AND ADAPTIVE DIRECTIONAL SYSTEMS

The first hearing aid systems with directional microphone options had a directional mode that had to be activated by the user via a manual control (usually via a rocker switch or button). Thus the instruments had two very distinct modes; one being omnidirectional and the other being directional. However, some authors have suggested that a significant proportion of wearers were not willing/able to switch between the microphone settings and often did not know how best to use the directional feature in real-life situations.[15] The issue is complex as directional microphone polar plot patterns are not beneficial in all challenging situations, i.e. if speech is originating from behind the user or if the desired input signal has a high ratio compared to background noise.[16]

In order to overcome this problem, automatic directional switching was introduced that enabled the hearing instrument to determine what directionality mode would be most suitable for the environment that the user encountered. In order for this to work switching algorithms were designed to analyze certain characteristics of the environment and then make a decision regarding how to transition between directionality options. This advancement has led to the development of adaptive directional systems where polar plots can change, in a much more dynamic fashion, enabling the null region to be moved to the angle where the most disruptive environmental noise signal is detected (Fig. 14.6). The polar plot changes can also occur independently and simultaneously within different frequency ranges (multiband directionality) in order to maximize speech intelligibility (Fig. 14.7). This means that different unwanted noise signals that possess a distinct spectrum from speech, emerging from different directions, can be reduced simultaneously while directionality remains fixed on signals of interest like speech. Multiband directionality also has been utilized by some manufacturers to enable low-frequency inputs to be picked up in a more natural omnidirectional fashion, similar to what occurs for unaided ears, while mid-high frequency signals can be processed by a directional polar plot. This low-frequency omnidirectionality has been reported by some authors as being preferable to the majority of users when compared to traditional directional systems.[16]

In very recent years, certain manufacturers have made algorithms to enable the instrument's directional polar plot width to automatically

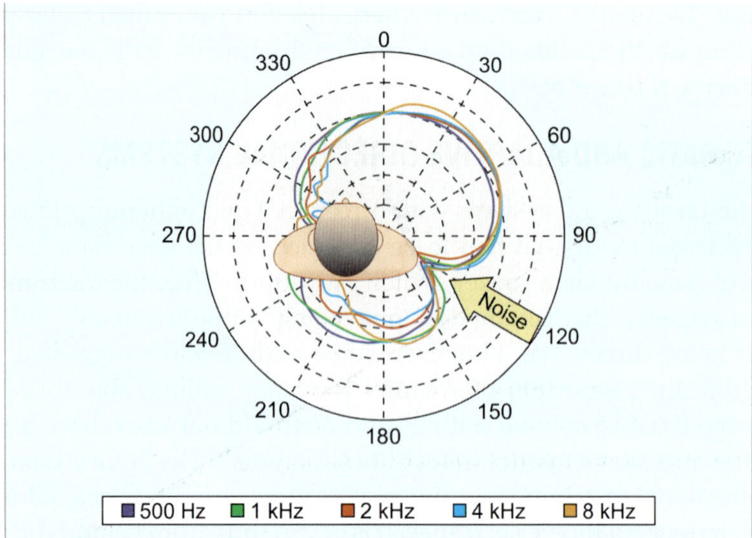

Fig. 14.6: Multifrequency polar plot altering in order to attenuate a static noise signal. *Courtesy*: Sivantos Erlangen, Germany.

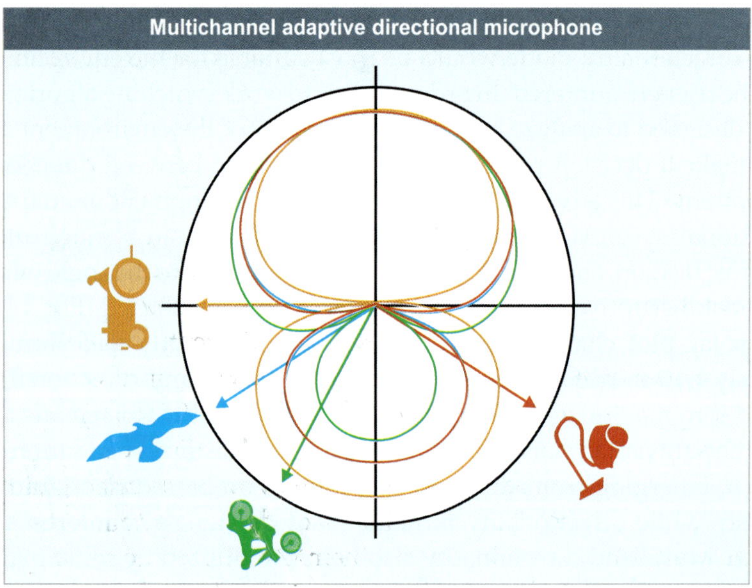

Fig. 14.7: Polar plot changes can occur independently and simultaneously within different frequency ranges (multiband directionality) in order to maximize noise reduction and signal to noise ratio. *Courtesy*: Sivantos Erlangen, Germany.

or manually alter depending upon the dynamics of the input signal. For example, for a salient static signal the directional plot can narrow, in order to increase focus, as opposed to widen for weaker moving

81. Vogl TJ, Bisdas S. Differential diagnosis of jugular foramen lesions. Skull Base. 2009;19:3-16.
82. Murphy TP, Brackmann DE. Effects of preoperative embolization on glomus jugulare tumors. Laryngoscope. 1989;99:1244-7.
83. Tasar M, Yetiser S. Glomus tumors: therapeutic role of selective embolization. J Craniofac Surg. 2004;15:497-505.
84. Brito JP, Asi N, Gionfriddo MR, et al. The incremental benefit of functional imaging in pheochromocytoma/paraganglioma: a systematic review. Endocrine. 2015;50:176-86.
85. Telischi FF, Bustillo A, Whiteman ML, et al. Octreotide scintigraphy for the detection of paragangliomas. Otolaryngol Head Neck Surg. 2000;122:358-62.
86. Bustillo A, Telischi F, Weed D, et al. Octreotide scintigraphy in the head and neck. Laryngoscope. 2004;114:434-40.
87. Bustillo A, Telischi FF. Octreotide scintigraphy in the detection of recurrent paragangliomas. Otolaryngol Head Neck Surg. 2004;130:479-82.
88. Hoegerle S, Ghanem N, Altehoefer C, et al. 18F-DOPA positron emission tomography for the detection of glomus tumours. Eur J Nucl Med Mol Imaging. 2003;30:689-94.
89. Timmers HJ, Kozupa A, Chen CC, et al. Superiority of fluorodeoxyglucose positron emission tomography to other functional imaging techniques in the evaluation of metastatic SDHB-associated pheochromocytoma and paraganglioma. J Clin Oncol. 2007;25:2262-9.
90. Taieb D, Timmers HJ, Shulkin BL, et al. Renaissance of (18)F-FDG positron emission tomography in the imaging of pheochromocytoma/paraganglioma. J Clin Endocrinol Metab. 2014;99:2337-9.
91. Lenders JW, Duh QY, Eisenhofer G, et al. Pheochromocytoma and paraganglioma: an endocrine society clinical practice guideline. J Clin Endocrinol Metab. 2014;99:1915-42.
92. Young AL, Baysal BE, Deb A, et al. Familial malignant catecholamine-secreting paraganglioma with prolonged survival associated with mutation in the succinate dehydrogenase B gene. J Clin Endocrinol Metab. 2002;87:4101-5.
93. Luchetti A, Walsh D, Rodger F, et al. Profiling of somatic mutations in phaeochromocytoma and paraganglioma by targeted next generation sequencing analysis. Int J Endocrinol. 2015;2015:138573.
94. Toledo RA, Dahia PL. Next-generation sequencing for the diagnosis of hereditary pheochromocytoma and paraganglioma syndromes. Curr Opin Endocrinol Diabetes Obes. 2015;22:169-79.
95. Drucker AM, Houlden RL. A case of familial paraganglioma syndrome type 4 caused by a mutation in the SDHB gene. Nat Clin Pract Endocrinol Metab. 2006;2:702-6; quiz following 6.
96. Brackmann DE. Ear Research Foundation of Florida, House Ear Institute. Neurological Surgery of the Ear and Skull Base. New York: Raven Press; 1982. pp. xviii, 408.
97. Jackson CG, Glasscock ME, 3rd, Harris PF. Glomus tumors. Diagnosis, classification, and management of large lesions. Arch Otolaryngol. 1982;108:401-10.
98. Powell S, Peters N, Harmer C. Chemodectoma of the head and neck: results of treatment in 84 patients. Int J Radiat Oncol Biol Phys. 1992;22:919-24.
99. Chino JP, Sampson JH, Tucci DL, et al. Paraganglioma of the head and neck: long-term local control with radiotherapy. Am J Clin Oncol. 2009;32:304-7.

100. Boyle JO, Shimm DS, Coulthard SW. Radiation therapy for paragangliomas of the temporal bone. Laryngoscope. 1990;100:896-901.
101. Tran Ba Huy P. Radiotherapy for glomus jugulare paraganglioma. Eur Ann Otorhinolaryngol Head Neck Dis. 2014;131:223-6.
102. Lalwani AK, Jackler RK, Gutin PH. Lethal fibrosarcoma complicating radiation therapy for benign glomus jugulare tumor. Am J Otol. 1993;14:398-402.
103. Hinerman RW, Mendenhall WM, Amdur RJ, et al. Definitive radiotherapy in the management of chemodectomas arising in the temporal bone, carotid body, and glomus vagale. Head Neck. 2001;23:363-71.
104. Gabriel EM, Sampson JH, Dodd LG, et al. Glomus jugulare tumor metastatic to the sacrum after high-dose radiation therapy: case report. Neurosurgery. 1995;37:1001-5.
105. Niemeijer ND, Alblas G, van Hulsteijn LT, et al. Chemotherapy with cyclophosphamide, vincristine and dacarbazine for malignant paraganglioma and pheochromocytoma: systematic review and meta-analysis. Clin Endocrinol. 2014;81:642-51.
106. van Hulsteijn LT, Niemeijer ND, Dekkers OM, et al. (131)I-MIBG therapy for malignant paraganglioma and phaeochromocytoma: systematic review and meta-analysis. Clin Endocrinol. 2014;80:487-501.
107. Martucci VL, Pacak K. Pheochromocytoma and paraganglioma: diagnosis, genetics, management, and treatment. Curr Probl Cancer. 2014;38:7-41.
108. Moe KS, Li D, Linder TE, et al. An update on the surgical treatment of temporal bone paraganglioma. Skull Base Surg. 1999;9:185-94.
109. Poe DS, Jackson G, Glasscock ME, et al. Long-term results after lateral cranial base surgery. Laryngoscope. 1991;101:372-8.
110. Pareschi R, Righini S, Destito D, et al. Surgery of glomus jugulare Tumors. Skull Base. 2003;13:149-57.
111. Fayad JN, Keles B, Brackmann DE. Jugular foramen tumors: clinical characteristics and treatment outcomes. Otology Neurotol. 2010;31:299-305.
112. Pensak ML, Jackler RK. Removal of jugular foramen tumors: the fallopian bridge technique. Otolaryngol Head Neck Surg. 1997;117:586-91.
113. Oghalai JS, Leung MK, Jackler RK, et al. Transjugular craniotomy for the management of jugular foramen tumors with intracranial extension. Otol Neurotol. 2004;25:570-9; discussion 9.
114. Sanna M, Fois P, Pasanisi E, et al. Middle ear and mastoid glomus tumors (glomus tympanicum): an algorithm for the surgical management. Auris Nasus Larynx. 2010;37:661-8.
115. Schick B, Draf W, Kahle G. Jugulotympanic paraganglioma: therapy concepts under development. Laryngorhinootologie. 1998;77:434-43.
116. Gstoettner W, Matula C, Hamzavi J, et al. Long-term results of different treatment modalities in 37 patients with glomus jugulare tumors. Eur Arch Otorhinolaryngol. 1999;256:351-5.
117. Woods CI, Strasnick B, Jackson CG. Surgery for glomus tumors: the Otology Group experience. Laryngoscope. 1993;103:65-70.
118. Carlson ML, Sweeney AD, Pelosi S, et al. Glomus tympanicum: a review of 115 cases over 4 decades. Otolaryngol Head Neck Surg. 2015;152:136-42.

subject's ease of listening by increasing their cognitive listening capacity and auditory memory ability.[22,23]

One additional reduction technique that is ubiquitous within all current hearing aid systems is a process known as expansion. One potential issue with modern instruments is that sophisticated compression systems have increased a user's ability to perceive very soft environmental sounds. This may be disagreeable to subjects who have speech in noise perception issues as the audibility of unusual softer sound can act as a potential distraction; particularly if they have not experienced amplification previously. Also individuals with some degree of normal residual hearing can often become aware of circuit noise from the instrument itself that is usually perceived as being a low-intensity white noise. Expansion serves to reduce the audibility of very soft input sounds (e.g. below 40 dBSPL) by applying less amplification for softer sounds, in comparison to louder sounds, below a set TK. As a result of this, unwanted circuit noise and very low-level external noises (e.g. the low hum from a computer hard drive etc.) should be rendered inaudible. However, it has been reported that if expansion TKs are set too high, this may result in soft speech phonemes, like consonants, becoming lost.[24] It is, therefore, essential to ensure that expansion does not result in decrease of speech audibility performance while striving to insulate patients from potentially distracting low-level inputs. As a result of this issue, some manufacturers have recently provided clinicians with the ability to alter instrument expansion parameters in order to meet patient's requirements to a closer degree.

IMPROVING SNR WITH WIRELESS EAR-TO-EAR PROCESSING

Since 2004, hearing instruments, which are fitted as a pair for binaural use, have been able to wirelessly exchange data (Fig. 14.9) that enables bilateral acoustic situation detection so that features like directional/ noise reduction algorithms can operate in synchrony based upon the environmental characteristics detected by each instrument. This, so-called ear-to-ear connection, also allows for microphone polar plots to alternate, independently, for each ear in order to enable the greatest SNR for speech irrespective of its direction of origin. Small-scale laboratory-based studies have reported of linked hearing aid systems as being beneficial to test subjects when trying to discriminate/detect speech and noise sources that originate from different directions.[25] While surveys from users comparing linked to unlinked hearing aids in everyday use situations demonstrated a significant higher preference for binaurally linked devices.[26]

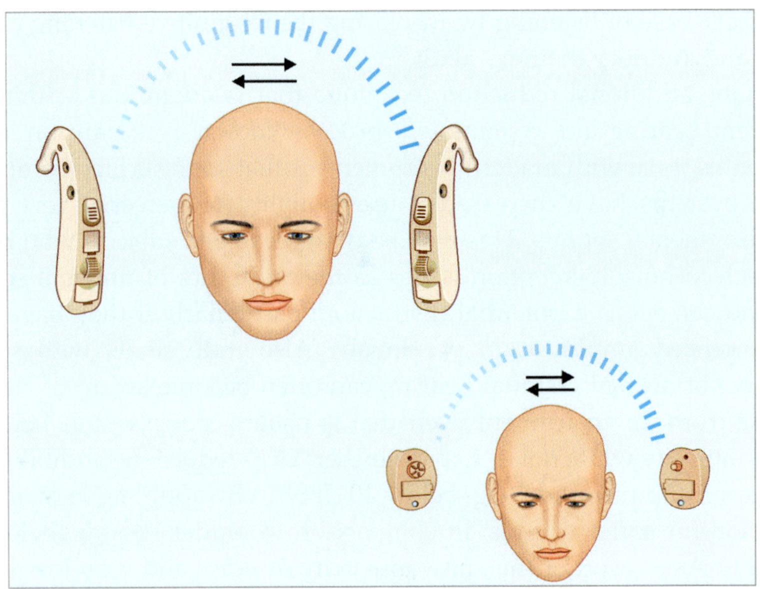

Fig. 14.9: Hearing instruments wirelessly exchanging data to enable bilateral acoustic situation detection.
Courtesy: Sivantos Erlangen, Germany.

FEEDBACK REDUCTION SYSTEMS

Acoustic feedback occurs in hearing aids when sound from the instrument's speaker is transduced by the microphone and subsequently amplified causing a looping between the device output and input. Hearing aid feedback usually manifests as an undesirable high-pitched signal (usually described as a whistling noise) that can dramatically reduce user satisfaction.[27] Since the early 1990s manufacturers and researchers have strived to develop more effective ways of enabling instruments to control feedback production[28] that would allow for more acceptable and open hearing aid fittings. The most successful and prolifically applied strategy, to date, relies upon inverting the phase of the feedback signal thus enabling the cancellation of the unwanted signal without reducing instrument gain. In practice, the instrument performs a correlation analysis between the input and output signals. The differential between the two signals enables the instrument to evaluate the frequency content of the feedback signal (Fig. 14.10). To enable cancellation, a phase inverted signal is generated with the same frequency characteristics as the feedback noise.

The advent of this technology has enabled the utilization of open ear instrument fittings that has revolutionized the way that milder hearing losses are aided.

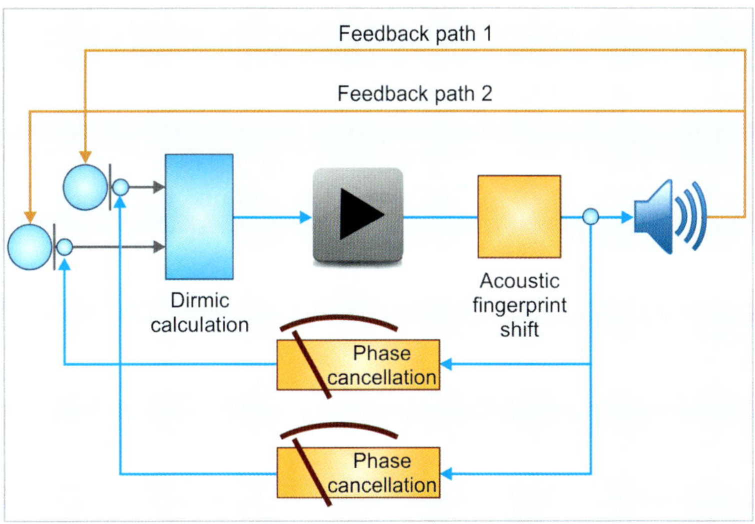

Fig. 14.10: Hearing aid digital feedback suppression circuit enabling the cancellation of a generated feedback signal by a phase cancellation algorithm.
Courtesy: Sivantos Erlangen, Germany.

WIRELESS CONNECTIVITY AND HEARING AID ACCESSORIES

History

Even some of the earliest hearing aid systems possessed the ability to wirelessly connect to a sound source via the use of audio induction loop systems that are still commonly utilized in public areas that could present challenging audibility issues. However, while this technology undoubtedly benefits hearing aids users, it does have limitations with respect to sound audibility (prone to magnetic interference, frequency range <3.5 kHz, etc.). As a result of this, over the past 30 years, manufacturers have developed innovative alternative connectivity solutions for assistive listening devices and external microphones. Frequency modulation (FM) signal transmission products were originally designed, over 30 years prior, for the application in the education of children with hearing loss in order to improve SNR in reverberant classroom environments.[29] This technology also became available for personal amplification use via the utilization of external microphone systems. This technology started to be used more prolifically by clinicians with the advent of reasonably discreet FM hearing aid receivers in mid-1990s.[30] However, these products can experience radio interference and as there are no internationally agreed frequency ranges for transmission it is unlikely that these systems will ever be used in public spaces. Presently, the new technology trend in wireless connectivity revolves around the utilization of Bluetooth ultra-high frequency radio waves (2.4–2.485 GHz) to enable direct audio streaming from devices and external mics. Most of these systems utilize a streamer (or gateway) that serves as a bridge between the hearing aid and the Bluetooth signal. This is mainly because translation of a classic Bluetooth signal would require far too much power from the hearing aid battery cell. The streamers convert the Bluetooth signal into a low-power radio signal that can then be translated by the hearing aid with greater "ease". As most manufacturers' streamers are approximately the size of an mp3 player, they can accommodate a rechargeable battery system that can provide the power requirements for the translation process. However, as a result of the introduction of Bluetooth 4.0 low energy technology in 2010, the power requirements for translation have reduced dramatically. This has enabled a number of manufacturers to engineer hearing aids that can directly stream audio information from Bluetooth 4.0 enabled devices like iPhone. Examples of these systems include the GN Resound LiNX and Starkey Halo instruments that were released to market in 2014.

Clinical Applications

The modern application of wireless connective functionality in hearing aid systems has allowed for the development of a useful assortment of accessories and instrument features that clinicians can utilize in order to overcome patient specific audibility issues.

Audio Streaming

Recently specific Bluetooth streamer systems have evolved that also act as remote control systems for hearing aid functions. These not only enable users to alter hearing aid amplification parameters and program but also provide the direct streaming of audio information, from external devices, to the hearing instruments with the stereo transmission of signal and no audible delay. In this way, hearing aids are able to act as a bespoke personal headset for telephone conversation, television, and music while simultaneously providing amplification. Figure 14.11 provides an example of how multifunctional modern instrument systems have become with an array of connectivity options available. While this technology provides superior functionality and convenience compared to traditional FM systems, the fact that most manufacturer streamers have to be within 1 m of the hearing aids to enable communication is a disadvantage. However, as referenced previously, this technology is likely to be vastly improved by low-energy Bluetooth in the years to come.

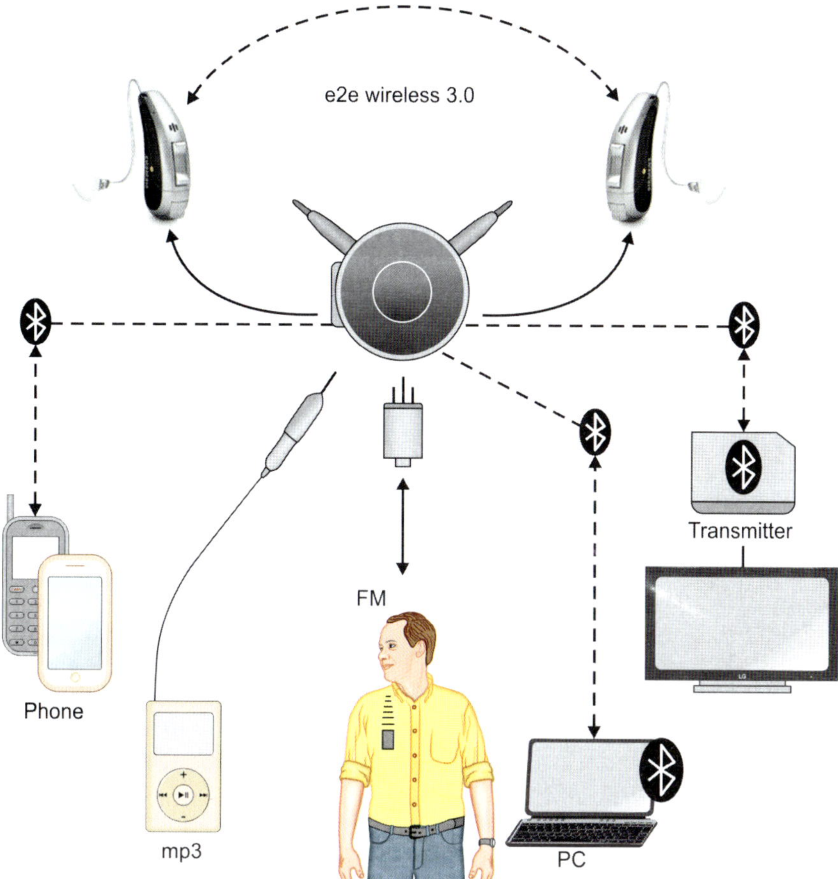

Fig. 14.11: Connectivity options with wireless hearing aid systems utilizing Bluetooth enabled technology.
Courtesy: Sivantos Erlangen, Germany.

SNR Improvement

Even though instruments imply sophisticated directional/noise reduction systems, they can still fail to provide clarity for speech information in challenging listening situations, especially when individuals are afflicted with either complex hearing loss or auditory processing disorders. Signal deterioration also occurs with distance between the listener and the sound source; the intensity of a signal of interest will decrease, by 6 dB, every time the distance between the user and the sound source is doubled pursuant to the inverse square law.

The majority of manufacturers currently provide external microphone solutions that are of key importance to hearing aid users who experience severe problems with speech in noise intelligibility. These systems, once again, are designed to improve the SNR for the listener

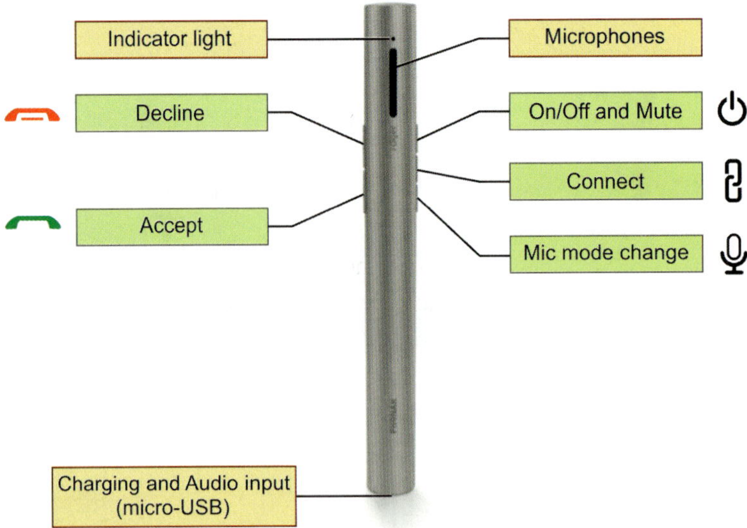

Fig. 14.12: The Roger Pen from Phonak is a contemporary example of an adaptive external microphone system.
Courtesy: Phonak Stäfa, Switzerland.

by reducing the distance between the listener and the signal of interest. Some modern-day external microphone systems also utilize adaptive directional microphone algorithms, much in the same way as hearing aids, in order to provide an even greater chance of making speech more prominent than noise (Fig. 14.12). Some of the most modern examples are actually integrated into hearing aid remote control systems for convenience of use.

The streaming of information from audio devices also has a clear role to play in SNR improvement in a user's everyday life. The wireless connection serves to exclude ambient noise by only processing the target signal, which is then transmitted directly into the hearing instruments. This listening improvement could be very relevant for effective telephone communication when users are fitted with instruments binaurally as the signal will be conveyed to both ears providing a binaural integration advantage that can improve the SNR by up to 3 dB.[31]

Frequency Lowering Systems

Frequency lowering algorithms have been developed specifically for individuals who experience speech perception challenges when using standard amplification strategies. This usually occurs due to an instrument exhibiting an unacceptable level of acoustic feedback as a result of either achieving, or striving to achieve, a required gain level (this is much more likely to occur with open ear canal instrument fittings). Another reason for this could be due to the user not possessing adequate high-frequency hearing functionality. High-frequency hearing loss can be linked to the death of cochlea inner hair cells that can cause a complete dysfunction of the affected organ area; these areas are referred to as "dead regions."[32] The provision of amplification to dead regions can result in hearing aid users experiencing distortion of input sounds that can have a negative impact upon a subject's speech discrimination ability and overall auditory comfort.[33] An alternative way of providing audibility of speech sounds that cannot be amplified is to reduce the frequency at which they are perceived. This involves the instrument utilizing an algorithm that serves to shift high-frequency sounds to a lower frequency band, in real time, that correlates with better cochlea function and hearing ability. This method is predominantly applied by clinicians in order to help individuals with very poor high-frequency hearing acuity.

Over the last 10 years, interest in frequency reduction technologies has grown dramatically. At this moment in time, all but one of the six main hearing aid manufacturing companies provide instruments with frequency lowering algorithms that are specifically designed for use with high-frequency hearing loss. Each company has developed its own distinct algorithm with different adaptable parameters to enable appropriate redistribution of high-frequency information to a lower frequency bandwidth. Most contemporary algorithms lower input frequencies by broadly utilizing one of two following techniques:

1. *Linear frequency transposition*: This strategy works by shifting high-frequency signal content from a source region to a lower frequency target region. The source and target regions both have a predefined frequency range that can be influenced by the clinician in order to cater for the extent of the high-frequency loss. The algorithms then search for intense spectral peaks within the source regions and select a range (up to one octave) of information around these signals of interest to resynthesize into the lower target range. Signals with high spectral peaks are selected for transposition in order to hopefully prioritize signals that would be of interest. This is done in order to try to ensure that the least important signals are removed so that the target area does not become saturated with acoustic information (Fig. 14.13). As the frequency distribution of the information that is lowered from the source region remains unchanged, the resulting sound will be perceived as being very similar to the original signal, albeit at a lower pitch. However, as the

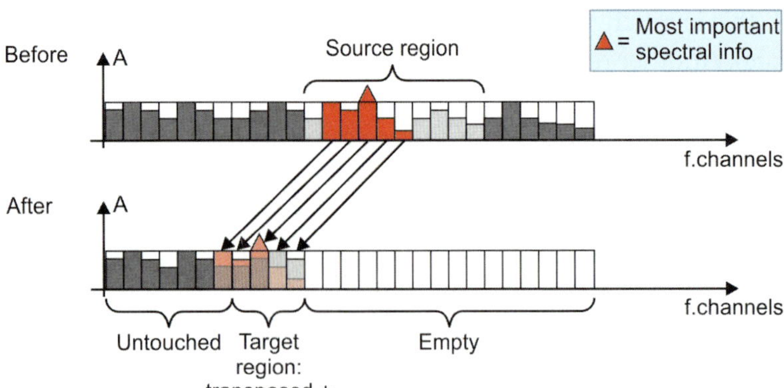

Fig. 14.13: An example of a frequency transposition system in action: the most salient acoustic information along within an octave range bandwidth is shifted from the source onto the target region. After transposition, the target region contains both the peaks form the source region and the original sound (illustrated in red).
Courtesy: Sivantos Erlangen, Germany.

information is lowered in pitch by a fairly substantial degree, this can lead to high-frequency speech sounds, like fricatives, sounding dramatically different to what a user is accustomed to. Transposition is, therefore, considered to be the most effective when applied with audiometric configurations that have a severe loss component.[34]

2. *Nonlinear frequency compression*: This approach to frequency reduction does not rely upon transposing high-frequency signals to a lower frequency region as in the above method. Instead, the method serves to reduce the bandwidth of the speech signal by applying frequency lowering compression to high-pitched input signals.[35] Frequency compression works in very similar fashion to gain compression in that the compression of information only occurs above a predefined knee point or start frequency. The part of the frequency spectrum below the start frequency is left untouched. This can be seen in Figure 14.14 and is designated F_{min}. As with linear transposition systems, certain manufacturer algorithms will analyze the device input and prioritize the compression of high spectral peak signals in order to prioritize the most salient acoustic information.[36] However, the application of frequency compression to a speech signal can alter the natural formant ratios that can result in the production of an output signal that is rather different from the original input signal.[37] Therefore, when using this frequency lowering method, clinical outcomes are most likely to be influenced by how the algorithm's adaptive parameters, like start frequency and compression ratio, are configured.[38]

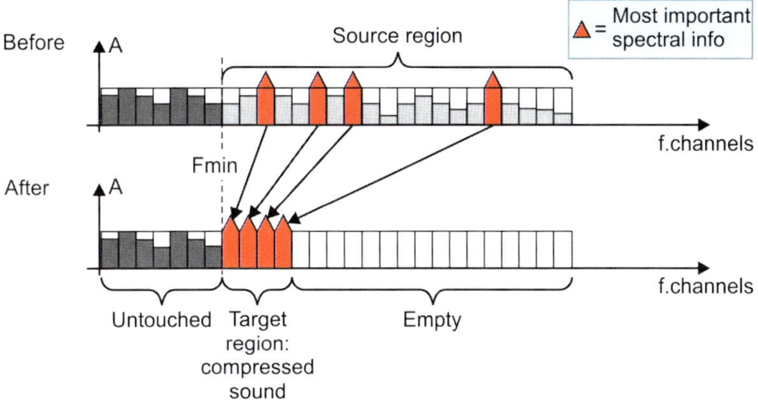

Fig. 14.14: An example of a nonlinear frequency compression system in action: the most salient acoustic information, from the source region, is selected so that the most important spectral information is reduced in pitch for improved audibility (illustrated in red). *Courtesy*: Sivantos Erlangen, Germany.

Clinical Benefits

A number of authors have reported that modern frequency lowering technology can provide benefits to both adult[39,40] and pediatric[41-43] device users. However, it is important to note that there is a high degree of variation between these studies relating to the nature of the algorithms that were applied and how frequency lowering parameters were selected for studying participants. Therefore, at the time of writing, it is still difficult to predict how frequency lowering algorithms will perform when utilized in real-life situations. However, as it has been reported that the efficacy of frequency lowering systems, typically, improves over time[44] then it is clinically important that users are appropriately supported and provided with realistic expectations from the start of the process. This is particularly important because as transposition/compression systems transfer high-frequency signals to lower frequency areas, the user's initial listening experience may be perceived as being unnatural compared to their auditory memory.

TINNITUS THERAPY FEATURES

All major hearing instrument manufacturers currently provide aids with tinnitus sound therapy features that have become known as combination devices (i.e. a combination between a hearing aid and a wearable noise generator). The sound therapy signals can be utilized for a number of different therapeutic purposes with some models having the potential to be used in order to support traditional structured therapy techniques like tinnitus retraining therapy. Certain features are designed to reduce the user's autonomic reaction to the tinnitus percept by providing signals that are conducive to relaxation; alternatively, others can be applied in order to provide masking. All instruments are able to provide noise signals and amplification simultaneously, within one shared program, thus enabling the concurrent provision of sound therapy and hearing acuity optimization. Most companies provide devices that are preprogrammed with a variety of sound therapy signals (like white noise, pink noise, nature sounds, fractal tones, etc.) with the clinician being able to vary the output and frequency composition of the noises in order to suit the patient's hearing loss and tinnitus profile. Certain companies also provide "environmental steering" functionality algorithms that serve to modulate the volume of the sound therapy signal in order to ensure that the output level is appropriate with the ambient noise level (i.e. the sound therapy signal output will reduce when there is high environmental noise and vice versa).

The advent of Bluetooth connectivity technology in hearing aids has also started to impact the way in which manufacturers are providing sound therapy options for tinnitus with a number having developed tinnitus specific applications that store an expansive library of noise files. These noise files can be streamed directly to the hearing instruments and serve to provide a much more varied selection of sound therapy options for the user. The disadvantage of this is that the signals cannot be customized by the clinician so are less bespoke for the user's auditory profile.

A low number of small scale studies have suggested that these systems can be useful for the management of tinnitus, with the supplementation of appropriate support/counseling; however, larger controlled studies are required in order to obtain greater clarity with regard to combination device efficacy.[45,46]

REFERENCES

1. Mortality and Burden of Diseases, WHO; 2011 Estimates for disabling hearing loss (DHL). Available from: http://www.who.int/pbd/deafness/news/Million-slivewith hearingloss.pdf [Accessed: 18th November 2015].
2. Mathers, C., Smith, A., & Concha, M. 2003. Global burden of hearing loss in the year 2000 (online). Geneva: World Health Organization. Available from: http://www.who.int/healthinfo/statistics/bod_hearingloss.pdf. [Accessed: 18th November 2015].
3. Mulrow CD, Aguilar C, Endicott JE, et al. Quality-of-life changes and hearing impairment. A randomized trial. Ann Intern Med. 1990;113:188-94.
4. Dalton DS, Cruickshanks KJ, Klein BE, et al. The impact of hearing loss on quality of life in older adults. Gerontologist. 2003;43(5):661-8.
5. Li CM, Zhang X, Hoffman HJ, et al. Hearing impairment associated with depression in US adults, National Health and Nutrition Examination Survey 2005-2010. JAMA Otolaryngol Head Neck Surg. 2014;140(4):293-302.

6. Mulrow CD, Tuley MR, Aguilar C. Sustained benefits of hearing aids. J Speech Hear Res. 1992;35:1402-05.

7. Chisolm TH, Johnson CE, Danhauer JL, et al. A systematic review of health-related quality of life and hearing aids: final report of the American Academy of Audiology Task Force on the Health-Related Quality of Life Benefits of Amplification in Adults. J Am Acad Audiol. 2007;18:151-83.

8. Plude DJ, Enns JT, Brodeur D. The development of selective attention: a life-span overview. Acta Psychol. 1994;86(2–3):227-72.

9. Hawley ML, Litovsky RY, Culling JF. The benefit of binaural hearing in a cocktail party: effect of location and type of interferer. J Acoust Soc. 2004;115(2):833-43.

10. Moore BCJ. Psychophysics of normal and impaired hearing. Br Med Bull. 1987;43:887-908.

11. Moore BCJ. Perceptual consequences of cochlear hearing loss and their implications for the design of hearing aids. Ear Hear. 1996;17(2):133-61.

12. McCay V. Psychosocial aspects of hearing impairment. In: Schow RL, Nerbonne MA, (eds). Introduction to Audiologic Rehabilitation. Boston: Allyn & Bacon; 1996. pp. 229-63.

13. Valente M, Mispagel KM, Tchorz J, et al. Effect of type of noise and loudspeaker array on the performance of omnidirectional and directional microphones. J Am Acad Audiol. 2006;17:398-412.

14. Cord MT, Surr RK, Walden BE, et al. Relationship between laboratory measures of directional advantage and everyday success with directional microphone hearing aids. J Am Acad Audio. 2004;15(5):353-64.

15. Walden B, Surr R, Cord M, et al . Predicting hearing aid microphone preference in everyday listening. J Am Acad Audiol. 2004;15:353-64.

16. Groth J, Laureyns M, Piskosz M. Double-blind study indicates sound quality preference for surround sound processor. Hear Rev. 2010;17(3):36-41.

17. Nyffeler M. Auto ZoomControl: Automatic change of focus to speech signals of interest. Field Study News 2010;September, www.phonakpro.com.

18. Chung K. Challenges and recent developments in hearing aids. Part I. Speech understanding in noise, microphone technologies and noise reduction algorithms. Trends Amplif. 2004;8:83-124.

19. Nordrum S, Erler S, Garstecki D, et al. Comparison of performance on the hearing in noise test using directional microphones and digital noise reduction algorithms. Am J Audiol. 2006;15:81-91.

20. Loizou PC, Kim G. Reasons why current speech-enhancement algorithms do not improve speech intelligibility and suggested solutions. IEEE Trans Audio Speech Lang Process. 2011;19:47-56.

21. Bentler RA. Effectiveness of directional microphones and noise reduction schemes in hearing aids: a systematic review of the evidence. J Am Acad Audiol. 2005;16:473-84.

22. Desjardins JL, Doherty KA. The effect of hearing aid noise-reduction on listening effort in hearing impaired adults. Ear Hear. 2014;35(5):600-10.

23. Ng EHN, Rudner M, Lunner T, et al. Effects of noise and working memory capacity on memory processing of speech for hearing aid users. Int J Audiol. 2013;52:433-41.

24. Brennan M, Souza P. Effects of expansion on consonant recognition and consonant audibility. J Am Acad Audiol. 2009;20:119-27.

25. Hornsby BW, Ricketts TA. Effects of noise source configuration on directional benefit using symmetric and asymmetric directional hearing aid fittings. Ear Hear. 2007;28(2):177-86.

26. Smith P, Davis A, Day J, et al. Real-world preferences for linked bilateral processing. Hear J. 2008;61(7):33-8.

27. Kochkin S. Customer satisfaction with hearing aids in the digital age. Hear J. 2005;58(9):30-37.

28. Drylund O, Bisgaard N. Acoustic feedback margin improvements in hearing instruments using a prototype DFS (digital feedback suppression system). Scand Audiol. 1991;39:147-61.

29. Ross M. FM Auditory Training Systems. Timonium, MD: York Press, 1992.

30. Phonak. (2009) The History of FM [Online]. Available from: http://www.phonak. com/uk/b2c/en/products/fm/what_is_fm/the_history_of_fm.html. [Accessed: 18th November 2015].

31. Keys JW. Binaural versus monaural hearing. J Acoust Soc Am. 1947;19(4): 629-31.

32. Moore BC, Huss M, Vickers DA, et al. A test for the diagnosis of dead regions in the cochlea. Br J Audiol. 2000;34(4):205-24.

33. Moore BC. Dead regions in the cochlea: diagnosis, perceptual consequences, and implications for the fitting of hearing aids. Trends Amplif. 2001;5(1):1-34.

34. Kuk F, Keenan D, Auriemmo J, et al. Re-evaluating the efficacy of frequency transposition. ASHA Leader. 2009;14(1):14-7.

35. Simpson A. Frequency-lowering devices for managing high-frequency hearing loss: a review. Trends Amplif. 2009;13(2):87-106.

36. Serman M, Hannemann R, Kornagel U. Siemens Hearing Instruments White Paper: Frequency Compression. 2013. Available from: https://www.bestsound-technology.co.uk/nhs/media/2014/07/Octiv_WhiteP-FreqComp.pdf.

37. Glista D, Scollie S, Bagatto M, et al. Evaluation of nonlinear frequency compression: clinical outcomes. Int J Audiol. 2009;48(9):632-44.

38. Kuk F, Keenan D, Auriemmo J, et al. Interpreting the efficacy of frequency-lowering algorithms. Hear J. 2010;63(4):30-40.

39. McCreery RW, Brennan MA, Hoover B, et al. Maximizing audibility and speech recognition with nonlinear frequency compression by estimating audible bandwidth. Ear Hear. 2012;20:1-4.

40. Glista D, Scollie S, Bagatto M, et al. Evaluation of nonlinear frequency compression: Clinical outcomes. Int J Audiol. 2009;48:632-44.

41. Miller-Hansen DR, Nelson PB, Widen JE, et al. Evaluating the benefit of speech recoding hearing aids in children. Am J Audiol. 2003;12(2):106-13.

42. Wolfe J, John A, Schafer E, et al. Evaluation of nonlinear frequency compression for school-age children with moderate to moderately severe hearing loss. J Am Acad Audiol. 2010;21(10):618-28.

43. Wolfe J, John A, Schafer E, et al. Long-term effects of non-linear frequency compression for children with moderate hearing loss. Int J Audiol. 2011;50 (6):396-404.

44. Kuk F, Keenan D, Korhonen P, et al. Efficacy of linear frequency transposition on consonant identification in quiet and in noise. J Am Acad Audiol. 2009;20: 465-79.

45. Henry JA, Frederick M, Sell S, et al. Validation of a novel combination hearing aid and tinnitus therapy device. Ear Hear. 2015;36(1):42-52.

46. Sweetow RW, Sabes JH. Effects of acoustical stimuli delivered through hearing aids on tinnitus. J Am Acad Audiol. 2010;21(7):461-73.

Chapter 15

Mastoid Cavity Obliteration with Bioactive Glass Granules

Goesta Schimanski, Esther Schimanski

INTRODUCTION

Mastoid cavities are generally formed during cholesteatoma surgery with the aim to get an ear safe and free of infection, and especially to avoid future recurrent cholesteatoma. To eliminate a mastoid cholesteatoma, there are two kinds of techniques: canal wall up (CWU) technique and canal wall down (CWD) technique. Canal wall up is performed in all types of cholesteatoma surgery when the cholesteatoma is limited to the middle ear structures or in the region of the epitympanum and/or attic [alternatively named intact wall technique (IWT)]. In these cases, the posterior wall of the outer ear canal (OEC) can be preserved. Bone will be reduced till the cholesteatoma can be removed completely. A special kind of CWU is the combined approach-technique (CAT or bilateral): the cholesteatoma is removed through the OEC and after opening the planum mastoideum. This procedure is chosen in cases of acute or chronic mastoiditis, too. The postoperative finding is an intact OEC, eventually widened and/or partially reconstructed with a suitable material (favored autogenous) in the region where bone was removed.

The risk of CWU after cholesteatoma surgery is a residual (remaining epithelium) and/or a retraction cholesteatoma (recurrent retraction pocket mostly in the epitympanum).

Canal wall down (alternatively named open technique [OPT]) will be performed if the cholesteatoma is extended in the mastoid, in case of severe chronic mastoiditis and of rare benign tumors. The posterior wall of the OEC will be removed completely and the whole mastoid area can be visualized: a mastoid cavity is formed.

Canal wall down avoids a recurrent retraction cholesteatoma due to the wide opening of the mastoid. Residual cholesteatoma might occur in the mastoid. This is not precarious because it will be detected during the regular visits within the first months postoperatively. It can

be recognized as whitish pearls (epithelium cysts) and can be removed easily. In order to achieve a clear, self-cleansing mastoid cavity, following surgical guidelines must be followed:
- Widening the OEC (meatoplasty), especially the entry
- Lowering the facial ridge
- Avoiding any bony overhang in the edges of the cavity (saucerized cavity)
- Thinning out the bony covering of middle fossa and sinus sigmoideus if necessary to avoid overhangs (without exposing them)
- Open sinodural angle and terminal cell.

Blind spots and deep dips left after these procedures are obliterated with soft tissue (fascia, connective tissue graft or flap) or autologous cartilage combined with bone pâté.[1-4] If there is a region with the risk of remaining epithelium, especially deep dips, we recommend to cover it by a thin plate of cartilage. While doing the second look 6–12 months later, the plate can be lifted or removed more easily than soft tissue, which may alternatively be used to fill the recess. An angled endoscope can be supportive.

Moreover, we recommend always to cover the bony wall of the cavity with a fascia graft or suitable flap unless an obliteration is planned in a one-stage procedure. For future revision surgery, it is rather more comfortable to lift this kind of connective tissue layer than a transparent thin epithelium layer.

Various criteria must be considered when choosing the type of technique (CWU or CWD):
- Dimension of pneumatization of the mastoid
- Extensiveness of the disease
- Patient characteristics (age, reliability, compliance, lifestyle habits, etc.)
- Training, preferences, and experience of the surgeon.

The analysis of our data from mastoid surgeries between 1983 and 2014 (31 years) shows the following partition: 8,912 (86.4%) CWU (including tympanoplasty without cholesteatoma), 316 (3.1%) CAT, 1,091 (10.6%) CWD, completed by 213 revisions of mastoid cavities (radical cavities).

Causes for Failures in CWD

- The above-mentioned recommendations are not respected, mainly high facial ridge and meatus too narrow, especially the entry of the OEC
- Extended cavity cholesteatoma in combination with a huge cavity due to a vast pneumatization

- Low dura (middle fossa)and/or high sinus sigmoideus
- Deep sinodural angle and/or terminal cell
- New grown bone formation (similar to exostosis) in "old" mastoid cavities performed during childhood or youth.

Impact of Mastoid Cavities after CWD

- Audiological
  - *Change of the acoustic characteristics of the external ear because of the enlarged volume*: The mean resonant frequency was significantly decreased compared to a normal ear.[5-8]
  - 5–10 dB reduced sound transmission after staged ossiculoplasties compared to CWU procedures.[9,10]
- Middle ear pressure (MEP)
  - *The mastoid is an active counter-regulator*: It is related to continuous regulation of smaller changes of MEP, whereas the Eustachian tube is related to intermittent regulation of higher pressures. Vascularization and gas exchange of the mastoid mucosa might play an important role in MEP.[11,12]
- Quality of life
  - Caloric stimuli (wind, cold water, suction cleaning) induce vertigo because there is no protection of the semicircular canals. The labyrinthine organ is covered by thin epithelial lining only.[13]
  - Accumulation of keratin debris followed by recurrent infections, drainage (often foul-smelling), and hearing loss. Patients with these conditions, often ongoing for decades, become socially withdrawn and professionally inhibited.[14]
  - Difficulty with the use of conventional hearing aids.[15]
- Aesthetic aspect
  - After an extensive meatoplasty, patients are bothered by an extreme wide entry of the OEC.
- Economic impact
  - Frequent clinic visits and treatments for aural toilet and plethora of topical medications in case of a chronically draining cavity.[16]
  - Multiple surgeries in an attempt to curing.

Obliteration of Mastoid Cavities

Using an obliteration technique can ease most of the mentioned effects. Therefore, for the patient the obliteration of a mastoid, whether partially or completely, is suitable to ease negative consequences deriving from an open mastoid. By using a mathematical model to predict the development of gas pressure balance in the function of different middle ear volumes there was the conclusion that, typical in cholesteatoma cases, mastoid obliteration as a surgical reduction of mucosal surface for gas exchange can improve middle ear gas pressure balance resulting in better long-term outcome.[17]

If not indicated primarily, the obliteration can be performed in a second stage procedure, although it has to be considered that the surgeon has to challenge a distorted anatomy where the landmarks are difficult to identify, especially after several pre-operations.

Until today, numerous techniques with various obliteration and reconstruction materials have been published. Similar to the choice of the cholesteatoma surgery technique (CWU vs. CWD) the decision for mastoid obliteration (MO) is influenced by the school, routine and last but not least by the individual personality and sensitivity of the surgeon. My teacher in otosurgery used to say that patients with decades of complaints and after multiple pre-operations should be treated with sensitive and tender care, but "Keep the expectations low". It is essential that the patient should be thoroughly informed in detail prior to this challenging operation. This includes the expected benefit, the advantages and disadvantages of various materials and techniques and of course alternative treatment options. Finally, the experience of the surgeon is decisive for the result of the entire procedure.

Materials for Mastoid Obliteration

There are biological (normally autologous) and nonbiological (alloplastic) materials. Homologous materials are no longer allowed due to medicolegal reasons.

Biological material
- Soft tissue[18] and numerous flaps with various kind of techniques[19-26]
- Bone (chips, pâté, demineralized bone matrix),[27-38] sometimes combined with flaps[39-41] or ceramics[42]
- Fat,[43,44] sometimes simultaneously with Cochlea Implant (CI)[45,46] or Vibrant Sound Bridge (VSB)[47]
- Cartilage (harvested from cavum conchae, tragus, cymba).[48-51]

Alloplastic (nonbiological) material
- Methylmethacrylat[52]
- Ceramics (various kind of composition and manufacturing process as powder, cement, granules, block)[53-67]
- Silicone[68]
- Bioactive glass.[69-73]

Cartilage or soft tissue like fascia or perichondrium is regularly used as coverage of other materials. Many surgeons use fibrin glue to keep the obliteration material in place and seal it.

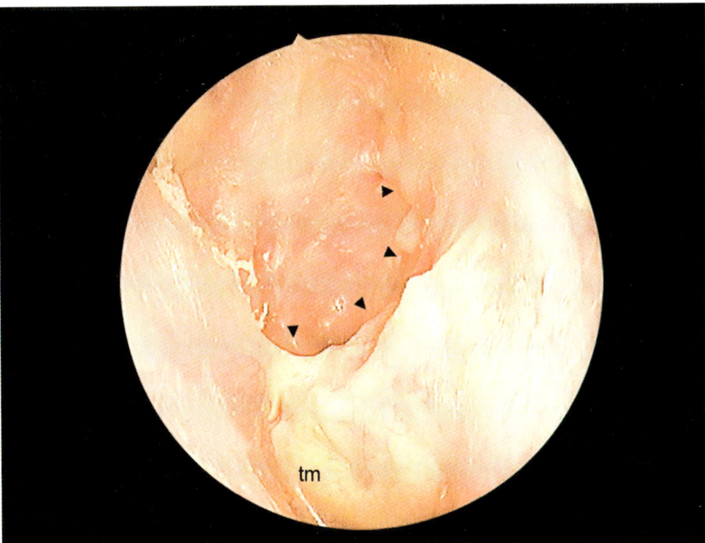

Fig. 15.1: Five years after obliteration with Palva flap and cartilage (left ear). (tm: Tympanic membrane; black arrow heads: cartilage pulled into the mastoid because of shrinking of the soft tissue).

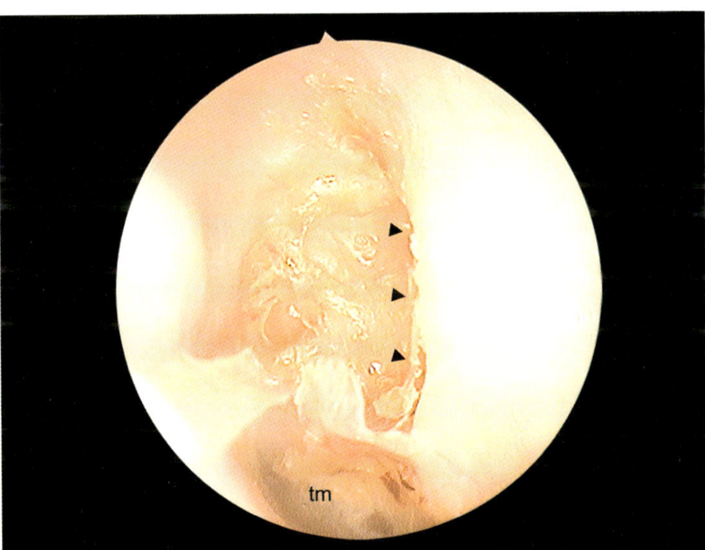

Fig. 15.2: Six years postoperatively (left ear). Same technique of surgery as Figure 5.1.

Results of Mastoid Obliteration

Soft tissue flaps tend to induce shrinking, atrophy and fibrosis. The result is a partly or re-established cavity and retraction pockets (Figs. 15.1 and 15.2).[31,22,40] To minimize this effect, vascularized flaps were created[26,27] or the flap was used in combination with bone pâté.

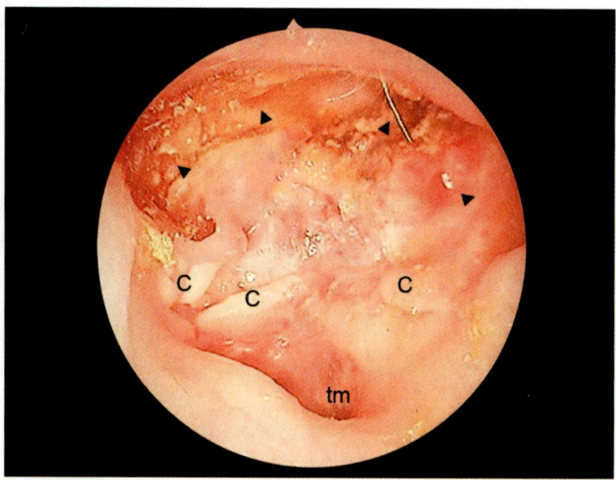

Fig. 15.3: Six years after obliteration with cartilage and bone pâté (left ear). (tm: Tympanic membrane; C: Cartilage; black arrow heads: retractions with effusion).

Bone pâté, as well as *ceramics* that is a foreign material, has a tendency to get infected and being partly rejected and resorbed will result in some cases to revision surgery because of recurrent pocket formation (Fig. 15.3).[33,35,42,62,65-67] To prevent infection, the obliteration material is sometimes mixed with antibiotic, e.g. Cloramphenicol,[33] Rifamycin,[37] and Augmentin.[75,62] Because of resorption and a certain loss of bone pâté an attempt has been made to over-obliterate the cavity to compensate for volume loss.[30]

Cartilage plates tend to bend, especially close to the edges. The result is a gap between overlapping plates into which epithelium will migrate underneath the plates and/or into the mastoid. Figures 15.4A and B show an example of a 12-year-old boy 1.5 years after two pre-operations performed elsewhere.

Our own results after 859 MOs (1983–2014) confirm mainly the results of the studies mentioned above (Table 15.1).

The use of HA granules was stopped after 18 cases due to the increased infection/rejection rate. Since 2012, BAG S53P4 (BonAlive granules) has been used regularly. The granules are covered by sliced cartilage plates and free graft of fascia. We have not prescribed any antibiotics except in those cases with pre-operatively proven bacteria-like proteus, pseudomonas, or any specific multiresistant strains.

Bioactive Glass

History[76]

The first Larry Hench (University of Florida) invented bioactive glass (BAG) in 1969. All implant materials available at the time, e.g. metals

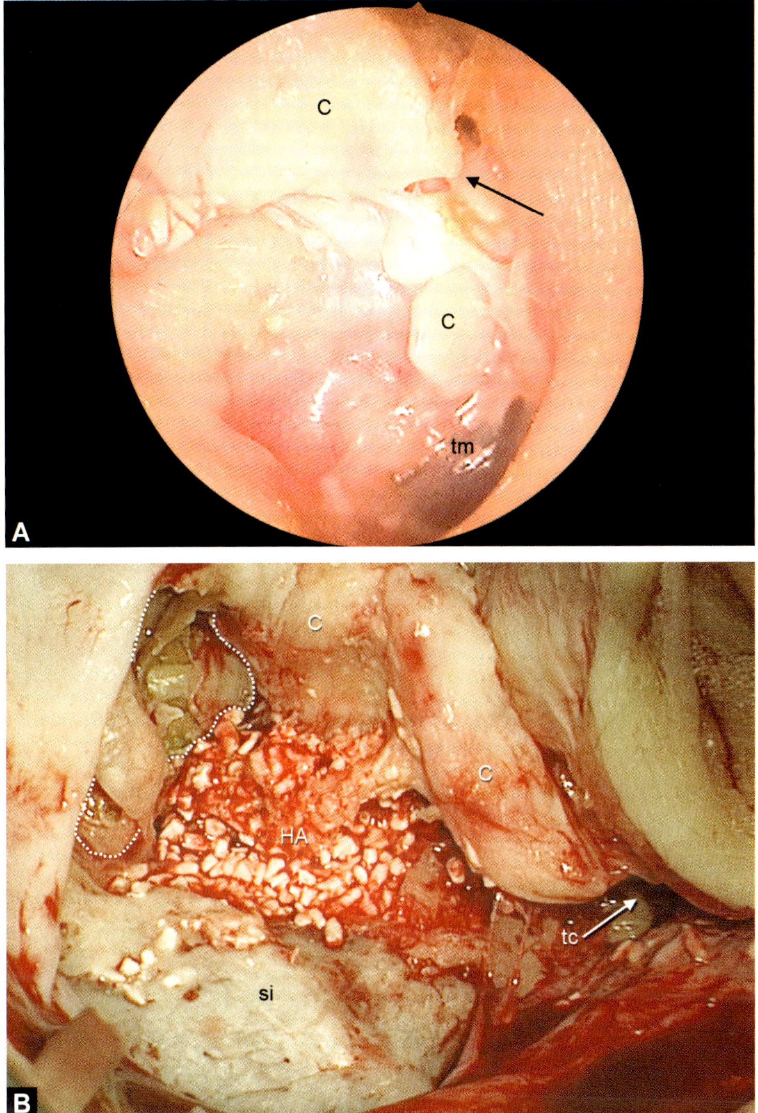

Figs. 15.4A and B: (A) 1.5 years after obliteration with HA (right ear) covered by cartilage. Black arrow: retraction between two plates of cartilage. (B) Mastoid opened (dotted white line: Cholesteatoma epithelium; tc with white arrow: Terminal cell; si: Sinus sigmoideus; C: Cartilage; HA: Hydroxyapatit).

and polymers that were designed to be bioinert, triggered fibrous encapsulation after implantation, rather than forming a stable interface or bond with tissues. The main discovery was that a glass of the composition 46.1% SiO_2, 24.4% Na_2O, 26.9% CaO, and 2.6% P_2O_5, later termed 45S5 and Bioglass, formed a strong bond with bone. This launched the field of many new bioactive materials such as ceramics

Table 15.1: Pathological findings after mastoid obliteration (1983–2014) mean follow-up 33 months (std +/-27.8).

	Total n (%)	Infection rejection	Granulation post. wall	Retraction pocket	Shrinking fibrosis	Patholog. finding total n (%)
Cartilage/bone	516 (61)	—	11 (2%)	32 (6%)	—	43 (8)
Bone pâté (BP)	33 (4)	4 (12%)	1 (3%)	2 (6%)	—	7 (21)
Hydroxyapatit (HA)	18 (2)	3 (20%)	—	2 (13%)	—	5 (33)
Palva flap (PF)	145 (17)	—	7(5%)	14 (10%)	10 (7%)	31 (21)
BAG S53P4	133 (16)	—	—	3 (3%)	—	3 (3)
Combin. BP/HA/PF	14 (2)	—	—	—	—	—

[synthetic hydroxyapatite (HA), calcium phosphate and others]. They are defined as materials that stimulate a beneficial response from the body, particularly bonding to host tissue (usually bone).

Mechanism of bioactivity

- Bone bonding is attributed to the formation of a hydroxycarbonate-apatite (HCA) layer, which interacts with collagen fibrils of damaged bone to form a bond.[77] Bone bonding to the HCA layer is thought to involve protein adsorption, incorporation of collagen fibrils, attachment of bone progenitor cells, cell differentiation, and the excretion of bone extracellular matrix, followed by its mineralization.
- Osteogenesis is related to the action of dissolution products of the glasses on osteoprogenitor cells, stimulating new bone growth. However, the HCA layer also provides a surface suitable for osteogenic cell attachment and proliferation.[78]

Mechanism of HCA layer formation

There are five proposed stages for HCA formation in body fluid in vivo or in simulated body fluid in vitro.[64,79]

1. Rapid cation exchange of Na^+ and/or Ca^{2+} with H^+ from solution, creating silanol bonds (Si–OH) on the glass surface: $Si - O - Na^+ + H^+ + OH^- \rightarrow Si - OH^+ + Na^+ (aq) + OH^-$

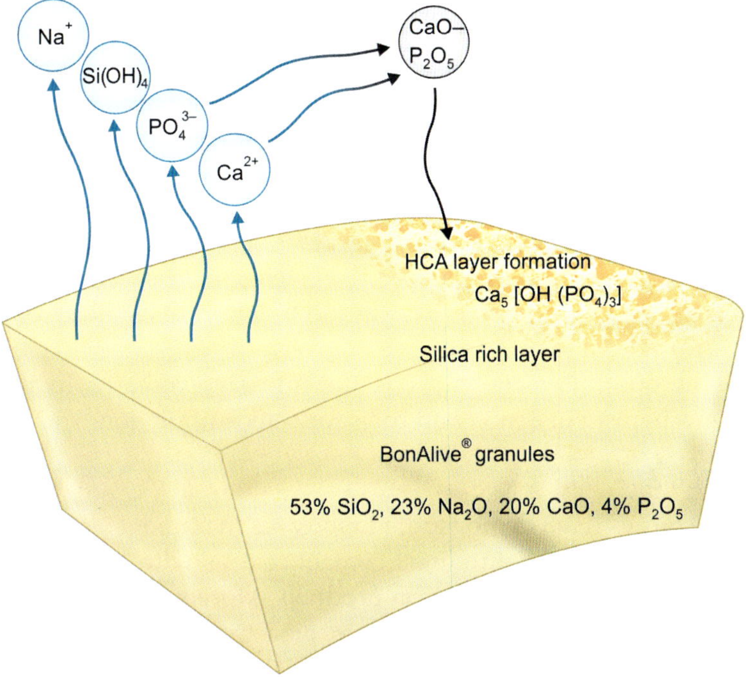

Fig. 15.5: Chemical cascade of ion migration of BAG S53P4.

The pH of the solution increases and a silica-rich (cation-depleted) region forms near the glass surface. Phosphate is also lost from the glass if present in the composition.

2. High local pH leads to attack of the silica glass network by OH$^-$, breaking Si–O–Si bonds. Soluble silica is lost in the form of Si(OH)$_4$ to the solution, leaving more Si–OH (silanols) at the glass–solution interface: Si–O–Si + H$_2$O → Si–OH + OH–Si

3. Condensation of Si–OH groups near the glass surface: repolymerization of the silica-rich layer.

4. Migration of Ca^{2+} and PO$_4^{3-}$ groups to the surface through the silica-rich layer and from the solution, forming a film rich in amorphous CaO–P$_2$O$_5$ on the silica-rich layer.

5. Incorporation of hydroxyls and carbonate from solution and crystallization of the CaO–P$_2$O$_5$ film to HCA (Fig. 15.5).

Glass composition is the variable that has the greatest influence on rate of HCA layer formation and bone bonding. Bioactivity has been shown to be directly related to the activation energy of silica dissolution in the glass.[80] As a rule of thumb, melt-derived glasses with compositions containing >60% SiO$_2$ do not bond and are bioinert.[76]

Stimulation of Osteogenesis

Once the HCA layer has formed, proteins adsorb to the HCA layer,[81] cells attach, differentiate, and produce bone matrix. Human osteoblasts cultured on bioactive glasses produce collagenous extracellular matrix (ECM) that mineralizes to form bone nodules without the usual supplements of hormones present in the culture.[82-84] The dissolution of calcium ions and soluble silica from bioactive glass was shown to stimulate osteoblast cell division, production of growth factors, and ECM proteins. Other bioceramics need osteogenic supplements added to the media such as dexamethasone and b-glycerophosphate, for bone nodule formation to occur.

Numerous publications prove the intensive research in respect to the mechanism of action and basis for osteostimulation.[85-91]

Neovascularization

In vitro studies have demonstrated increases in angiogenic indicators through both direct and indirect contact of cells with bioactive glass particles or with their dissolution products. Moreover, in vivo studies have confirmed the ability of certain bioactive glasses to stimulate neovascularization. The incorporation of Bioglass into bone tissue-engineered scaffolds is thus perceived to be widely beneficial in biomaterial-based regenerative medicine strategies.[92]

Antibacterial Effect

The antibacterial action of a BAG is influenced by its chemical composition and the dissolution conditions in its surroundings. It has been suggested to be based on several factors, including high pH and osmotic effects caused by the nonphysiological concentration of ions dissolved from the glass.[93-95] It was proven against periodontal pathogens, *Klebsiella ozaenae*, *Hemophilus influenza*, and *Streptococcus pneumonia*.[96-99] In an extensive work the efficacy of six powdered BAGs and two sol-gel derived materials against 29 clinically important bacterial species was shown, e.g. *Acinetobacter* sp, *Corynebacter*, various *Enterococcus* sp, *Escherichia coli*, *Proteus*, *Pseudomonas aeruginosa*, various *Staphylococcus* (including methicillin-resistent Staphylococcus aureus MRSA),[100] as well as by comparing three bioactive glasses.[101] The same result was demonstrated by tests with 17 bacterial species: there was no significant difference seen between gram-positive and gram-negative bacteria.[102]

Antibiofilm Effect

Biofilms are multicellular networks of bacteria encased in a matrix.[103] The role of mastoid biofilm in chronic otitis media was confirmed.[104]

The most recent research results indicate that the bioactive glass S53P4 has antibiofilm properties where the mechanism is thought to be that the high pH and osmotic pressure can penetrate the biofilm structure and kill the bacteria.[105]

Excretion of Dissolution Products

As natural levels of Si in the human body are low (0.6 μmL^{-1} for serum and 41 μmL^{-1} for muscle), it is important to be sure of the route of excretion of the dissolution products. Harmless Si excretion in urine was observed in rabbits up to 7 months after implantation of Bioglass 45S5 particles in the tibia[106] and muscle.[107] For 750 mg of Bioglass 45S5 implanted in the tibia, Si levels in the urine were below saturation, and histology of the brain, heart, kidney, liver, lung, lymph nodes, spleen, and thymus showed no elevation of Si levels. In addition, results were presented on a long-term evaluation of blood silicon and ostecalcin in humans that have been treated with BAG S53P4 due to benign bone tumors and no elevated values were found.[10]

Animal Research

The results of the animal research support the effectiveness of BAG S53P4 as bone-graft substitute.[109,110] Autogenous bone was compared to BAG[111] and HA in frontal sinus obliteration[112] and as filler material in combination with BAG around titanium.[113] BAG S53P4 cones and granules were compared in a long-term study.[114]

BAG S53P4

BAG S53P4 consists of 53% SiO_2, 23% Na_2O, 20% CaO, and 5% P_2O_5. It is manufactured in Turku (Finland).

This material was the most effective BAG in respect to the antibacterial action, which had a clear growth-inhibitory effect and fastest killing on all pathogens tested.[100] Lower concentrations were needed compared to the other (tested) BAGs.[102]

In 1994, it was used for obliteration of frontal sinuses for the first time.[115] and afterwards in several other studies including craniomaxillofacial surgery (CMF) all with positive results up to 9 years follow-up.[116-122] At the same time, the implantation of BAG S53P4 started in orthopedics.[123] In the following years, studies were published describing the treatment of benign bone tumors,[124,125] bone cysts,[126] and the delicate and often resistant to therapy chronic osteomyelitis.[127-130] In traumatology[131,132] and spinesurgery,[133,134] BAG S53P4 was used for bone repairing, remodeling, and stabilization showing the antibacterial properties as well as vascularization effect.[135]

In otosurgery, the obliteration of the mastoid is the most relevant field for the use of BAG S53P4. Moreover, we have implanted the BAG granules in two cases with extensive cholesteatoma of the OEC (*see* below "Own experiences"). It was confirmed that this material gives extra support to antimicrobial properties even in closed cavities. Although BAG S53P4 is a resorbable material, it does not resorb before new bone has formed. It fulfills the criteria of being a good biomaterial for MO.[73] After previous failed efforts in achieving a dry, safe ear and to avoid a large cavity in CWD mastoidectomy, it was evaluated as a noteworthy material. To repair dural fistula or correcting dural protrusion after bony dehiscence at the middle cranial fossa BAG plates in combination with granules have been used successfully.[71] Because BAG is radiopaque, the implant can later be examined by radiography if necessary.[70] In a prospective study there was not observed any adverse reaction to BAG S53P4 granules by using it in mastoid obliteration.[136]

Own experience using BAG S53P4

Since 2012, we have regularly been using BAG S53P4 for obliteration of mastoid cavities.[137] In the following 3 years, it was implanted in 133 cases:

- Eight primary surgeries
  - Two extensive cholesteatoma of the outer canal (intrusion into the mastoid)
- 10 cases CWU (bilateral)
- 115 cases CWD.

Figure 15.6 shows the partition of pre-operations. In the group with >4 previous surgeries there were three cases with five and three cases with six, seven, and eight pre-operations each.

Fifty-four cases (43.2%) had one or more reconstructions of the posterior wall, that failed in achieving a dry and safe ear. The findings leading to revision surgery were retraction, mastoid cholesteatoma or extended granulation tissue in the mastoid causing effusion and fetid infections.

Figure 15.7 shows the distribution of patient age with an average age of 41.4 years (57% male, 43% female). The range of follow-up was between two cases <4 months and 23 patients >24 months (mean follow-up 17.3 months, std ± 8.72) (Fig. 15.8).

Postoperative findings and treatment

The first visit was regularly 3 weeks postoperatively for removal of the package (gel foam). Of the first 100 cases, 68% needed treatment with a Polyvinyl acetal (PVA)-stick and otologica during the first or

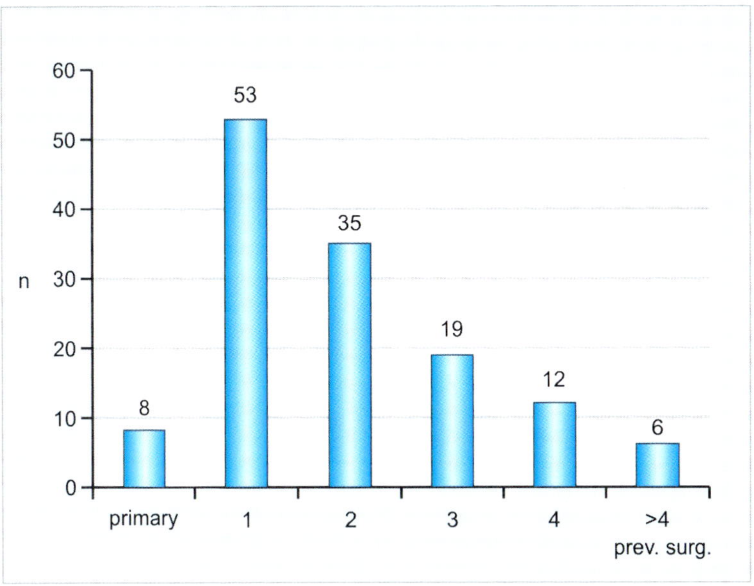

Fig. 15.6: Distribution of primary and previous surgeries.

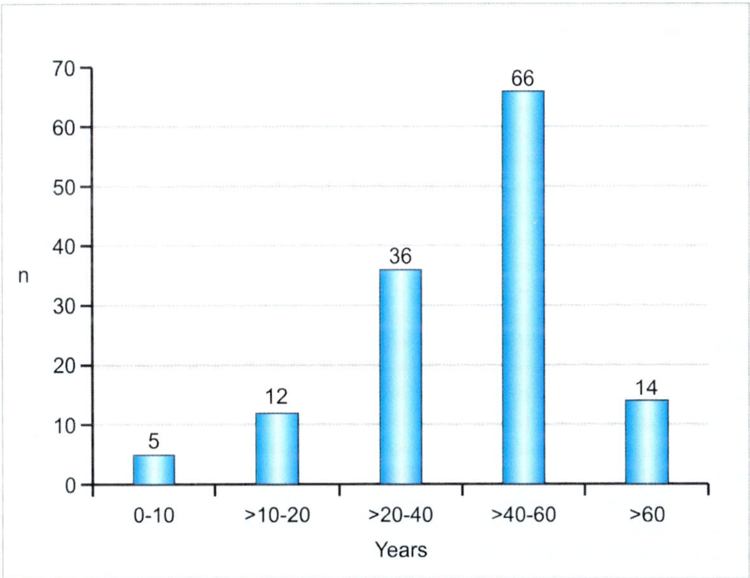

Fig. 15.7: Distribution of age.

second visit. Figure 15.9 (blue columns) shows that this treatment was necessary in 23% with 3–4 appointments, in 6% with 4–5 and in 4% with 6 or more appointments. The reason for these frequent treatments was a distinctive swelling of the posterior wall (reconstructed meatus with cartilage, fascia, and skin covering the BAG). We have left

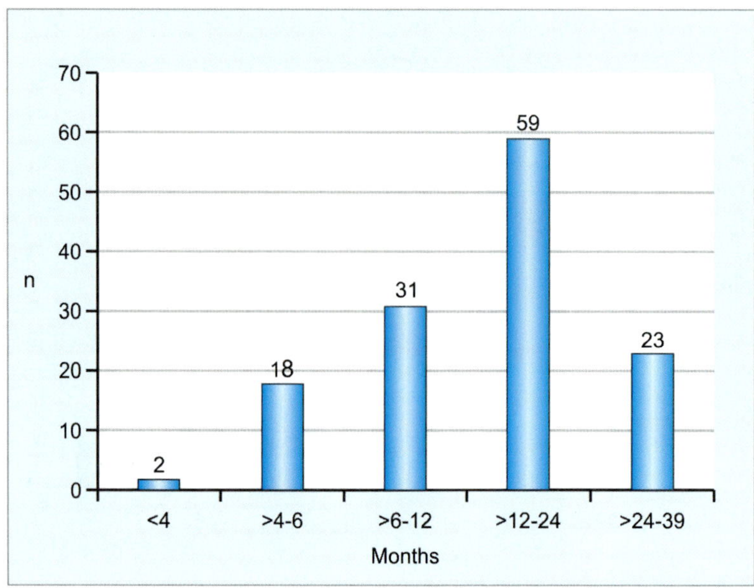

Fig. 15.8: Time of follow-up.

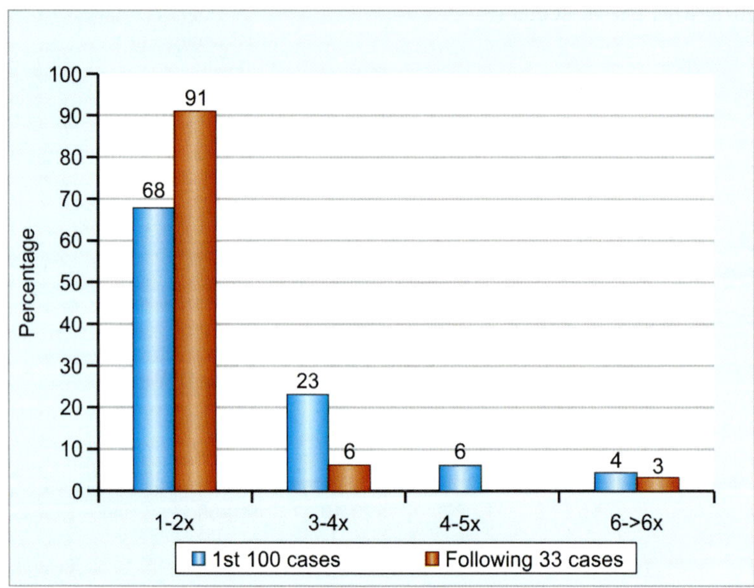

Fig. 15.9: Frequency of postoperative treatment with PVA-stick.

one or more sticks to expand for 8–10 days to prevent stenosis of the OEC (Fig. 15.10). The patient was instructed to use ear drops daily.

Moreover, we have seen three cases with a superficial retroauricular abscess few days after surgery, two of them with CWU (bilateral). Evaluating these findings, the theory was that the cystoid edematous

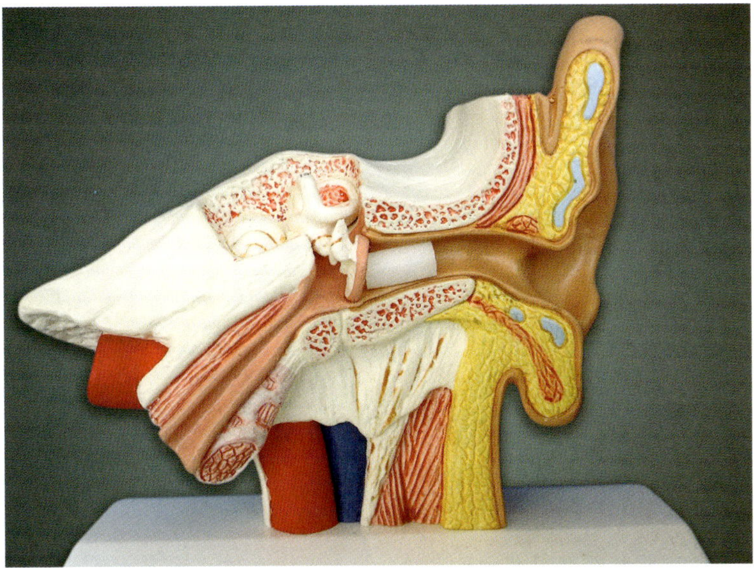

Fig. 15.10: Ear-model with expanded PVA-stick in the outer ear canal.

swelling and the abscess were caused by surplus fluid in the obliterated mastoid. This fluid is an ideal nutrition solution for bacteria. Staphylococcus aureus, a germ of the superficial skin, was detected in the cases with abscess. The histology of BAG probes of one of the three cases 4 weeks postoperatively proved that there was concentric fibrosis (Fig. 15.11A) and no sign of infection, e.g. granulocyte or histiocytic foreign body reaction (Fig. 15.11B). This is remarkable in consideration of the severe adjacent infection. Additionally, there is calcification beginning as a sign of appositional bone growth (arrows in Figs. 15.11A to C).

The consequence for the following 33 cases was to insert a drainage tube deep into the BAG granules (Figs. 15.12A and B). Within the first 2 days postoperatively, 2–3.5 mL fluid could be collected in the compressible reservoir. This procedure clearly reduced the necessity to use PVA sticks (*see* Fig. 15.9, red columns). According to this experience for us the explanation for the edematous swelling was that the surplus fluid is bulging the weakest area consisting of soft tissue: in case of CWD the reconstructed posterior wall and in case of CWU (bilateral) because of the preserved bony canal wall the retroauricular region.

Nevertheless there are two cases with long-lasting superficial problems: One case with chronic myringitis lasting >24 months and one case with chronic otitis of the external canal because of a resistant Enterobacter

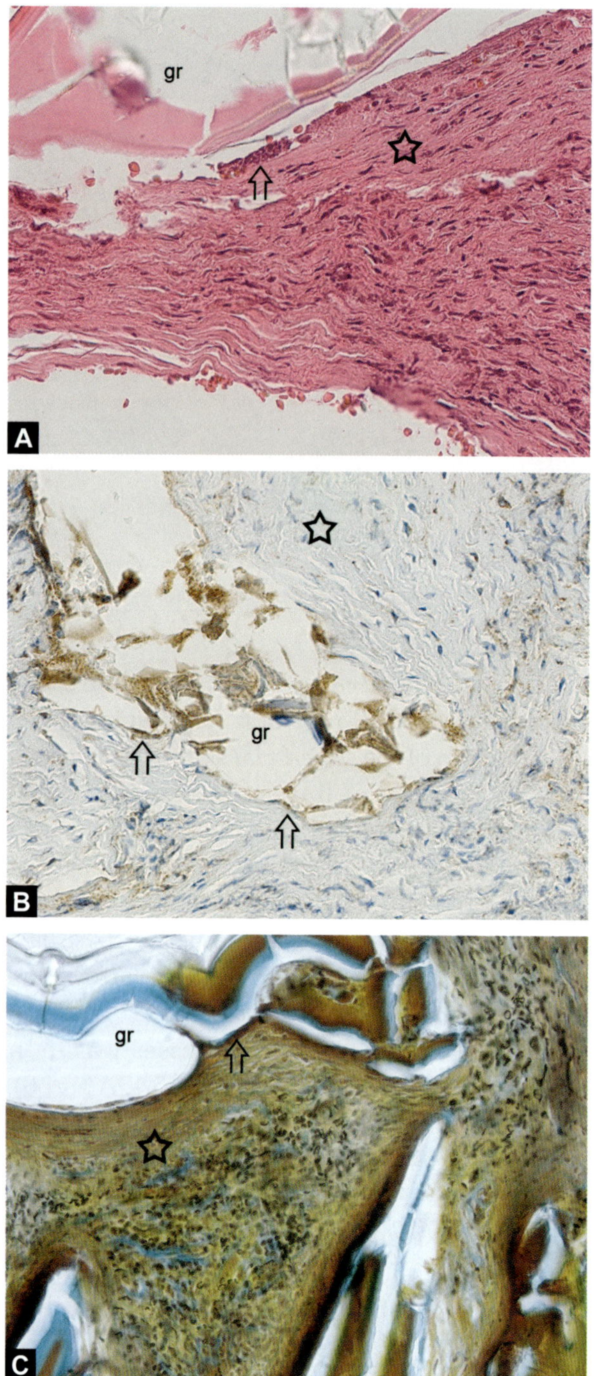

Figs. 15.11A to C: (A) Histology: HE staining (× 400): calcification (arrow), concentric fibrosis (asterisk), and BAG granule (gr). (B) CD 68 immunohistology (× 400): no foreign body reaction and no signs of inflammation. (C) Polarization histology.
Courtesy: (C) JT Silvola, Oslo, Norway.

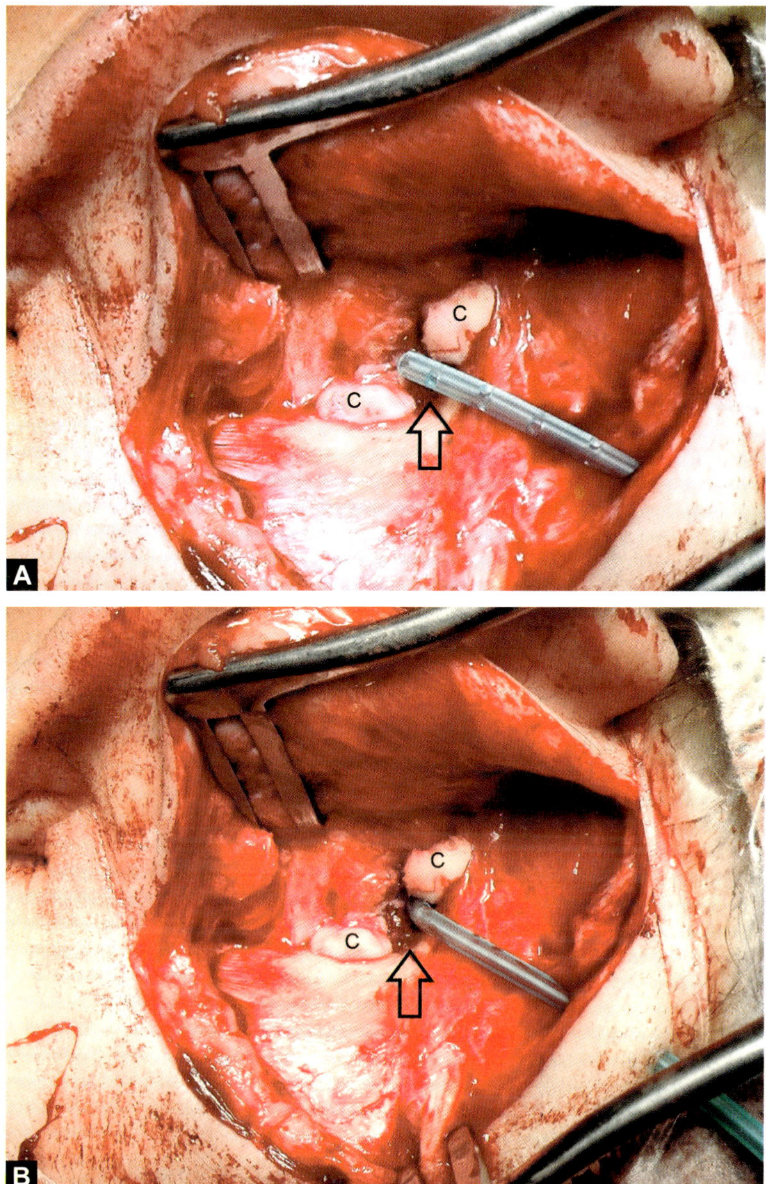

Figs. 15.12A and B: (A) Drainage tube (right ear) before inserting into the mastoid filled with bioactive glass granules. (c: Cartilage covering granules; arrow: entry to the mastoid). (B) Drainage tube placed deep in the obliterated mastoid.

affection lasting >32 months. We assume that some ears with severe altered skin in the cavity and complaint duration sometimes ongoing for decades maintained their problems after obliteration surgery. In those cases the unsatisfying healing is not due to the obliteration material.

Reasons for revisions

There were 12 cases requiring revision surgery:
- Six stenosis of the entry of the OEC or the whole OEC
- Three retraction pockets (transition zone of the OEC to BAG granules)
- One abscess retroauricular
- One bleeding (temporalis muscle) 1 day postoperatively.

Consequences due to the revision findings

The revisions show that even after three decades of surgical practice, there is still a learning curve when using new material. The ambition to achieve an end result where the OEC has a close to normal anatomy can lead to overload the mastoid. The result will be a meatus too narrow. A sufficient aeration of the OEC is essential for a good healing of the altered OEC skin without major problems. Therefore, a meatoplasty and widening of the bony OEC especially the anterior wall is recommended. The anterior tympanomeatal angle should be as visible as possible.

Retraction pockets occurred in two cases because we lifted the skin of the cavity in the transition zone to the bony OEC not wide enough especially in the area of the facial ridge. The problem was solved in a short time by lining the retraction pocket with suitable cartilage pieces. The third case showed two retractions to the attic. The reason might be that during filling-in, the BAG granules did not reach this delicate structure. Intraoperatively accumulated fluid underneath the lining soft tissue and the skin will be resorbed in this area, which is not filled with granules: retractions will result. Figure 15.13 shows the 6 months postoperatively finding of the patient of *see* Figure 15.2. As a consequence, we now obliterate the attic with suitably thin cartilage plates under the skin and lining with fascia before filling in BAG granules into the mastoid.

Another revision was necessary because of a retroauricular abscess 6 days postoperatively. The infected seroma was limited to the subcutaneous region. Antibiotic intravenous therapy was done for 5 days. The other two abscesses were treated conservatively: reopening of two single knot sutures in the lower part of the retroauricular incision and aspiration of the small quantity of seroma followed by local control of the finding and oral antibiotic therapy for 5 days. All three cases healed within 1 week. We did not see the necessity of removing BAG S53P4 in either of the cases. After introducing the mini drainage into the routine of the obliteration surgeries using BAG S53P4 these findings have so far not reoccurred.

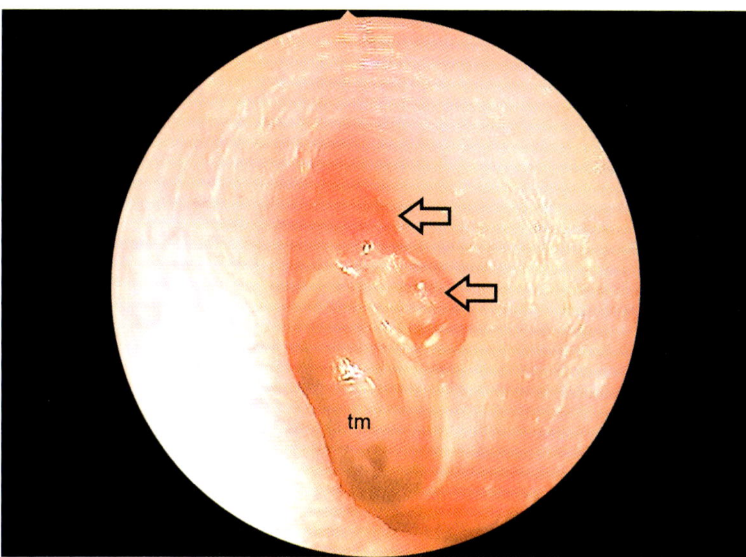

Fig. 15.13: Six months after obliteration with BAG S53P4 (left ear), same patient as Figure 15.2. Arrows: retractions due to postoperative surplus of fluid and following resorption. (tm: Tympanic membrane).

To evaluate the audiological result we excluded all cases in which a tympanoplasty was performed simultaneously, e.g. closure of a perforation, ossiculoplasty, underlay of an adhesive tympanic membrane. Eighty-eight cases remained of which we excluded another five cases with deafness or inner ear damage near to deafness.

There was no difference between the pre- and postoperatively bone conduction. The air conduction from 0.5 kHz up to 2 kHz remained unimproved. 4 kHz improved significantly (65.0–59.2 dB, std ± 26.9) and there was a slight, not significant improvement at 8 kHz (69.1–65.9 dB, std ± 25.6).

SUMMARY

- Soft tissues like fascia and perichondrium grafts are suitable to cover a small mastoid cavity, which can be formed when there is poor pneumatization.
- All kinds of flaps tend to shrink because a flap is not a solid obliteration material. To what extent this process will develop cannot be predicted. Therefore, the intraoperative obliteration finding is not the same as the future finding several years later. There is no difference when it is used in combination with a solid material like bone, HA, or BAG. The quality and the size of a flap depends on how often pre-operations were done. To create a flap needs time and depends on the skill of the surgeon.

- Cartilage is easy to harvest (cavum conchae, tragus, cymba). It is relatively stable because of its metabolism: it is nourished by diffusion. Problems will occur when there is not enough material available after several pre-operations.
- Due to the tendency of cartilage to bend, gaps can occur between the plates. Into these gaps epithelium will migrate behind or into the mastoid (*see* Figs. 15.4A and B). In combination with soft tissue flaps covering cartilage can be retracted due to the shrinking process of the soft tissue (*see* Figs. 15.1 and 15.2). Moreover, rejection, e.g. because of infection cannot generally be avoided.
- Bone pâté is harvested by a burr. The amount might be too little especially after preoperation(s) to obliterate a cavity completely. In these cases it can be used to fill deep dips to achieve a saucerized cavity. There is a high risk of infection and rejection if germs have colonized and shown a presence in the cavity for many years (*see* Fig. 15.3).
- Harvesting bone pâté needs a specific skill of the surgeon. Collecting epithelium must be avoided in any circumstance. Otherwise, the result will be a residual cholesteatoma hidden somewhere deep in the mastoid. The quality of the harvested bone pâté and the vitality of the bony ground are dependent on the rinsing intensity, as well as on the size of the burr, the drilling speed, the pressure of the burr on the bone surface. Bone material, which has become too hot, through friction forces will increase the risk of rejection. Finally, the surgeon influences that as well.
- HA is a synthetic ceramic material manufactured in various combinations of chemical molecular compounds. According to our experiences and to various reports, infection and following rejection occur time and time again. The reason might be that there is a difference in the osmotic pressure and the ion migration in the solvent compared to BAG. Furthermore, the properties of a synthetic HA are not the same as the natural bone mineral in regard to calcium phosphate crystallization.[138] To avoid the tendency of infection it was proposed to add antibiotic to ceramics prophylactically (and to bone pâté as well). Besides that the use of oral or even intravenous antibiotic treatment is quite normal, often as "one shot" therapy. In this context the economic aspect and the problem of antibiotic resistance as a global problem is to be regarded.[139] The decreasing effectiveness of antibiotics has quickened in recent years, and with the arrival of more and more untreatable strains of bacteria "we are at the dawn of post-antibiotic era".[140] Therefore, any antibiotic treatment should be considered individually and critically.

- Some authors prefer a strongly stimulated osteogenesis within a few months, e.g. highly porous HA matrix (76% HA, 24% silicone dioxide).[65] In maxillofacial surgery, this property is beneficial especially in implantology and augmentation of the mandible (periodontology). In cases when following procedures demanding a stable bone structure are to be done in a clear time frame. In otosurgery, this is not necessary and might be rather a disadvantage. If further surgeries are planned because of implantation of CI or VSB after 6–12 months postoperatively, it is advantageous to find an obliteration material that can be handled easily. If a more or less complete solid ossification occurs in the mastoid, landmarks are difficult to identify needing more time because of burring with a higher risk to sensible structures.

After using BAG S53P4 during the indicated time of 3 years, the reported experiences of various specialties (orthopedic, spine surgery, traumatology, dental surgery, and CMF) up to more than a decade related to our clinical outcome can be confirmed. The clinical performance, safety, and efficacy in regard to osteostimulation were proven as well as the effect of preventing the growth of clinically relevant bacteria (gram positive and gram negative). In this study, failures, especially the longer lasting treatments, could be resolved to a large extend due to a detailed documentation, evaluation, and critical handling of the postoperative findings. A longer term follow-up and multicenter studies including a broader number of cases with MO should be initiated to reassure the outcome of our experience.

Recommendations for Using BAG S53P3 in MO

By considering the experience of other surgeons, the individual learning curve can be shortened. This is the primary reason why we hereby summarize our surgical technique by using BAG S53P4 in revision MO surgery and try to put it in a nutshell.

Retroauricular opening of the mastoid area and preparation of the connective tissue:

- *Retroauricularly*: Superficial skin incision at least 1–1.5 cm behind the angle of the auricle and lifting the skin together with the subcutaneous tissue. Cave: perforation because of extended scar after pre-operations.
- Semicircular incision of the connective tissue/periosteum layer of the mastoid surface as far behind as possible. Dissecting the bony mastoid surface by lifting this tissue ("collar flap") in direction to the meatus/entry of the cavity (Fig. 15.14). Cave: free sinus sigmoideus, dura (middle crania fossa).

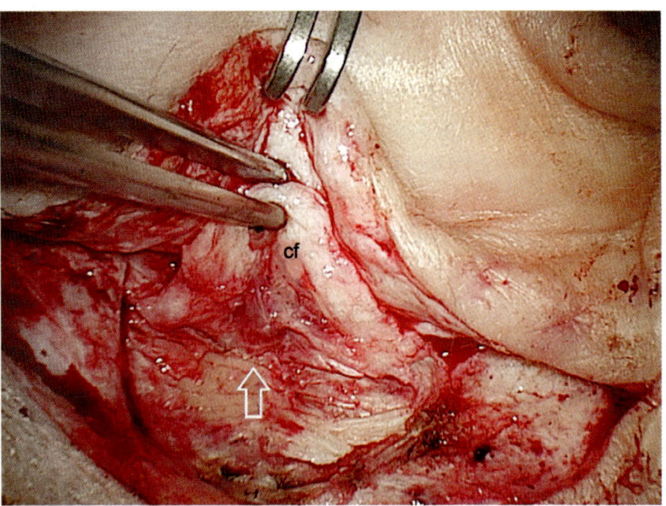

Fig. 15.14: "Collar flap" (cf) lifted (right ear) after retroincision. White arrow: bony ridge/entry of the mastoid cavity.

Preparation of mastoid cavity:
- Any bony overhang of the mastoid entry is reduced until there is a good overview to the cavity. Simultaneously the skin of the cavity is lifted continuously till the attic, labyrinth block and lower part of the OEC is reached. Cave: fistula of one of the semicircular canals (SCCF), dural and sinus dehiscence, free facial nerve (especially vertical mastoidal section).
- Removing any granulations and/or effusing mucosa and smoothing the bone at least by a diamond burr (large diameter).
- *Endaurally*: Control whether the skin of the cavity is lifted completely to prevent retraction pockets in the transition zone of the cavity and the lower part of the OEC or the attic.
- Meatoplasty: partial resection of the cartilage of cavum conchae, widening the OEC especially in the inferior and anterior area. The anterior tympanomeatal angle should be visible as clear as possible.

Reconstruction of the posterior wall of the ear canal:
- The cartilage is cut into thin slices (0.3–0.5 mm). If necessary, cartilage can be harvested from the tragus or cymba additionally. By slicing it with a suitable device (Fig. 15.15), you get a selection of sufficient numerous plates for the reconstruction of the posterior OEC.
- *Retroauricularly*: Lining the skin with pressed humid fascia or connective tissue graft (not wet or dry like parchment to obtain an ideal condition for modeling) starting from the attic. Cave: higher risk of necrosis if the graft consists of solid scar tissue.

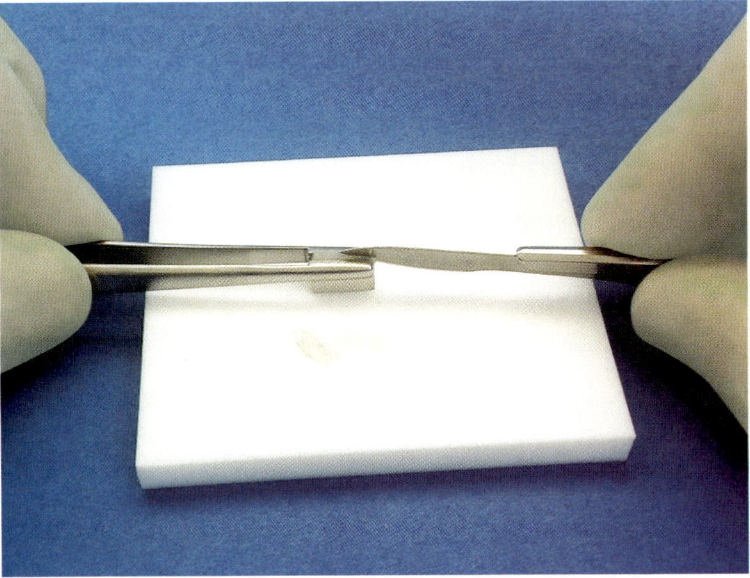

Fig. 15.15: Cartilage forceps (Schimanski design).

- Filling up the attic with small sliced pieces of cartilage and covering, e.g. free facial nerve or SCCF with cartilage in combination with tissue graft and dura or sinus as well.
- Reconstruction of the posterior OEC by lining the connective tissue with overlapping pieces of cartilage. The multiple sliced plates are slightly curved in various shapes and can be placed in a suitable way. Multiple slicing diminishes a further bending effect (Fig. 15.16).

 Stepwise obliteration with BAG S53P4 and shaping of the external auditory canal:

- Filling up the cavity with BAG S53P4 granules moistened well with saline solution to one-third or not more than half of the cavity volume especially in the region of the attic and terminal cell or any deep dip to prevent future liquid in excavations not filled with granules.
- *Endaurally*: Modeling the skin of the reconstructed posterior wall. Covering with silastic sheets in a circular way first to use the elastic properties of the silastic for dilating. Filling up the OEC with gelfoam package. This will guarantee the wideness of the OEC and prevent a bulging of the posterior wall during the following implantation of the BAG granules (Fig. 15.17).
- Now the mastoid is filled up with BAG granules up to the level of the cortical bone.

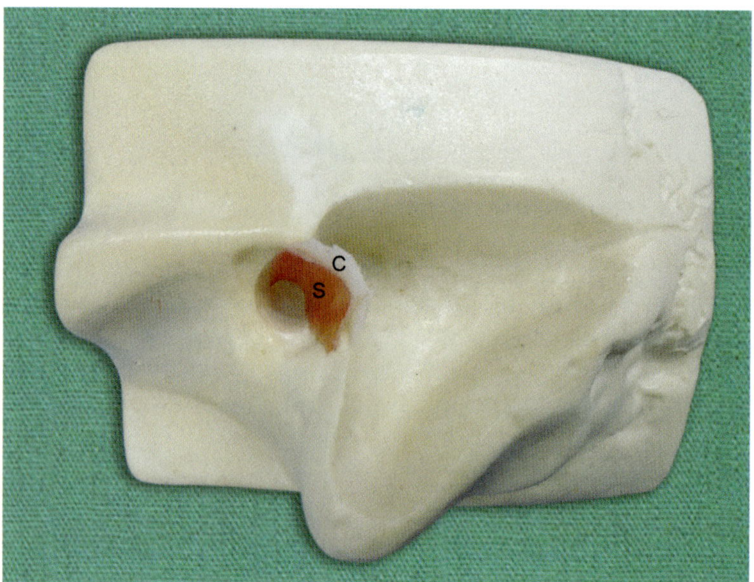

Fig. 15.16: Model (left ear): reconstructed post. Wall. (s: Skin; c: Cartilage).

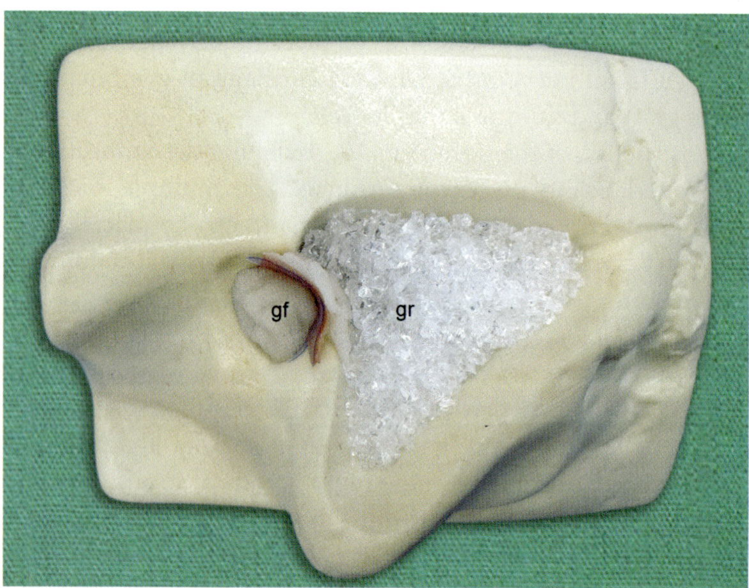

Fig. 15.17: Model (left ear): mastoid filled half with bioactive glass granules (gr), outer ear canal filled with gelfoam (gf) package and blue silastic sheets.

- If there are any retractions in the outer part of the posterior OEC because of solid scar, the "collar flap" can be used for lining at least partially by slicing it.

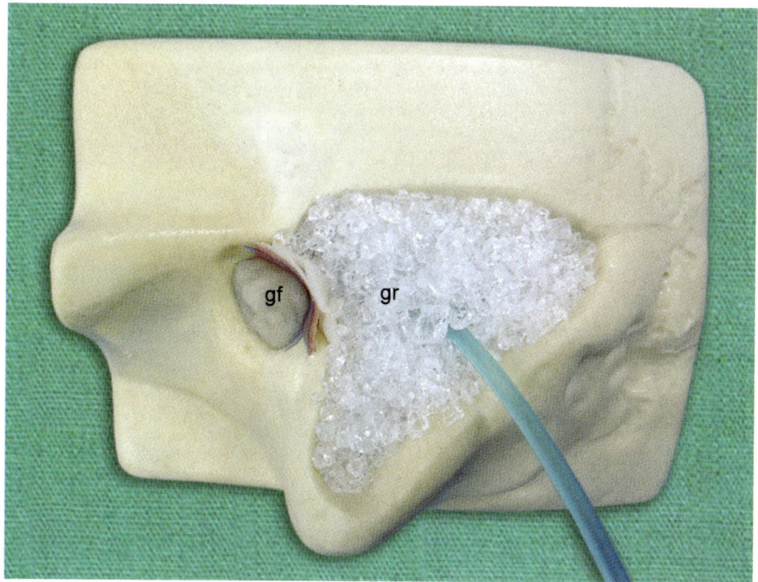

Fig. 15.18: Model (left ear): mastoid filled with bioactive glass granules (gr) and inserted drainage tube. (gf: Gelfoam).

Inserting the retroauricular drainage:
- The tube of the drainage system, which is shortened to the depth of the mastoid is introduced deep into the BAG granules (Fig. 15.18) and the surface of the granules is covered by remnant cartilage plates (*see* Figs. 15.12A and B) or/and the "collar flap" (Fig. 15.19).

Closing of the wound and immediate postoperative treatment:
- The incisions are closed by sutures and the drainage is fixed firmly before the circular bondage.
- The collecting bottle of the drainage remains accessible. Before the bottle is connected to the tube the suction system of the operation room will extract surplus of blood and serous liquid first. During the first few hours postoperatively, the vacuum will release frequently due to leakage of the incisions.
- The vacuum is to be renewed regularly. The amount of the collected fluid is noted.
- The drainage tube can be removed when the vacuum maintains for 8–12 hours. In general this will be after 36–48 hours.

DISCLOSURES

None of the authors has a financial interest concerning materials or products presented in this article.

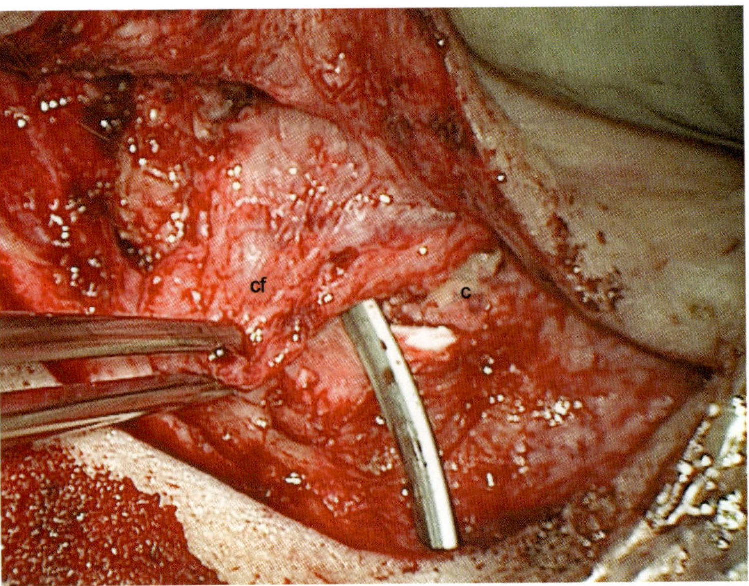

Fig. 15.19: "Collar flap" (cf) pulled back by a sharp forceps (right ear). (c: Cartilage).

REFERENCES

1. Sade J, Weinberg J, Berco E, et al. The marsupialised (radical) mastoid. J Laryngol Otol. 1982;96:869-75.
2. Fisch U. Tympanoplasty, Mastoidectomy and stapes surgery. Stuttgart: Thieme; 1994. p. 195.
3. Hildmann H, Sudhoff H, Jahnke K. Principles of an individualized approach to cholesteatoma surgery. In: Jahnke K (Ed). Middle Ear Surgery—Recent Advances and Future Directions. Stuttgart: Thieme; 2004. pp. 73-93.
4. Sanna M, Khrais T, Falcioni M, et al. The Temporal Bone—A Manual for Dissection and Surgical Approaches. Stuttgart: Thieme; 2006. pp. 27-8.
5. Evans RA, Day GA, Browning GG. Open-cavity mastoid surgery: its effect on the acoustics of the external ear canal. Clin Otolaryngol. 1989;14:317-21.
6. Hartwein J. The acoustics of the open mastoid cavity (so-called "radical cavity") and its modification by surgical measures. I. Physical principles, experimental studies. Laryngorhinootologie. 1992;19:551-7.
7. Jang C-H. Changes in external ear resonance after mastoidectomy: open cavity mastoid versus obliterated mastoid cavity. In: Rosowski JJ, Merchant SN (Eds). The Function and Mechanics of Normal, Diseased and Reconstructed Middle Ears. Amsterdam: Kugler Publications; 2000. pp. 291-6.
8. Jang C-H. Changes in external ear resonance after mastoidectomy: open cavity mastoid versus obliterated mastoid cavity. Clin Otolaryngol. 2002;27:509-11.
9. Shelton C, Sheehy JL. Tympanoplasty: review of 400 staged cases. Laryngoscope. 1990;100:679-81.
10. Whittemore KR Jr, Merchant SN, Rosowski JJ. Acoustic mechanisms: canal wall-up versus canal wall-down mastoidectomy. Otolaryngol Head Neck Surg. 1998;118:751-61.

11. Gaihede M, Dirckx JJ, Jacobsen H, et al. Middle ear pressure regulation—complementary active actions of the mastoid and the Eustachian tube. Otol Neurotol. 2010;31:603-11.
12. Dirckx JJJ, Marcosohn Y, Gaihede ML. Quasi-static pressures in the middle ear cleft. In: Puria S, Fay RR, Popper AN (Eds). The Middle Ear-Science, Otosurgery and Technology. Berlin Heidelberg: Springer; 2013. pp. 93-133.
13. Beutner D, Helmstaedter V, Stumpf R, et al. Impact of partial mastoid obliteration on caloric vestibular function in canal wall down mastoidectomy. Otol Neurotol. 2010;31:1399-403.
14. Dornhoffer JL, Smith J, Richter G, et al. Impact on quality of life after mastoid obliteration. Laryngoscope. 2008;118:1427-32.
15. Kurien G, Greeff K, Gomaa N, et al. Mastoidectomy and mastoid obliteration with autologous bone graft: a quality of life study. J Otolaryngol Head Neck Surg. 2013;42:49.
16. Black B. Mastoidectomy elimination. Laryngoscope. 1995;105:1-3.
17. Csakanyi Z, Katona G, Konya D, et al. Middle ear gas pressure regulation: the relevance of mastoid obliteration. Otol Neurotol. 2014;35:944-53.
18. Mosher HP. A method of filling the excavated mastoid with a flap from the back of the auricle. Laryngoscope. 1911;21:1158-63.
19. Kirsch H. Temporalis muscle grafts in the radical mastoid operation. J Laryngol Otol. 1928;43:735-6.
20. Palva T. Reconstruction of the ear canal in surgery for chronic ear. Arch Otolaryngol. 1962;75:329-34.
21. Palva T, Palva A, Karja J. Musculoperiosteal flap in cavity obliteration: histopathological study seven years postoperatively. Arch Otolaryngol. 1972;95:172-7.
22. Gopalakrishnan S, Chadha SK, Gopalan G, et al. Role of mastoid obliteration in patients with persistent cavity problems following modified radical mastoidectomy. J Laryngol Otol. 2001;115:967-72.
23. Ramsey MJ, Merchant SN, McKenna MJ. Postauricular periosteal-pericranial flap for mastoid obliteration and canal wall downtympanomastoidectomy. Otol Neurotol. 2004;25:873-8.
24. Uçar C. Canal wall reconstruction and mastoid obliteration with composite multifractured osteoperiosteal flap. Eur Arch Otorhinolaryngol. 2006;263: 1082-6.
25. Singh V, Atlas M. Obliteration of the persistently discharging mastoid cavity using the middle temporal artery flap. Otolaryngol Head Neck Surg. 2007;137:433-8.
26. Yung M, Smith P. Mid-temporal pericranial and inferiorly based periosteal flaps in mastoid obliteration. Otolaryngol Head Neck Surg. 2007;137: 906-12.
27. Shiller A . "Mastoid osteoplasty" using autologous cancellous bone. J Laryngol Otol. 1962;75:647-68.
28. Shea MC Jr, Gardner G Jr. Mastoid obliteration using homograft bone. Arch Otolaryngol. 1970;92:358-65.
29. Shea MC Jr, Gardner G Jr, Simpson ME. Mastoid oblieation using homogenous bone chips and autogenous bone paste. Trans Am Acad Ophthalmol Otolaryngol. 1972;76:160-72.
30. Solomons NB, Robinson JM. Obliteration of mastoid cavities using bone pâté. J Laryngol Otol. 1988;102:783-4.
31. Moffat DA, Gray RF, Irving RM. Mastoid obliteration using bone pâté. Clin Otolaryngol. 1994;19:149-57.

32. Shinkawa A, Sakai M, Tamura Y, et al. Canal-Down tympanoplasty; one-stage tympanoplasty with mastoid obliteration; for non-cholesteatomous chronic otitis media associated with osteitis. Tokai J Exp Clin Med. 1998;23:19-23.

33. Roberson JB, Mason TP, Stidham KR. Mastoid obliteration: autogenous cranial bone pâté reconstruction. Otol Neurotol. 2003;24:132-140.

34. Leatherman BD, Dornhoffer JL. The use of demineralized bone matrix for mastoid cavity obliteration. Otol Neurotol. 2004; 25:22-6.

35. Takahashi H, Iwanaga T, Kaieda S, et al. Mastoid obliteration combined with soft-wall reconstruction of posterior ear canal. Eur Arch Otorhinolaryngol. 2007; 264:867-71.

36. Beutner D, Stumpf R, Zahnert T, et al. Long-term results following mastoid obliteration in canal wall downtympanomastoidectomy. Laryngo-Rhino-Otol. 2007;86:1-6.

37. Vercruysse JP, De Foer B, Somers T, et al. Mastoid and epitympanic bony obliteration in pediatric cholesteatoma. Otol Neurotol. 2008;29:953-60.

38. Kuo CY, Huang BR, Chen HC, et al. Surgical results of retrograde mastoidectomy with primary reconstruction of the ear canal and mastoid cavity. Biomed Res Int. 2015;2015:517-35.

39. Palva T. Operative technique in mastoid obliteration. Acta Otolaryngol. 1973; 75:289-90.

40. Silvola J, Palva T. Pediatric one-stage cholesteatoma surgery: long term results. Int J Pediatr Otorhinolaryngol. 1999;19:87-90.

41. Ghiasi S. Mastoid cavity obliteration with combined palva flap and bone pâté. Iran J Otorhinolaryngol. 2015;27:23-8.

42. Park JS, Kang MY, Hong JC, et al. Result of mastoid obliteration according to the graft materials: autogenous bone, allogenic bone, hydroxylapatite. Int Adv Otol. 2011;7:305-10.

43. Delcanizo SR. Radical surgical treatment of the ear with implantation of free fat grafts. Rev Clin Esp. 1949;34:403-8.

44. Ringenberg JC, Fornatto EJ. The fat graft in middle ear surgery. Arch Otolaryngol. 1962;76:407-13 .

45. Gray RF, Ray J, McFerran DJ. Further experience with fat graft obliteration of mastoid cavities for cochlear implants. J Laryngol Otol. 1999;113:881-4.

46. Bernardeschi D, Nguyen Y, Smail M, et al. Middle ear and mastoid obliteration for cochlear implant in adults: indications and anatomical results. Otol Neurotol. 2015;36:604-9.

47. Ihler F, Koehler S, Meyer AC, et al. Mastoid cavity obliteration and vibrant soundbridge implantation for patients with mixed hearing loss. Laryngoscope. 2014;124:531-7.

48. Levinson RM. Cartilage-perichondrial composite graft tympanoplasty in the treatment of posterior marginal and attic retraction pockets. Laryngoscope. 1987; 97:1069-74.

49. Brask T. Obliteration of the mastoid cavities with crushed homograft cartilage in patients with cholesteatoma. In: Tos M, Thomsen J, Peitersen E (Eds). Cholesteatoma and Mastoid Surgery. Amsterdam: Kugler and Ghedini; 1989. pp. 931-3.

50. Dornhoffer JL. Surgical modification of the difficult mastoid cavity. Otolaryngol Head Neck Surg. 1999;120:361-7.

51. Kuo C-L, Lien C-F, Shiao A-S. Mastoid obliteration for pediatric suppurative cholesteatoma: long-term safety and sustained effectiveness after 30 years' experience with cartilage obliteration. Audiol Neurotol. 2014;19:358-69.
52. Meuser W. Permanent obliteration of old radical mastoid cavities combined with tympanoplasty. J Laryngol Otol. 1984;9:31-4.
53. Zoellner C, Buesing C-M. How useful is tricalcium phosphate ceramic in middle ear surgery? Am J Otol. 1986;7:289-93.
54. Reck R, Storkel S, Meyer A. Bioactive glass ceramics in middle ear surgery. Ann N Y Acad Sci. 1988;523:100-106.
55. Reck R, Bernal-Sprekelsen M. The effect of fibrin glue on the healing of hydroxyapatite ceramics. An animal experiment study. HNO. 1989;37:112-6.
56. Hartwein J, Hoermann K. A technique for the reconstruction of posterior canal wall and mastoid obliteration in radical cavity surgery. Am J Otol. 1990;11: 169-73.
57. Yung MW, Karia KR. Mastoid obliteration with hydroxyapatite—the value of high resolution CT scanning in detecting recurrent cholesteatoma. Clin Otolaryngol. 1997;22:553-7.
58. Estrem SA, Highfill G. Hydroxyapatite canal wall reconstruction/mastoid Obliteration. Otolaryngol Head Neck Surg. 1999;120:345-9.
59. Kupperman D, Tange RA. Ionomeric cement in the human middle ear cavity: long-term results of 23 cases. Laryngoscope. 2001;111:306-9.
60. Dornhoffer JL, Simmons O. Canal wall reconstruction with Mimix hydroxyapatite cement: results in an animal model and case study. Laryngoscope. 2003; 113:2123-8.
61. Bagot D'Arc M, Daculsi G, Emam N. Biphasic ceramics and fibrin sealant for bone reconstruction in ear surgery. Ann Otol Rhinol Laryngol. 2004;113:711-20.
62. Mahendran S, Yung MW. Mastoid obliteration with hydroxyapatite cement: the Ipswich experience. Otol Neurotol. 2004;25:19-21.
63. Minoda R, Hayashida M, Masuda M, et al. Preliminary experience with ß-tricalcium phosphate for use in mastoid cavity obliteration after mastoidectomy. Otol Neurotol. 2007;28:1018-21.
64. Clark AE, Pantano CG, Hench LL. Auger spectroscopic analysis of Bioglass corrosion films. J Am Ceram Soc. 1976;59:37-9.
65. Punke C, Zehlicke T, Boltze C, et al. Experimental studies on a new highly porous hydroxyapatite matrix for obliterating open mastoid cavities. Otol Neurotol. 2008;29:807-11.
66. Lee H-B, Lim HJ, Cho M, et al. Clinical significance of β-tricalcium phosphate and polyphosphate for mastoid cavity obliteration during middle ear surgery: human and animal study. Clin Exp Otorhinolaryngol. 2013;6:127-34.
67. Yung M, Bennett A. Use of mastoid obliteration techniques in cholesteatoma. Curr Opin Otolaryngol Head Neck Surg. 2013;21:455-60.
68. Cho SW, Cho Y-B, Cho H-H. Mastoid obliteration with silicone blocks after canal wall down mastoidectomy. Clin Exp Otolaryngol. 2012;5:23-7.
69. Jang C-H, Cho YB, Bae CS. Evaluation of bioactive glass for mastoid obliteration: a guinea pig model. in vivo 2007;21:651-6.
70. Stoor P, Pulkkinen J, Grénman R. Bioactive glass S53P4 in the filling of cavities in the mastoid cell area in surgery for chronic otitis media. Ann Otol Rhinol Laryngol. 2010;119:377-82.

71. Sarin JS, Grénman R, Aitasalo K, et al. Bioactive glass S53P4 in mastoid obliteration surgery for chronic otitis media and cerebrospinal fluid leakage. Ann Otol Rhinol Laryngol. 2012;121:563-9.

72. Shokry S, Hossieni Al`Sayed, Zidan MF, et al. Avoiding mastoid cavity problems: mastoid obliteration using Bioactive glass. The Egyptian Journal of Hospital Medicine. 2012;47:321-33.

73. Silvola JT. Mastoidectomy cavity obliteration with bioactive glass: a pilot study. Otolaryngol Head Neck Surg. 2012;20:1-8.

74. Walker PC, Mowry SE, Hansen MR, et al. Long-term results of canal wall reconstruction tympanomastoidectomy. Otol Neurotol. 2014;35:e24-e30.

75. Yung MW. The use of hydroxyapatite granules in mastoid obliteration. Clin Otolaryngol. 1996;21:480-4.

76. Jones JR. Review of bioactive glass: from Hench to hybrids. Acta Biomater. 2013;9:4457-86.

77. Hench LL, Paschall HA. Direct chemical bonding of bioactive glass-ceramic materials and bone. J Biomed Mater Res Symp. 1973;4:25-42.

78. Hench LL, Polak JM. Third-generation biomedical materials. Science. 2002;295:1014-7.

79. Hench LL. Bioceramics—from concept to clinic. J Am Ceram Soc. 1991;74:1487-510.

80. Arcos D, Greenspan DC, Vallet-Regi M. A new quantitative method to evaluate the in vitro bioactivity of melt and sol–gel-derived silicate glasses. J Biomed Mater Res Part A. 2003;65A:344-51.

81. Brink M, Söderling E, Turunen T, et al. Protein adsorption properties of bioactive glasses compared to their behaviour in rabbit tibia. Bioceramics. 1995;8:471-6.

82. Kaufmann E, Ducheyne P, Shapiro IM. Evaluation of osteoblast response to porous bioactive glass (45S5) substrates by RT-PCR analysis. Tissue Eng. 2000;6:19-28.

83. Gough JE, Jones JR, Hench LL. Nodule formation and mineralisation of human primary osteoblasts cultured on a porous bioactive glass scaffold. Biomaterials. 2004;25:2039-46.

84. Bosetti M, Cannas M. The effect of bioactive glasses on bone marrow stromal cells differentiation. Biomaterials. 2005;26:3873-9.

85. Virolainen P, Heikkilä J, Yli-Urpo A, et al. Histomorphometric and molecular biologic comparison of bioactive glass granules and autogenous bone grafts in augmentation of bone defect healing. J Biomed Mater Res. 1997;35A:9-17.

86. Loty C, Sautier JM, Tan MT, et al. Bioactive glass stimulates in vitro osteoblast differentiation and creates a favorable template for bone tissue formation. J Bone Miner Res. 2001;16:231-9.

87. Dieudonné SC, van den Dolder J, de Ruijter JE, et al. Osteoblast differentiation of bone marrow stromal cells cultured on silica gel and sol-gel-derived titania. Biomaterials. 2002;23:3041-51.

88. Lindfors NC, Aho AJ. Granule size and composition of bioactive glasses affect osteoconduction in rabbit. J Mater Sci Mater Med. 2003;14:265-372.

89. Wilson T, Parikka V, Holmbom J, et al. Intact surface of bioactive glass S53P4 is resistant to osteoclastic activity. J Biomed Mater Res. 2005;77A:67-74.

90. Välimäki VV, Aro HT. Molecular basis for action of bioactive glasses as bone graft substitute. Scand J Surg. 2006;95:95-102.

91. Meretoja VV, Malin M, Seppälä JV, et al. Osteoblast response to continuous phase macroporous scaffolds under static and dynamic culture conditions. J Biomed Mater Res. 2008;89A:317-25.

92. Gorustovich AA, Perio C, Boccaccini AR. Effect of bioactive glasses on angiogenesis: a review of *in vitro* and *in vivo* evidences. Tissue Eng. Part B Rev. 2010;16:199-207.

93. Zhang D, Munukka E, Hupa L, et al. Factors controlling antibacterial properties of bioactive glasses. Key Engineering Materials. 2007;330-2:173-6.

94. Zhang D, Hupa M, Hupa L. In situ pH within particle beds of bioactive glasses. Acta Biomater. 2008;4:1498-505.

95. Zhang D, Leppäranta O, Munukka E, et al. Antibacterial effects and dissolution behavior of six bioactive glasses. J Biomed Mater Res. 2010;93A:475-83.

96. Stoor P, Kirstilä V, Söderling E, et al. Interactions between bioactive glass and periodontal pathogens. Microb Ecol Health Dis. 1996;9:109-14.

97. Stoor P, Söderling E, Salonen JI. Antibacterial effects of a bioactive glass paste on oral micro-organisms. Acta Odontol Scand. 1998;56:161-5.

98. Stoor P, Söderling E, Grenman R. Interactions between the bioactive glass S53P4 and the atrophic rhinitis–associated microorganism Klebsiella ozaenae. J Biomed Mater Res. 1999;48:869-74.

99. Stoor P, Söderling E, Grénman R. Bioactive glass S53P4 in repair of septal perforations and its interactions with the respiratory infection-associated microorganisms Haemophilus influenzae and Streptococcus pneumoniae. J Biomed Mater Res. 2001;58:113-20.

100. Munukka E, Leppäranta O, Korkeamäki M, et al. Bactericidal effects of bioactive glasses on clinically important aerobic bacteria. J Mater Sci Mater Med. 2008; 19:27-32.

101. Zhang D, Munukka E, et al. Comparison of antibacterial effect on three bioactive glasses. Key Engineering Materials. 2006;309-11:345-8.

102. Leppäranta O, Vaahtio M, Peltola T, et al. Antibacterial effect of bioactive glasses on clinically important anaerobic bacteria in vitro. J Mater Sci Mater Med. 2008;19:547-51.

103. Kania R, Ars B (Eds). Biofilms in Otitis Media. Amsterdam: Kugler Publications; 2015.

104. Lampikoski H, Aarnisalo AA, Jero J, et al. Mastoid biofilm in chronic otitis media. Otol Neurotol. 2012;33:785-8.

105. Drago L, Vassena C, Fenu S, et al. In vitro antibiofilm activity of bioactive glass S53P4. Future Microbiol. 2014;9:593-601.

106. Lai W, Garino J, Ducheyne P. Silicon excretion from bioactive glass implanted in rabbit bone. Biomaterials. 2002;23:213-17.

107. Lai W, Garino J, Flaitz C, et al. Excretion of resorption products from bioactive glass implanted in rabbit muscle. J Biomed Mater Res Part A. 2005;75A:398-407.

108. Lindfors NC, Heikkilä JT, Aho AJ. Long-term evaluation of blood silicon and ostecalcin in operatively treated patients with benign bone tumors using bioactive glass and autogenous bone. J Biomed Mater Res. 2008;87:73-6.

109. Heikkilä J, Mattila KT, Andersson ÖH, et al. Behavior of bioactive glass in human bone. Bioceramics. 1995;8:35-40

110. Lindfors NC, Tallroth K, Aho AJ. Bioactive glass as bone-graft substitute for posterior spinal fusion in rabbit. J Biomed Mater Res. 2002;63:237-44.

111. Lindfors NC, Aho AJ. Tissue response to bioactive glass and autogenous bone in the rabbit spine. Eur Spine J. 2000;9:30-5.
112. Peltola MJ, Aitasalo KM, Suonpää JT, et al. In vivo model for frontal sinus and calvarial bone defect obliteration with bioactive glass S53P4 and hydroxyapatite. J Biomed Mater Res. 2001;58:261-9.
113. Turunen T, Peltola J, Helenius H, et al. Bioactive glass and calcium carbonate granules as filler material around titanium and bioactive glass implants in the medullar space of the rabbit tibia. Clin Oral Impl Res. 1997;8:96-102.
114. Heikkilä JT, Salonen H, Yli-Urpo A, et al. Long term behaviour of bioactive glass cone and granules in rabbit bone. Bioceramics. 1996;9:123-6.
115. Aitasalo K, Peltola M, Suonpää J, et al. Obliteration of frontal sinuses with bioactive glass after chronic suppurative sinusitis. One year follow up. Bioceramics. 1994;7:409-14.
116. Suominen E, Kinnunen J. Bioactive glass granules and plates in the reconstruction of defects of the facial bones. Scand J Plast Reconstr Surg Hand Surg. 1996;30:281-9.
117. Aitasalo K, Suonpää J, Peltola M, et al. Behaviour of bioactive glass (S53P4) in human frontal sinus obliteration. Bioceramics. 1997;10:429-32.
118. Peltola M, Suonpää J, Aitasalo K, et al. Obliteration of the frontal sinus cavity with bioactive glass. Head Neck. 1998;20:315-9.
119. Aitasalo K, Peltola M, Suonpää J, et al. Bioactive glass S53P4 in frontal sinus obliteration. A 9-year experience. Key Engineering Materials. 2001;192-195: 877-880.
120. Turunen T, Peltola J, Yli-Urpo A, et al. Bioactive glass granules as a bone adjunctive material in maxillary sinus floor augmentation. Clin Oral Impl Res. 2004; 15:135-41.
121. Peltola M, Aitasalo K, Suonpää J, et al. Bioactive glass S53P4 in frontal sinus obliteration: A long-term clinical experience. Head Neck. 2006;28:834-41.
122. Aitasalo K, Peltola M. Bioactive glass hydroxyapatite in fronto-orbital defect reconstruction. Plast Reconstr Surg. 2007;120:1963-72.
123. Heikkilä JT, Aho HJ, Yli-Urpo A, et al. Bone formation in rabbit cancellous bone defects filled with bioactive glass granules. Acta Orthop. 1995;66:463-7.
124. Lindfors NC, Heikkilä JT, Koski I, et al. Bioactive glass and autogenous bone as bone graft substitutes in benign bone tumors. J Biomed Mater Res. 2009; 90:131-6.
125. Lindfors NC, Koski I, Heikkilä JT, et al. A prospective randomized 14-year follow-up study of bioactive glass and autogenous bone as bone graft substitutes in benign bone tumors. J Biomed Mater Res. 2010;94B:157-64.
126. Lindfors NC. Treatment of a recurrent aneurysmal bone cyst with bioactive glass in a child allows for good bone remodelling and growth. Bone. 2009;45: 398-400.
127. Lindfors NC, Hyvönen P, Nyyssönen M, et al. Bioactive glass S53P4 as bone graft substitute in treatment of osteomyelitis. Bone. 2010;47:212-8.
128. Singh H, Wang MY. Bioglass for the treatment of osteomyelitis. Neurosurgery. 2010;67:20-1.
129. Drago L, Romanò D, De Vecchi E, et al. Bioactive glass BAG-S53P4 for the adjunctive treatment of chronic osteomyelitis of the long bones: an in vitro and prospective clinical study. BMC Infect Dis. 2013;13:584.

130. Romanò CL, Logoluso N, Meani E, et al. A comparative study of the use of bioactive glass S53P4 and antibiotic-loaded calcium-based bone substitutes in the treatment of chronic osteomyelitis. Bone Joint J. 2014;96:845-50.
131. Heikkilä JT, Kukkonen J, Aho AJ, et al. Bioactive glass granules: a suitable bone substitute material in the operative treatment of depressed lateral tibial plateau fractures: a prospective, randomized 1 year follow-up study. J Mater Sci Mater Med. 2011;22:1073-80.
132. Pernaa K, Koski I, Mattila K, et al. Bioactive glass S53P4 and autograft bone in treatment of depressed tibial plateau fractures. A prospective randomized 11-year follow-up. J Long-term Eff Med Impl. 2011;21:139-48.
133. Frantzén J, Rantakokko J, Aro H, et al. Instrumented spondylodesis in degenerative spondylolisthesis with bioactive glass and autologous bone. A prospective 11-year follow-up. J Spinal Disorder Tech. 2011;24:455-61.
134. Rantakokko J, Frantzén J, Heinänen J, et al. Posterolateral spondylodesis using bioactive glass S53P4 and autogenous bone in instrumented unstable lumbar spine burst fractures—a prospective 10-year follow-up study. Scand J Surg. 2012;101:66-71.
135. Lindfors N. Clinical experience on bioactive glass S53P4 in reconstructive surgery in the upper extremity showing bone remodelling, vascularization, cartilage repair and antibacterial properties of S53P4. J Biotechnol Biomaterial. 2011;1 (electronic version).
136. Bernardeschi D, Nguyen Y, Russo FY, et al. Cutaneous and labyrinthine tolerance of bioactive glass S53P4 in mastoid and epitympanic obliteration surgery: prospective clinical study. BioMed Research International Volume 2015 (2015), Article ID 242319, 6 pages.
137. Schimanski G, Schimanski E. Obliteration of mastoid cavities. 30 years of experience with recommendations for surgical strategy. HNO 2015;63:538-45 (German).
138. Dey A, Bomans PHH, Mueller FA, et al. The role of prenucleation clusters in surface-induced calcium phosphate crystallization. Nat Mater. 2010;9:1010-4.
139. Laxminarayan R, Duse A, Wattal C, et al. Antibiotic resistance—the need for global solutions. Lancet Infect Dis. 2013;13:1057-98.
140. Centers for Disease Control and Prevention (CDC). Vital signs: carbapenem-resistant Enterobacteriaceae. MMWR Morb Mortal Wkly Rep. 2013;62:165-70.

Chapter 16

Nonsurgical Remodeling Techniques of the Face

Nikul Amin, Alwyn D'Souza

INTRODUCTION

Remodeling techniques of the face involve both surgical and nonsurgical/minimally invasive options. Public demands for nonsurgical options are forever on the increase because of minimal or no downtime, cost implications, and its safety in conjunction with excellent outcome. In this chapter, we focus on the nonsurgical/minimally invasive options currently in use in the remodeling of the face. These include the use of botulinum toxins for neuromodulation, commonly used filler techniques and fat transfer. In this chapter, we discuss the global assessment of the patient's facial aging, clinical documentation as well as scientific basis for using various treatment options, based on current literature and personal experience.

AGING

Aging is commonly assessed and defined in society by observing changes in facial aesthetics. Our face is the part of the body most on show, and therefore facial aesthetics and its modulation is a huge industry that is constantly growing.

The original thinking that facial aging was related to loss of facial elasticity and gravity induced facial descent has been proven to be an oversimplistic concept.

A youthful facial appearance has several key factors. Understanding the process of aging helps us understand what makes us look youthful. When considering the aging process and therefore also approaches to remodeling of the face, it is vital to understand that the face is made up for four key structures: *skin, fat, muscle,* and *bone.* Facial aging is a multifactorial process composing of all of these components and anatomic zones; therefore, correction of one without the other will often lead to suboptimal outcomes (Figs. 16.1A and B).

The common concerns related to aging as reported by patients are as follows:

- Forehead lines
- Crow's feet
- Glabellar lines
- Eyebrow ptosis
- Loss of cheek volume/full midface
- Nasolabial folds
- Marionette lines
- Perioral wrinkling
- Thinning of lips
- Sagging necklines
- Loss of chin and jawline definition

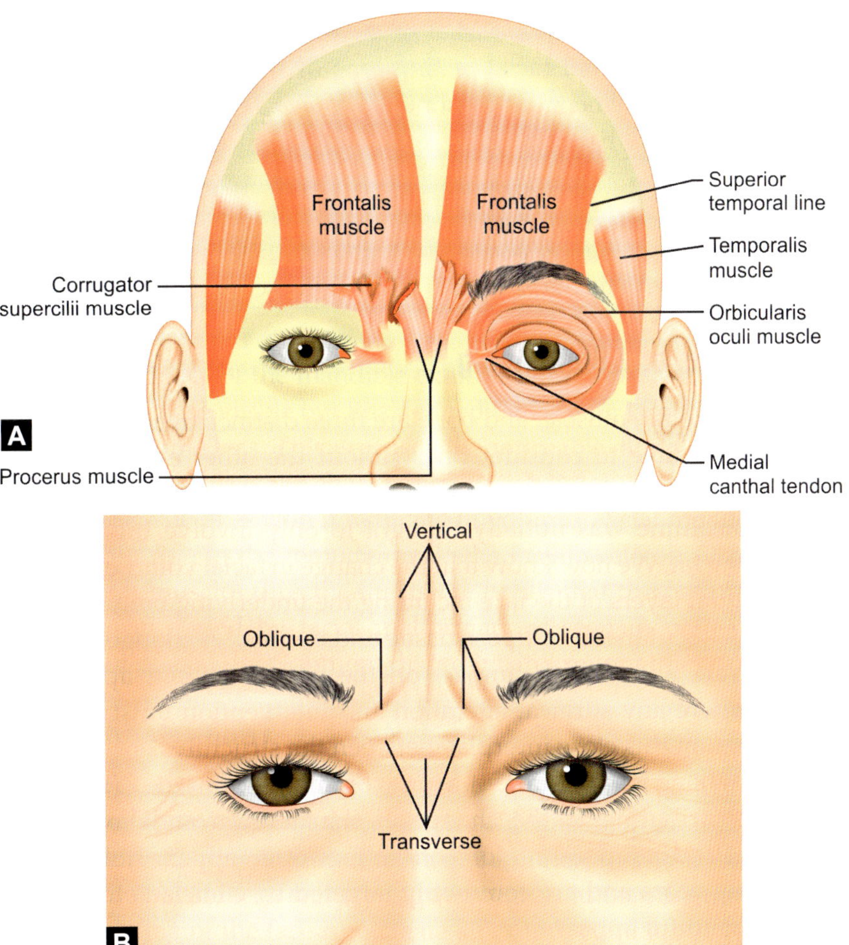

Figs. 16.1A and B: Forehead aging.

The Skin Aging and Its Effects

The skin's surface should be smooth and without blemishes. There should be very little laxity in the skin giving an equal, symmetrical light reflex.

masculine and feminine features is important. It is important to explain the aging process to patients to aid their understandings and define their expectations.

History

One of the most important parts of any consultation is the interaction between the patient and the surgeon. Patients' desired outcomes greatly vary from one another and a close understanding between surgeon and patient is vital in managing patients' ideas, concerns and expectations. An open approach with open questions is vital to allow the patient to express the exact sites of their concern without coercing personal views. An open free conversation will encourage the patient to present their ideas, and as the clinical expert it is our role to offer opinions and options available to that patient based on the skills, resources, and experience of the clinician. Asking patients why they have sought your care at this point in their life will give an indication as to what element of their aging process is affecting them most.

Pre-existing medical conditions should be considered. This includes known skin conditions, immunosuppressive conditions, and autoimmune conditions, which can all affect outcomes and healing, therefore guiding the clinician on the most appropriate technique for nonsurgical remodeling. History of trauma should be explored.

Social history including smoking history, alcohol consumption, occupation, and family support is useful in determining a tailored treatment plan.

Examination

A stepwise approach to the examination is necessary but one should naturally focus on the area of most concern to the patient. Absolute symmetry is often desired by patients, but generally is not achievable and this should be explained to the patient emphasizing asymmetric nature of normal face. Understanding the process and pattern of volume loss is important in allowing the clinician to target appropriate areas. It should be stressed that generalized volume replacement would lead to swollen appearance that will not provide an aesthetically pleasing outcome. Conversely, it may not be possible to correct one specific facial subunit without remodeling an adjacent subunit. Explaining the process of aging to the patient will aid their understanding, co-cooperativeness, and treatment compliance.

A useful tool when undertaking facial analysis is the use of old photographs from the patient's youth. These can often be used to

Table 16.1: The five-point wrinkle assessment scale.

Score	Findings
0	No wrinkles
1	Fine wrinkles
2	Moderate wrinkles
3	Deep wrinkles
4	Extremely deep wrinkles

identify areas of aging to be addressed. A three-way mirror and photography are crucial. When undertaking facial analysis, it is important to assess for both surgical and nonsurgical remodeling options. In certain patients, their desired outcome may require a surgical intervention either as sole treatment or in combination with other nonsurgical options. The skin should be closely analyzed and findings documented. There are very few widely accepted validated tools for assessing and grading facial aging. The five-point wrinkle assessment scale (WAS) can use high-resolution digital photographs or dermoscopy in the clinic to make clinical assessment.[12] The five-point WAS ranges from 0 to 4 and its use allows for quantifiable assessment pre- and postprocedural (Table 16.1).[13]

Specific validated assessment scales are available for each specific facial region if required that follow a similar five-point rating scale.[14-16] Scoring scales based on clinical signs of photoaging have also been developed and the appropriate scale should be used depending on the aspect of remodeling being addressed.[17]

Discussion

Upon undertaking the history and examination an informed discussion should be had with the patient to formulate a treatment plan to create the youthful appearance desired by the patient while avoiding the unnatural plastic appearance dreaded by patients. Patients may present with very minor cosmetic flaws and it is the duty of the clinician to highlight and demonstrate achievable outcomes and the areas of the face in which remodeling may occur. Where appropriate the clinician should also highlight areas, which may be remodeled and augmented that may not have been identified by the patient but can help to achieve the desired outcome for the patient. This can be demonstrated by using case examples from patients who have previously consented to their case being used for such purposes. There is also an array of available easy-to-use computer software that can be used to demonstrate facial augmentation using standard and 3D images. These also form an important part of patient's clinical notes.

Table 16.2: FDA-approved fillers and Botulinum toxins.

Hyaluronic acid	• Restylane lyft
	• Restylane silk
	• Restylane gel
	• Restylane-L gel
	• Prevelle silk
	• Belotero balance
	• Juvéderm
	• Juvéderm voluma XC
	• Elevess
	• Captique gel
	• Hylaform
	• Perlane
Calcium hydroxylapatite	• Radiesse
Poly-L-lactic acid	• Sculpta
Collagen based	• Evolence
	• Cosmoderm 1
	• Fibrel
	• Zyplast
	• Zyderm
	• ArteFill
Botulinum toxins	
Botulinum toxin type A	• Botox
	• Dysport
	• Xeomin
Botulinum toxin type B	• Myobloc

The postoperative length of recovery and appropriate postoperative care should be explained preoperatively to avoid any unexpected surprises for the patient. Occasionally, counseling may be necessary to assess their desired outcomes and to ensure realistic expectations. Formal psychological assessment may be utilized in cases as deemed appropriate. Patients should also be informed about the cost implications of planned treatment as well as future costs.

Based on these discussions, nonsurgical remodeling techniques commonly offered include neuromodulation with botulinum toxins and volume replacement using various modalities. It is worth noting that there are a large number of commercial preparations available, and we have listed some of them here (Table 16.2).

BOTULINUM TOXIN

The role of botulinum toxin in the face has been extensively described and utilized over many years. Since the 1990s its use has steadily increased and is utilized not only by facial plastic/plastic surgeons but general practitioners, dentists as well as aesthetic practitioners and beauty therapists.

Botulinum toxin is a neurotoxin produced by *Clostridium botulinum,* a gram-positive anaerobic bacterium. There are currently seven known distinct serotypes (type A–type G). Only type A and type B are used in clinical practice and the most commonly used by far is botulinum toxin type A. It is marketed variably as OnabotulinumtoxinA (Botox), AbobotulinumtoxinA (Dysport), or IncobotulinumtoxinA (Xeomin). Botulinum toxin inhibits the release of acetylcholine at motor end plates of presynaptic neuromuscular junctions resulting in a flaccid paralysis. The chemical denervation lasts approximately 3 months when regeneration of the motor axons occurs (Figs. 16.3A to D).[18]

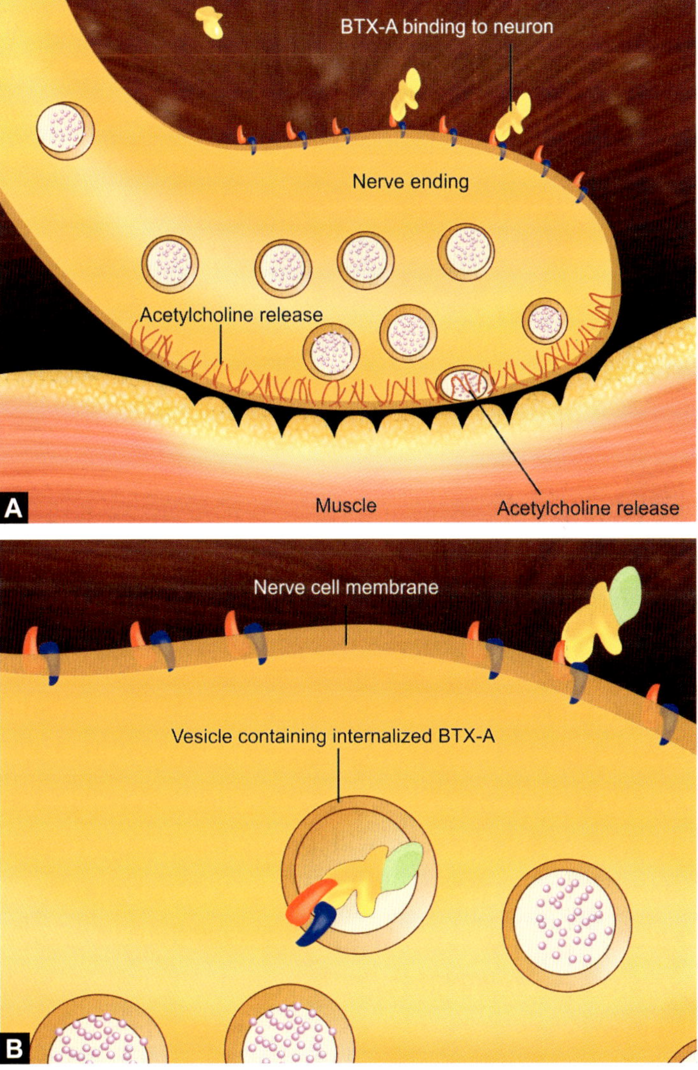

Figs. 16.3A and B: Diagram: Mechanism of action of botulinum toxin. (A) Toxin binds to nerve ending. (B) Toxin internalized.

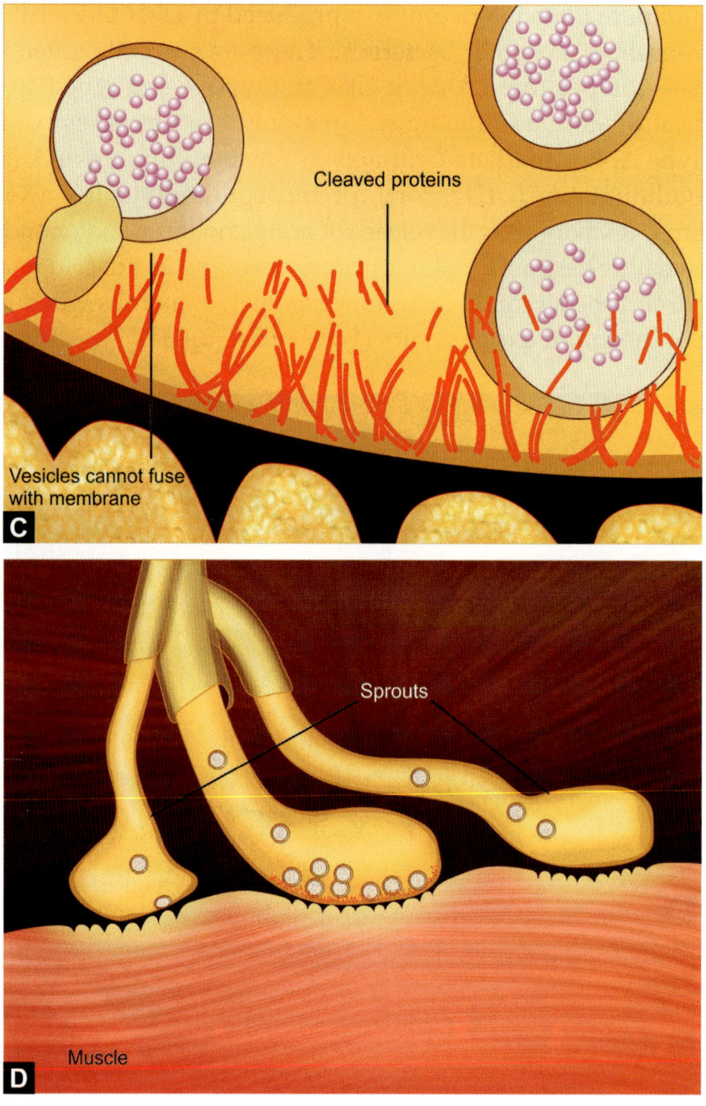

Figs. 16.3C and D: Diagram: Mechanism of action of botulinum toxin. (C) Light chain freed–blocks ACh release. (D) Sprouts eventually form.

Botulinum toxin injections will provide better outcomes when applied to facial zones affected by dynamic wrinkles as opposed to static wrinkles and this should be explained to the patient preprocedurally. The degree of paralysis required depends on the site of injection and the desired effect. Wrinkling in the glabellar region is associated with negative emotions such as anger and sadness, therefore is often completely paralyzed.[19] Conversely, areas associated with positive emotions, such as lateral canthal and forehead/brow, should not be completely paralyzed to avoid an emotionless, unnatural face, which can have significant social and emotional impact. Botulinum toxin also has an important role in aesthetic and functional correction of facial asymmetry.[20-22] Botulinum toxin injections can be used in synergy with injectable fillers. As well as improving the aesthetic outcome and results, the duration of the effects of fillers may thus be significantly increased.[23]

Technique

Facial upper third is the commonly targeted zone for botulinum toxin treatment. Treatment is often undertaken as a staged procedure where a further top up is offered at 2 weeks. Prior to injection the botulinum toxin of choice is reconstituted with sterile preservative free saline (Normal saline 0.9%), generally following manufacturer's guidelines. The dilution used will determine the volume injected. This is an important consideration when injecting into areas of the face as pain, bruising, and undesired side effects secondary to diffusion with larger volumes. Upon reconstitution the contents of the vial should be stored in a refrigerator (2°–8°), and ideally used within 24 hours. We recommend using a 1 mL luer lock syringe with a subdivided measurement scale and a 30 or 32 Gauge needle for injections.

The exact injection technique used will vary depending on the site of injection. The injection site can be marked out preinjection, if the clinician is inexperienced, to aid accurate deliverance of the toxin (Fig. 16.4). The injection site should be sterilized and the procedure carried out using an aseptic technique. The botulinum toxin should be slowly avoiding blood vessels. The depth of injection is dependent on the facial area. The forehead and glabella region often require deeper intramuscular injections, in comparison to the periorbital region where injections are generally subcutaneous. To get a uniform outcome, multiple injection sites are often required and a higher dose is often required in males due to increased muscle mass. The contraindications and side effects are described in Tables 16.3 and 16.4.

INJECTABLE FILLERS

Minimally invasive soft tissue remodeling with the use of synthetic and autologous fillers has been an increasingly popular treatment option in facial rejuvenation and remodeling in recent years. Injectable fillers can be used as sole treatment or in combination with other technique to achieve the desired volume replacement. Fillers may be classified as temporary and permanent. We recommend the use of temporary fillers,

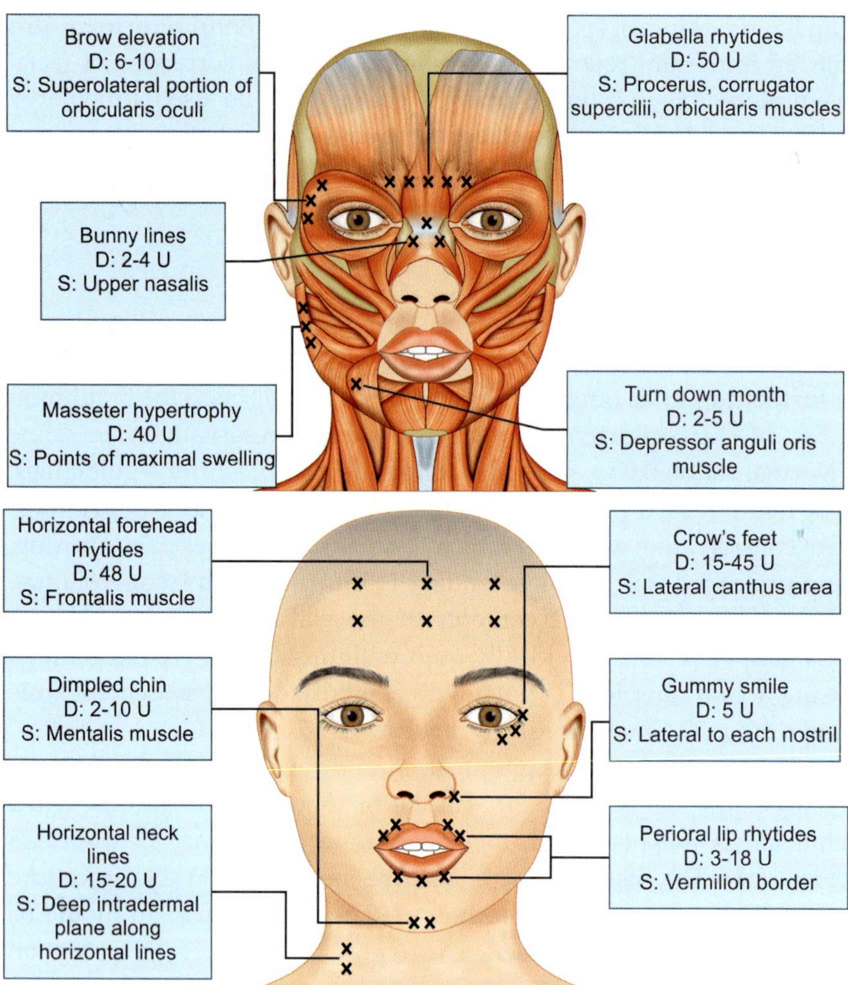

Fig. 16.4: Diagram shows the potential sites and doses, which may vary.

Table 16.3: Absolute and relative contraindications of botulinum toxin injection.	
Absolute contraindications	*Relative contraindications*
Allergy/hypersensitivity to botulinum toxin or components in formulation	Pre-existing cardiovascular disease, e.g. arrhythmia and myocardial infarction
Injection site infection	Pre-existing neuromuscular disorders
	Pre-existing compromised respiratory function or dysphagia
	Concurrent use of aminoglycosides, anticholinergics, muscle relaxants
	Pregnancy/Breastfeeding
	Pediatric patients (<18 years)

Table 16.4: The potential side effect of botulinum toxin injection.

Site	Side effect
Local	Pain, bruising, hematoma, infection, erythema, rash, swelling, muscle atrophy, muscle twitching, nonresponse, alopecia, madarosis
Nonspecific	Headache, nausea, vomiting, fatigue, flu-like symptoms
Glabellar region	Upper lid ptosis
Forehead	Brow ptosis
Brow	Cock-eyed appearance
Periocular	Diplopia, strabismus, ectropion, keratitis, corneal ulceration, brow asymmetry, blepharoptosis
Lacrimal	Decreased tear production, xerophthalmia
Perioral	Smile asymmetry, oral incompetence

Table 16.5: Properties of the ideal filler.

Biocompatible

Nonantigenic

Nontoxic

Easy to use

Long-lasting

Inexpensive

Reversible

Demonstrate a high safety profile

Predictable result with minimal downtime

as discussed below. The use of fillers has grown from being initially used to treat wrinkles and minor loss of volume to greater augmentation and remodeling of the face.

There has been a long history in the use of fillers in the face with many different substances being injected including paraffin, mineral oils and later on silicone.[24] The first injectable filler widely available was based on bovine collagen in the late 1970s, which had the drawbacks of short acting effect, allergy, and hypersensitivity reactions resulting in patients requiring skin testing.[25] Increased public hesitancy toward bovine-based products during the period of fear related to bovine spongiform encephalopathy led to their decline further. This decline promoted further research into the development of newer fillers. Table 16.5 summarized the properties of the ideal filler.[26,27] Though autologous fat was the earliest injectable filler first documented in Germany over a century ago, its initial popularity waned.[28] Multiple inorganic substances including silicone gel and polyethylene have been previously trialed, but issues concerning extrusion, granulomatous inflammation, and nodular palpability were documented.[29] This has led to the popularity of hyaluronic acid (HA)-based fillers, which fulfills many properties of the ideal filler.

Hyaluronic Acid

Hyaluronic acid fillers are currently the most widely used.[30] Initially isolated from the vitreous of cows' eyes, HA was subsequently identified in human tissues. Hyaluronic acid is a glycosaminoglycan composed of repeating disaccharide units of D-glucuronic acids and N-acetlyglucosamine.[28] It is a key component of connective tissue, cartilage, and fascia among other tissues.[31,32]

It has a structural role in the skin and helps to provide volume. During aging, there is loss of natural HA in the skin contributes to skin dehydration. Due to its anionic state it has an impressive ability to bind to water with studies showing that just 1 g of HA can bind to 6 liters of water.[33] It is this special ability of HA that allows it to create the required volumizing effect while helping maintain skin moisture and the appearance of rejuvenated skin.

Traditional HA fillers were derived from animals or nonanimal natural sources such as bacteria. There were reported cases of hypersensitivity and therefore modern HA based fillers are synthetic produced in laboratory. To prevent rapid degradation of the HA in vivo, it must undergo cross-linking to allow it to have a longer acting cosmetic outcome. Modulating the mechanical properties of HA by using hydrophobic ether-based cross-linking agents allows for enhancement and stabilization of its properties.[34] After cross-linking, the HA is modified into either a varying sized particle or nonparticle form depending on individual manufactures. Understanding the different rheological properties of these HA preparations allows the clinician to select the ideal HA filler based on the site of injection and desired outcome.

One great advantage of using HA-based fillers is that overfilling or unwanted aesthetic outcomes can be reversed with the use of hyaluronidase,[35] which is also used to reverse potentially serious complications of fillers such as injection site necrosis.[36]

The technique for injection of HA fillers and other fillers follow the same basic principles. An aseptic technique should be used throughout to minimize risk of infection. Prior to the filler injection local/regional anesthetic can be given separately or as part of premixed filler.

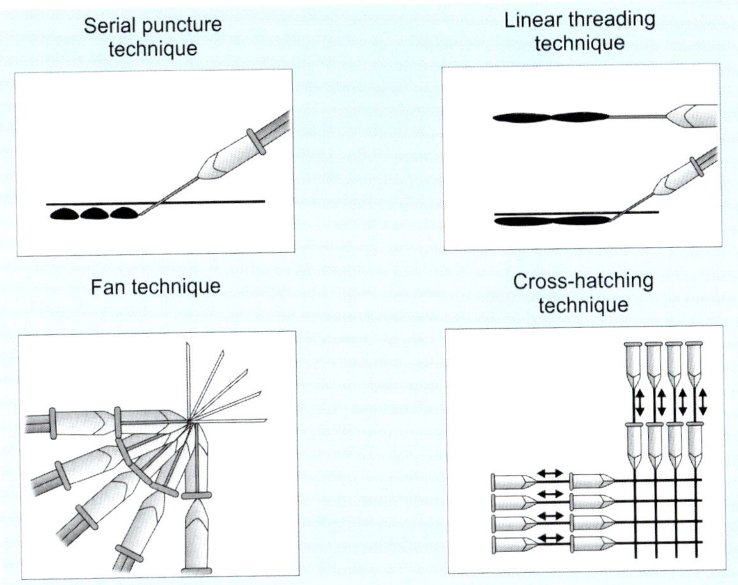

Fig. 16.5: Injection techniques.

There are several injection techniques (Fig. 16.5):

- Serial puncture technique
- Linear threading technique
- Fanning technique
- Cross-hatching technique.

Care is taken to administer the injectable filler slowly, being cognizant of surrounding neurovascular structures. For optimal cosmetic outcome, avoid large bolus injection to one site. Use of a cannula or handheld injector pump tends to provide further comfort during the procedure with improved cosmetic outcome (Figs. 16.6 and 16.7).

Calcium Hydroxylapatite

Synthetic calcium hydroxylapatite (CaHA) such as Radiesse are semi-solid fillers that are often blended with an aqueous carrier gel, which suspends the particle spheres allowing for it to be delivered as an injectable filler.[29,37] Although they are nonpermanent, their effects are often longer lasting and can be used both for subdermal and deep dermal filling. Calcium hydroxylapatite also has good biocompatibility and low immunogenicity due to its natural presence as a mineral component in human bones and teeth. There is an initial and immediate filling effect with synthetic CaHA-based fillers, which is in a large part associated with the gel carrier, which can be up to 70% of the constituent. The gel carrier is subsequently degraded and the CaHA

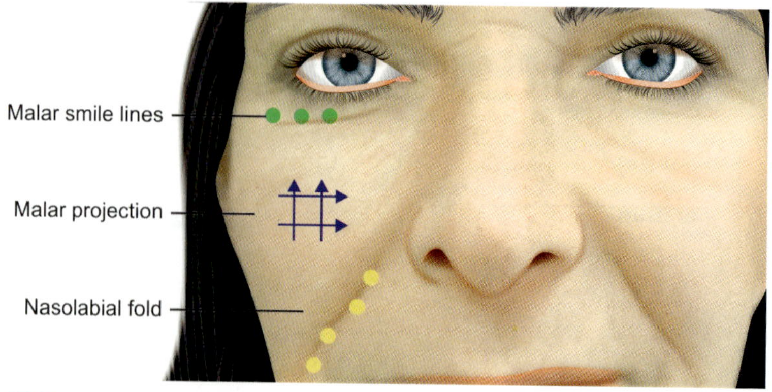

Fig. 16.6: Commonly treated areas of the mid-third of the face. Injection sites and patterning for hyaluronic acid fillers are shown.

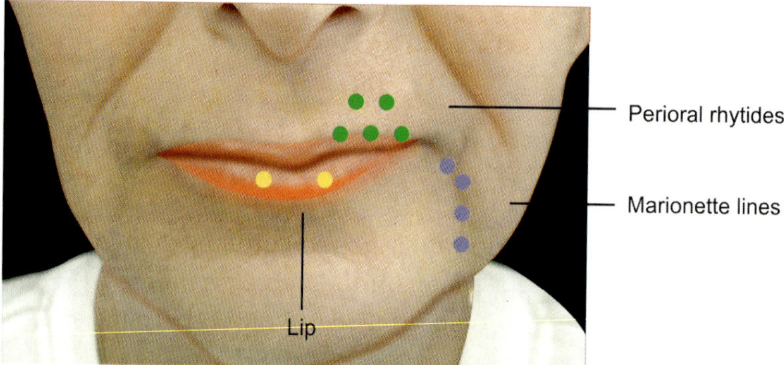

Fig. 16.7: Commonly treated areas of the lower third of the face. Injection sites and patterning for hyaluronic acid fillers are shown.

works by stimulation of new collagen production around the CaHA particles through fibroblast activation occurring up to 6 months postinjection.[38] The CaHA particles appear to remain in the skin for up to 12 months until reabsorption.[29] Calcium hydroxylapatite fillers can be used in rhytides and lipoatrophy associated with human immuno-deficiency virus (HIV).[39]

Poly-L-lactic Acid

Synthetic poly-L-lactic acid (PPLA) is used in a variety of medical implants and suture materials. It is also used as soft tissue filler (e.g. Sculptra). The PPLA particles are mixed with sodium carboxymethlycellulose mannitol and sterile water. As with CaHA, PPLA works as a direct filler initially but stimulates fibroblasts to promote collagen production and vascularization through biostimulation.[40,41] Patients should be coun-seled that the main effect is through a delayed action and it is therefore unsuitable for patients requiring immediate results. This delayed action of PPLA results in it being used with other faster acting fillers such as HA or CaHA. Three-four treatments are generally required at 3-month intervals. Studies have shown that the benefit may last up to 3 years, although the actual particles start to breakdown at 6 months.[42,43] Poly-L-lactic acid fillers are currently commonly used in HIV-associated lipoatrophy as it is licensed for such use.[44,45]

COMPLICATIONS

Although fillers have gained great popularity due to their low immuno-genicity and good bioavailability, there are still several documented cases of adverse events. Tyndall effect, delayed hypersensitivity/allergic reaction, granulomatous reaction and nodule formation have all been described.[46-48] Rare complications such as vascular occlusion causing blindness have been noted.[49] The complications are listed in Table 16.6.

PLATELET-RICH PLASMA (PRP)

Platelet-rich plasma (PRP) portrayed in media and often known to patients as "Dracula therapy or Vampire facelift" has gained recent popularity. It can be classified as "autologous blood with a concentration of platelets above baseline values". This concentration is often up to eight times more than within whole blood. This is delivered in a relatively small volume of plasma.[50]

The principle is based on platelets being a source of growth factors and immune modulators with a role in angiogenesis and tissue healing, in addition to coagulation.[51] The a granules of platelets contain many protein growth factors including platelet-derived growth factor, transforming growth factor, vascular endothelial growth factor (VEGF), and epidermal growth factor. Studies suggest that platelets release these growth factors, helping to recruit cells to aid soft tissue repair and rehabilitation facilitating healing.[50, 52]

Platelet-rich plasma therapy involves harvesting patient's own whole blood for centrifuging, primarily to separate the red blood cells. After this a second centrifugation acts to create a high concentration of platelets (PRP), to be separated from the platelet-poor plasma.[53] Upon delivery of this PRP, the relatively high concentration of growth factors will act locally on the soft tissues.

There are different platelet preparations including platelet-rich fibrin matrix (PRFM) and leukocyte-rich PRP (L-PRP), but we shall focus of PRP. The potential beneficial properties of PRP within facial plastic surgery include not only primary soft tissue augmentation, but

Table 16.6: Complications of fillers.

Complication	Prevention	Treatment options
Bleeding/Bruising	• Atraumatic injection • Avoiding aspirin and anticoagulants where possible	• Cooling • Self-limiting
Pain	• Atraumatic injection	• Analgesia
Pruritus	• Atraumatic injection	• Cooling • Antihistamines
Infection	• Aseptic technique • Cleaning skin preinjection	• Antibiotics
Hypersensitivity and anaphylaxis	• Skin tests	• Steroids • Antihistamines
Granulomatous reaction	• Avoid facial trauma • Ensure adequate depth of injection	• Intralesional steroid, antibiotics • Immunomodulators • Surgical excision
Nodule formation	• Ensure adequate depth of injection • Good technique of injection	• Intralesional steroid • Antibiotics • Immunomodulators • Hyaluronidase if appropriate • Surgical excision
Herpes infection	• Ask patients about history of oral herpes infections	• Antivirals
Tyndall effect (blue-gray discoloration)	• Ensure adequate depth of injection	• Laser treatment
Asymmetry	• Careful planning	• Touch-up secondary procedure
Misplacement	• Careful planning	• Hyaluronidase if appropriate
Vascular occlusion	• Good anatomical knowledge • Inject superficially • Prompt recognition	• Warm compression and massage. • Nitroglycerin paste • Oral aspirin • Heparin treatment • Hyaluronidase if appropriate

also improved wound healing and enhanced recovery postoperatively. In addition to facial plastic surgery, there has been an increase in use of PRP in orthopedics, sports medicine, and ophthalmology.[50,54] There have been several *in vitro* showing that PRP activates mesenchymal stem cell proliferation resulting in proliferation of human adipose-derived stem cells and human dermal fibroblasts through the release of large concentration of growth factors.[55-57] Studies suggest that these dermal fibroblasts undergo up regulation of matrix metalloproteinase -1 and type I collagen with differentiation into myofibroblasts helping to promote collagen remodeling and tissue contraction.[58,59] Platelet-rich plasma has also been used as an adjuvant treatment with fat grafting to improve graft survival as well as to minimize bruising and inflammation leading to decreased postoperative recovery time.[60-62] Other uses include surgical remodeling procedures such as facelift operations to reduce postoperative edema.[63] It also has been shown to aid epithelialization of split thickness skin grafts.[64] The role of PRP and PRFM as primary therapy for nonsurgical remodeling of the face is less well described but it has shown promising results in the management of rhytides when directly injected into the site of action.[65-67]

Platelet-rich plasma has also been shown to have a role in skin color homogeneity and could have a role in management of infraorbital dark circles.[68] Further research is essential to qualify these indications further.

FAT TRANSFER

Autologous fat transfer involves the harvesting patient's own fat from one part of the body with re-implantation to another site. Autologous fat transfer has been practiced for over a century but early enthusiasm for this approach waned with unpredictable long-term outcomes and poor graft survival.[28,69] The development of liposuction revolutionized the technique as large quantities of injectable fat were more easily available to harvest.[70] With the development of new techniques, concerns of bulky adipose tissue with unpredictable outcomes became less of an issue. Advances in technology, instrumentation and techniques have allowed us to gain more predictable outcomes.[71] Further filling compartmentalized facial zones allows for more precise and controlled remodeling of the face.[72]

Several theories have been postulated as to how the grafted fat integrates into the injected site. The "cell survival theory" is currently the most widely accepted. It states that the adipose tissue re-implanted integrates into the surround tissue in the same was as a skin graft. Following an initial period of polymorphonuclear leukocytic and lymphocytic infiltration with plasma imbibition there is a period of angiogenesis and neovascularization occurring approximately 4 days after implantation. The release of cytokines including VGEF as well as stem cells from the adipose tissue aids this process.

Local histiocytes remove the fat from the dead cells to allow creation of mature adipocytes.[69,73,74] Though the survival of transferred fat is variable, the main advantage of autologous fat grafting is biocompatibility and the lasting aesthetic effects over 7 years.[75]

The amount of fat to be harvested is dependent on the amount of facial remodeling required. A useful rule of thumb is that approximately half the aspirate will be fat suitable for injection with the rest of the content consisting of lysed adipocytes, blood, and local anesthetic.[76] Coleman described the use of centrifuging to remove the nonviable elements of the aspirate such as lysed cells, blood, and local anesthetic.[69,77,78] Some studies however, have shown, there to be no benefit to centrifuging the fat in comparison to simple filtering and washing in fat graft survival.[79,80] Regardless of technique it is important to carefully remove the lidocaine from the adipose tissues aspirates as studies have shown it to have a detrimental effect on adipocyte viability.[81]

The advantage of autologous fat transfer in facial remodeling surgery includes the vast availability of material, minimal scarring, little donor site morbidity, and speed of procedure.[82] The drawbacks include occasional nodule formation, fat hypertrophy, and prolonged edema and recovery time.[83,84]

DEOXYCHOLIC ACID

Synthetic deoxycholic acid (DCA) can be injected into subcutaneous fat causing focal adipocytolysis.[85] Injection of DCA induces an initial adipocytolysis through cell membrane disruption and a local inflammatory reaction. There is evidence of long-term tissue fibrosis, which may aid a reduction in the skin laxity.[86-88]

Excessive pre-platysmal submental fat leads to a loss of the cervicomental angles and therefore the appearance of a ageing and overweight profile.[87] Previous treatment options have included liposuction and "face-lift" surgery. DCA injections have been widely applied to the submental fat region, providing a pharmacological treatment option.

Kybella is a an FDA approved DCA injection that is available for clinical use. Caution should be taken injecting DCA too lateral due to potential risk of marginal mandibular nerve palsy resulting is asymmetrical facial appearance. There have also been reported cases of dysphagia which self-resolved. Care is advised when injecting near salivary glands or lymph nodes.

An important consideration is that with any subsequent global gain in adipose tissue due to weight gain, fat will not recur in the site of previous treatment resulting in uneven distribution, which may result in cosmetic asymmetry.[89]

The procedure can be performed once a month but care should be taken to avoid over treatment. The results are dose-specific and initial double-blinded randomized controlled studies have shown positive outcomes with improved patent and clinician reported outcome measures.[90,91] The effects of these DCA injections have been reported up to 5 years post treatment.[89]

CONCLUSION

Nonsurgical techniques provide an excellent platform for facial rejuvenation, with results vastly dependent on the executing clinician. The safety, minimal or no downtime and reasonable costs of the procedures have resulted in these being the first port of call among patients seeking aesthetic facial rejuvenation. Further research and development of new improved products will ascertain an increasingly higher demand for minimally invasive nonsurgical options.

REFERENCES

1. Bilac C, Sahin MT, Ozturkcan S. Chronic actinic damage of facial skin. Clin Dermatol. 2014;32:752-62.
2. Han A, Chien AL, Kang S. Photoaging. Dermatol Clin. 2014;32:vii, 291-9.
3. Beer K, Beer J. Overview of facial aging. Facial Plast Surg. 2009;25:281-4.
4. John HE, Price RD. Perspectives in the selection of hyaluronic acid fillers for facial wrinkles and aging skin. Patient Prefer Adherence. 2009;3:225-30.
5. Gonzalez-Ulloa M, Flores ES. Senility of the face—basic study to understand its causes and effects. Plast Reconstr Surg. 1965;36:239-46.
6. Rohrich RJ, Pessa JE, Ristow B. The youthful cheek and the deep medial fat compartment. Plast Reconstr Surg. 2008;121:2107-12.
7. Gibelli D, Codari M, Rosati R, et al. A Quantitative Analysis of Lip Aesthetics: The Influence of Gender and Aging. Aesthetic plastic surgery. 2015;39(5):771-6.
8. Calleja-Agius J, Muscat-Baron Y, Brincat MP. Skin ageing. Menopause Int. 2007;13:60-4.
9. Gerth DJ. Structural and volumetric changes in the aging face. Facial Plast Surg. 2015;31:3-9.
10. Staley RN, Bishara SE, Hanson JW, et al. Craniofacial development in myotonic dystrophy. Cleft Palate Craniofac J. 1992;29:456-62.
11. Kiliaridis S, Katsaros C. The effects of myotonic dystrophy and Duchenne muscular dystrophy on the orofacial muscles and dentofacial morphology. Acta Odontol Scand. 1998;56:369-74.
12. Tanaka H, Nakagami G, Sanada H, et al. Quantitative evaluation of elderly skin based on digital image analysis. Skin Res Technol. 2008;14:192-200.
13. Lee SJ, Kim JI, Yang YJ, et al. Treatment of periorbital wrinkles with a novel fractional radiofrequency microneedle system in dark-skinned patients. Dermatol Surg. 2015;41:615-22.
14. Narins RS, Carruthers J, Flynn TC, et al. Validated assessment scales for the lower face. Dermatol Surg. 2012;38:333-42.

15. Flynn TC, Carruthers A, Carruthers J, et al. Validated assessment scales for the upper face. Dermatol Surg. 2012;38:309-19.
16. Carruthers J, Flynn TC, Geister TL, et al. Validated assessment scales for the mid face. Dermatol Surg. 2012;38:320-32.
17. Glogau RG. Aesthetic and anatomic analysis of the aging skin. Semin Cutan Med Surg. 1996;15:134-8.
18. Holds JB, Alderson K, Fogg SG, et al. Motor nerve sprouting in human orbicularis muscle after botulinum A injection. Invest Ophthalmol Vis Sci. 1990;31:964-7.
19. Salti G, Ghersetich I. Advanced botulinum toxin techniques against wrinkles in the upper face. Clin Dermatol. 2008;26:182-91.
20. Haykal S, Arad E, Bagher S, et al. The role of botulinum toxin A in the establishment of symmetry in pediatric paralysis of the lower lip. JAMA Facial Plast Surg. 2015;17:174-8.
21. Klein FH, Brenner FM, Sato MS, et al. Lower facial remodeling with botulinum toxin type A for the treatment of masseter hypertrophy. An Bras Dermatol. 2014;89:878-84.
22. Cha YR, Kim YG, Kim JH, et al. Effect of unilateral injection of botulinum toxin on lower facial asymmetry as evaluated using three-dimensional laser scanning. Dermatol Surg. 2013;39:900-6.
23. Carruthers J, Carruthers A. A prospective, randomized, parallel group study analyzing the effect of BTX-A (Botox) and nonanimal sourced hyaluronic acid (NASHA, Restylane) in combination compared with NASHA (Restylane) alone in severe glabellar rhytides in adult female subjects: treatment of severe glabellar rhytides with a hyaluronic acid derivative compared with the derivative and BTX-A. Dermatol Surg. 2003;29:802-9.
24. Kontis TC, Rivkin A. The history of injectable facial fillers. Facial Plast Surg. 2009;25:67-72.
25. Glogau RG. Fillers: from the past to the future. Semin Cutan Med Surg. 2012;31:78-87.
26. Curi MM, Cardoso CL, Curra C, et al. Late-onset adverse reactions related to hyaluronic Acid dermal filler for aesthetic soft tissue augmentation. The Journal of craniofacial surgery. 2015;26(3):782-4.
27. Nettar K, Maas C. Facial filler and neurotoxin complications. Facial Plasti Surg. 2012;28:288-93.
28. Kim JE, Sykes JM. Hyaluronic acid fillers: history and overview. Facial Plast Surg. 2011;27:523-8.
29. Holzapfel AM, Mangat DS, Barron DS. Soft-tissue augmentation with calcium hydroxylapatite: histological analysis. Arch Facial Plast Surg. 2008;10:335-8.
30. Pierre S, Liew S, Bernardin A. Basics of dermal filler rheology. Dermatol Surg. 2015;41:S120-6.
31. Attenello NH, Maas CS. Injectable fillers: review of material and properties. Facial Plast Surg. 2015;31:29-34.
32. Beasley KL, Weiss MA, Weiss RA. Hyaluronic acid fillers: a comprehensive review. Facial Plast Surg. 2009;25:86-94.
33. Sutherland IW. Novel and established applications of microbial polysaccharides. Trends Biotechnol. 1998;16:41-6.
34. Choi SC, Yoo MA, Lee SY, et al. Modulation of biomechanical properties of hyaluronic acid hydrogels by crosslinking agents. Journal of biomedical materials research Part A. 2015;103(9):3072-80.

35. Cavallini M, Gazzola R, Metalla M, et al. The role of hyaluronidase in the treatment of complications from hyaluronic acid dermal fillers. Aesthet Surg J. 2013; 33:1167-74.

36. Cohen JL, Biesman BS, Dayan SH, et al. Treatment of Hyaluronic acid filler-induced impending necrosis with hyaluronidase: consensus recommendations. Aesthetic Surgery Journal/The American Society for Aesthetic Plastic Surgery. 2015;35(7):844-9.

37. Ahn MS. Calcium hydroxylapatite: Radiesse. Facial Plast Surg. 2007;15:vii, 85-90.

38. Marmur ES, Phelps R, Goldberg DJ. Clinical, histologic and electron microscopic findings after injection of a calcium hydroxylapatite filler. J Cosmet Laser Ther. 2004;6:223-6.

39. van Rozelaar L, Kadouch JA, Duyndam DA, et al. Semipermanent filler treatment of HIV-positive patients with facial lipoatrophy: long-term follow-up evaluating MR imaging and quality of life. Aesthet Surg J. 2014;34:118-32.

40. Gogolewski S, Jovanovic M, Perren SM, et al. Tissue response and in vivo degradation of selected polyhydroxyacids: polylactides (PLA), poly(3-hydroxybutyrate) (PHB), and poly(3-hydroxybutyrate-co-3-hydroxyvalerate) (PHB/VA). J Biomed Mater Res. 1993;27:1135-48.

41. Hyun MY, Lee Y, No YA, et al. Efficacy and safety of injection with poly-L-lactic acid compared with hyaluronic acid for correction of nasolabial fold: a randomized, evaluator-blinded, comparative study. Clin Exp Dermatol. 2015;40: 129-35.

42. Mest DR, Humble GM. Duration of correction for human immunodeficiency virus-associated lipoatrophy after retreatment with injectable poly-L-lactic acid. Aesthet Plast Surg. 2009;33:654-6.

43. Greco TM, Antunes MB, Yellin SA. Injectable fillers for volume replacement in the aging face. Facial Plast Surg. 2012;28:8-20.

44. Kates LC, Fitzgerald R. Poly-L-lactic acid injection for HIV-associated facial lipoatrophy: treatment principles, case studies, and literature review. Aesthet Surg J. 2008;28:397-403.

45. Gooderham M, Solish N. Use of hyaluronic acid for soft tissue augmentation of HIV-associated facial lipodystrophy. Dermatol Surg. 2005;31:104-8.

46. Cecchi R, Spota A, Frati P, et al. Migrating granulomatous chronic reaction from hyaluronic acid skin filler (Restylane): review and histopathological study with histochemical stainings. Dermatology. 2014;228:14-7.

47. Arron ST, Neuhaus IM. Persistent delayed-type hypersensitivity reaction to injectable non-animal-stabilized hyaluronic acid. J Cosmet Dermatol. 2007;6: 167-71.

48. Shahrabi Farahani S, Sexton J, Stone JD, et al. Lip nodules caused by hyaluronic acid filler injection: report of three cases. Head Neck Pathol. 2012;6:16-20.

49. Carruthers JD, Fagien S, Rohrich RJ, et al. Blindness caused by cosmetic filler injection: a review of cause and therapy. Plast Reconstr Surg. 2014;134:1197-201.

50. Hall MP, Band PA, Meislin RJ, et al. Platelet-rich plasma: current concepts and application in sports medicine. J Am Acad Orthop Surg. 2009;17:602-8.

51. Lubkowska A, Dolegowska B, Banfi G. Growth factor content in PRP and their applicability in medicine. J Biol Regul Homeost Agents. 2012;26:3s-22s.

52. Paoloni J, De Vos RJ, Hamilton B, et al. Platelet-rich plasma treatment for ligament and tendon injuries. Clin J Sport Med. 2011;21:37-45.

53. Sclafani AP, Azzi J. Platelet Preparations for Use in Facial Rejuvenation and Wound Healing: A Critical Review of Current Literature. Aesthetic plastic surgery. 2015;39(4):495-505.

54. Alio JL, Rodriguez AE, Wrobel Dudzinska D. Eye platelet-rich plasma in the treatment of ocular surface disorders. Curr Opin Ophthalmol. 2015;26:325-32.

55. Amable PR, Teixeira MV, Carias RB, et al. Mesenchymal stromal cell proliferation, gene expression and protein production in human platelet-rich plasma-supplemented media. PloS One. 2014;9:e104662.

56. Kakudo N, Minakata T, Mitsui T, et al. Proliferation-promoting effect of platelet-rich plasma on human adipose-derived stem cells and human dermal fibroblasts. Plast Reconstr Surg. 2008;122:1352-60.

57. Mishra A, Tummala P, King A, et al. Buffered platelet-rich plasma enhances mesenchymal stem cell proliferation and chondrogenic differentiation. Tissue Eng Part C Methods. 2009;15:431-5.

58. Kushida S, Kakudo N, Suzuki K, et al. Effects of platelet-rich plasma on proliferation and myofibroblastic differentiation in human dermal fibroblasts. Ann Plast Surg. 2013;71:219-24.

59. Shin MK, Lee JW, Kim YI, et al. The effects of platelet-rich clot releasate on the expression of MMP-1 and type I collagen in human adult dermal fibroblasts: PRP is a stronger MMP-1 stimulator. Mol Biol Rep. 2014;41:3-8.

60. Cho JM, Lee YH, Baek RM, et al. Effect of platelet-rich plasma on ultraviolet b-induced skin wrinkles in nude mice. J Plast Reconstr Aesthet Surg. 2011; 64: e31-9.

61. Modarressi A. Platlet rich plasma (PRP) improves fat grafting outcomes. World J Plast Surg. 2013;2:6-13.

62. Willemsen JC, van der Lei B, Vermeulen KM, et al. The effects of platelet-rich plasma on recovery time and aesthetic outcome in facial rejuvenation: preliminary retrospective observations. Aesthet Plast Surg. 2014;38:1057-63.

63. Powell DM, Chang E, Farrior EH. Recovery from deep-plane rhytidectomy following unilateral wound treatment with autologous platelet gel: a pilot study. Arch Facial Plast Surg. 2001;3:245-50.

64. Kakudo N, Kushida S, Minakata T, et al. Platelet-rich plasma promotes epithelialization and angiogenesis in a split thickness skin graft donor site. Med Mol Morphol. 2011;44:233-6.

65. Yuksel EP, Sahin G, Aydin F, et al. Evaluation of effects of platelet-rich plasma on human facial skin. J Cosmet Laser Ther. 2014;16:206-8.

66. Sclafani AP. Platelet-rich fibrin matrix for improvement of deep nasolabial folds. J Cosmet Dermatol. 2010;9:66-71.

67. Sclafani AP, Saman M. Platelet-rich fibrin matrix for facial plastic surgery. Facial Plast Surg Clin North Am. 2012;20: vi,177-86.

68. Mehryan P, Zartab H, Rajabi A, et al. Assessment of efficacy of platelet-rich plasma (PRP) on infraorbital dark circles and crow's feet wrinkles. J Cosmet Dermatol. 2014;13:72-8.

69. Billings E, Jr, May JW, Jr. Historical review and present status of free fat graft autotransplantation in plastic and reconstructive surgery. Plast Reconstr Surg. 1989;83:368-81.

70. Illouz YG. History and current concepts of lipoplasty. Clin Plast Surg. 1996;23: 721-30.

71. Coleman SR. Facial augmentation with structural fat grafting. Clin Plast Surg. 2006;33:567-77.
72. Rohrich RJ, Ghavami A, Constantine FC, et al. Lift-and-fill face lift: integrating the fat compartments. Plast Reconstr Surg. 2014;133:756e-67e.
73. Sommer B, Sattler G. Current concepts of fat graft survival: histology of aspirated adipose tissue and review of the literature. Dermatol Surg. 2000;26:1159-66.
74. Metzinger S, Parrish J, Guerra A, et al. Autologous fat grafting to the lower one-third of the face. Facial Plast Surg. 2012;28:21-33.
75. Buckingham ED. Fat transfer techniques: general concepts. Facial Plast Surg. 2015;31:22-8.
76. Lam SM, Glasgold RA, Glasgold MJ. Fat harvesting techniques for facial fat transfer. Facial Plast Surg. 2010;26:356-61.
77. Coleman SR. Facial recontouring with lipostructure. Clin Plast Surg. 1997;24:347-67.
78. Coleman SR. Structural fat grafts: the ideal filler? Clin Plast Surg. 2001;28:111-9.
79. Asilian A, Siadat AH, Iraji R. Comparison of fat maintenance in the face with centrifuge versus filtered and washed fat. J Res Med Sci. 2014;19:556-61.
80. Botti G, Pascali M, Botti C, et al. A clinical trial in facial fat grafting: filtered and washed versus centrifuged fat. Plast Reconstr Surg. 2011;127:2464-73.
81. Girard AC, Atlan M, Bencharif K, et al. New insights into lidocaine and adrenaline effects on human adipose stem cells. Aesthet Plast Surg. 2013;37:144-52.
82. Vico PG, Delange A, De Vooght A. Autologous fat transfer: an aesthetic and functional refinement for parotidectomy. Surg Res Pract. 2014;2014:873453.
83. Brodell LA, Gru AA, Haughey B, et al. Autologous fat transfer-induced facial nodule. J Am Acad Dermatol. 2013;69:e107-8.
84. Miller JJ, Popp JC. Fat hypertrophy after autologous fat transfer. Ophthal Plast Reconstr Surg. 2002;18:228-31.
85. Walker P, Fellmann J, Lizzul PF. A phase I safety and pharmacokinetic study of ATX-101: injectable, synthetic deoxycholic acid for submental contouring. Journal of Drugs in Dermatology: JDD. 2015;14(3):279-87.
86. Yagima Odo ME, Cuce LC, Odo LM, et al. Action of sodium deoxycholate on subcutaneous human tissue: local and systemic effects. Dermatologic Surgery: official publication for American Society for Dermatologic Surgery [et al]. 2007;33(2):178-88; discussion 88-9.
87. Wollina U, Goldman A. ATX-101 for reduction of submental fat. Expert opinion on pharmacotherapy. 2015;16(5):755-62.
88. Chung SJ, Lee CH, Lee HS, et al. The role of phosphatidylcholine and deoxycholic acid in inflammation. Life sciences. 2014;108(2):88-93.
89. Lowe NJ. Dissolving unwanted submental fat. The British journal of dermatology. 2014;170(2):237-8.
90. Ascher B, Hoffmann K, Walker P, et al. Efficacy, patient-reported outcomes and safety profile of ATX-101 (deoxycholic acid), an injectable drug for the reduction of unwanted submental fat: results from a phase III, randomized, placebo-controlled study. Journal of the European Academy of Dermatology and Venereology: JEADV. 2014;28(12):1707-15.
91. Rzany B, Griffiths T, Walker P, et al. Reduction of unwanted submental fat with ATX-101 (deoxycholic acid), an adipocytolytic injectable treatment: results from a phase III, randomized, placebo-controlled study. The British Journal of Dermatology. 2014;170(2):445-53.

Index

Note: Page numbers followed by f refer to figure and t refer to table respectively.